Current Research in

PHARMACEUTICAL TECHNOLOGY

Current Research in

PHARMACEUTICAL TECHNOLOGY

Edited By

Sabine Globig

Associate Professor of Biology, Hazard Community and Technical College, Kentucky, U.S.A.

William Hunter Jr.

Olean General Hospital, Olean, New York, U.S.A.

Apple Academic Press

TORONTO NEW YORK

Apple Academic Press Inc.
3333 Mistwell Crescent
Oakville, ON L6L 0A2
Canada

Apple Academic Press Inc.
1613 Beaver Dam Road, Suite # 104
Point Pleasant, NJ 08742
USA

Exclusive worldwide distribution by CRC Press, a Taylor & Francis Group

International Standard Book Number: 978-1-926692-68-5 (Hardback)

Library and Archives Canada Cataloguing in Publication

Current research in pharmaceutical technology/editors,
Sabine Globig and William Hunter.

ISBN 978-1-926692-68-5
1. Pharmaceutical technology. I. Globig, Sabine, 1949-
II. Hunter, William, 1946-

RS192.C87 2011 615'.19 C2011-905376-4

Preface

Pharmaceutical technology, a sub-specialty of the field of pharmaceutics, deals with the discovery, production, processing, and safe and effective delivery of medications to patients. Historically, it was the major component of the practice of medicine: the physician or healer was responsible for identifying medicinal plants or plant parts, determining the best method of extracting the active principle, and then producing and stocking the preparations as well as supplying them to patients, along with instruction as to their use. The earliest "technology", then, consisted of trial-and-error experimentation, extraction by boiling, steeping, drying, or grinding various plant parts, then mixing them with oils, creams, water, or wine, and administering the resultant preparations topically, orally, as poultices, or by inhalation of vapors, etc.

With the rise of the scientific age, however, and the resulting growth of knowledge in medicine, chemistry, and the biological sciences, a separate science of pharmacology was born: as the knowledge of human anatomy, physiology, and disease grew, along with ways to treat disease, physicians concentrated on treatment, and the discovery and production of medicines became a separate science. As more medicines were developed, and their use became more widespread, large-scale manufacturing and chemical synthesis of medicinal compounds was accompanied by marketing and distribution on a larger scale. These developments brought engineering, economic, and quality control issues into the mix. Today, technology is a key element in every aspect of pharmaceutics: discovery of new drugs, large-scale production, safety and efficacy testing, development of new and better delivery and diagnostic methods, even the tools for research into diseases and pharmaceuticals themselves. And yet the earliest methods of drug discovery and delivery have not been completely discarded: native herbalists and healers around the world, with traditional knowledge of the plant sources and preparations used in indigenous healing practices, are still being investigated as a promising source of new medicines.

Pharmaceutical research and production today includes considerations of cost-effectiveness and profitability, and pharmaceutical technology can contribute to cheaper, more cost-effective research and production methods. Technologies such as computer modeling for research, bioengineering for research instrumentation and for the scaling-up of production methods, and computing technology and biosystematics for the management and analysis of data, are all key components of today's pharmaceutical environment. At the forefront of present pharmaceutical research are such promising fields for future drug discovery and production as proteomics (the identification of all the proteins expressed by a genome and the determination of their role in physiological and pathological function) and pharmacogenomics (the study of the influence of genetic variation on drug response in patients). Other promising research areas are new techniques for determining safety and efficacy, such as high-throughput screening and cell culture modeling; more rapid and cost-effective molecular-scale diagnostics for both research and patient diagnosis; and new, more specific and effective drug delivery methods, such as nanoparticle encapsulation, *in vivo* gene splicing, and better extended/controlled-release delivery systems, which will allow the use of drugs that otherwise would not be effective or safe. The dream of personalized medicine (scanning a patient's genome in order to produce a precisely tailored remedy for whatever is amiss, with minimal, if any, side-effects and optimized effectiveness for their unique genetic make-up) may not yet be a realizable goal; but, along with technologies not yet imagined, it may well become a part of the field's future.

— **William Hunter Jr.**

List of Contributors

Alka Ahuja
Department of Pharmaceutics, Faculty of Pharmacy, Jamia Hamdard, Hamdard Nagar, New Delhi-110062, India.

M. Alagar
Department of Chemical Engineering, Alagappa College of Technology, Anna University, Chennai 600025, India.

Javed Ali
Department of Pharmaceutics, Faculty of Pharmacy, Jamia Hamdard, Hamdard Nagar, New Delhi-110062, India.

Jean-Pierre Andrieu
JP Ebel Institute of Structural Biology, CEA, CNRS, UJF, Grenoble, France.

Magnus A. Atemnkeng
Department of Pharmaceutical Technology and Physical Pharmacy, Faculty of Medicine and Pharmacy, Vrije Universiteit Brussel, Laarbeeklaan 103, B-1090 Brussels. Belgium.

Darlene Attiah
Department of Bioengineering, University of Illinois at Chicago, USA.

Sanjula Baboota
Department of Pharmaceutics, Faculty of Pharmacy, Jamia Hamdard, Hamdard Nagar, New Delhi-110062, India.

Hagit Bar
Department of Molecular Microbiology and Biotechnology, The George S. Wise Faculty of Life Sciences, Tel-Aviv University, Ramat Aviv 69978, Israel.
Department of Biological Chemistry, Weizmann Institute of Science, Rehovot 76100, Israel.

Itai Benhar
Department of Molecular Microbiology and Biotechnology, The George S. Wise Faculty of Life Sciences, Tel-Aviv University, Ramat Aviv 69978, Israel.

Xiu-Mei Cai
Department of Biochemistry and Molecular Biology, Shanghai Medical College, Fudan University, Shanghai, PR China.

Feng Cao
Molecular Imaging Program at Stanford (MIPS) and Bio-X Program, Department of Radiology, Stanford University, Stanford, CA 94305, USA.

Ana M. Carmona-Ribeiro
Department of Biochemistry, Institute of Chemistry, University of São Paulo, CP 26077, CEP 05513-970, São Paulo, Brazil.

Jadwiga Chroboczek
Institute of Biochemistry and Biophysics, Polish Academy of Sciences, Warsaw, Poland.
JP Ebel Institute of Structural Biology, CEA, CNRS, UJF, Grenoble, France.

Katelijne De Cock
Department of Pharmaceutical Technology and Physical Pharmacy, Faculty of Medicine and Pharmacy, Vrije Universiteit Brussel, Laarbeeklaan 103, B-1090 Brussels, Belgium.

Olivia Debrah
Department of Pharmaceutics, Ernest Mario School of Pharmacy, Rutgers University, 160 Frelinghuysen Road, Piscataway, New Jersey 08854-0789, USA.

Tejal A. Desai
Department of Bioengineering, University of Illinois at Chicago, USA.
Department of Biomedical Engineering, Boston University, 44 Cummington Street, Boston, MA 02215, USA.

Peng Wei Dong
State Key Laboratory of Biotherapy, West China Hospital, West China Medical School, Sichuan University, Chengdu, 610041, PR China.

Bernard Dublet
JP Ebel Institute of Structural Biology, CEA, CNRS, UJF, Grenoble, France.

Hicham Fenniri
National Institute of Nanotechnology, National Research Council (NINT-NRC) and Department of Chemistry, University of Alberta, 11421 Saskatchewan Drive, Edmonton, AB, T6G 2M9, Canada.

Brian S. Ford
Center for Gene Therapy, Tulane University Medical School, New Orleans, LA, 70115, USA.

Shao Zhi Fu
State Key Laboratory of Biotherapy, West China Hospital, West China Medical School, Sichuan University, Chengdu, 610041, PR China.

Sanjiv S. Gambhir
Molecular Imaging Program at Stanford (MIPS) and Bio-X Program, Department of Radiology, Stanford University, Stanford, CA 94305, USA.
Department of Medicine, Division of Cardiology, Stanford University School of Medicine, Stanford, CA 94305, USA.

Fariba Ghaidi
Department of Cellular and Physiological Sciences, Life Sciences Institute, University of British Columbia, Vancouver, British Columbia, Canada.
Department of Surgery, St. Paul's Hospital, University of British Columbia, Vancouver, British Columbia, Canada.

Oliver Gheysens
Molecular Imaging Program at Stanford (MIPS) and Bio-X Program, Department of Radiology, Stanford University, Stanford, CA 94305, USA.

Chang Yang Gong
State Key Laboratory of Biotherapy, West China Hospital, West China Medical School, Sichuan University, Chengdu, 610041, PR China.
School of Life Science, Sichuan University, Chengdu, 610064, PR China.

Carl A. Gregory
Center for Gene Therapy, Tulane University Medical School, New Orleans, LA, 70115, USA.
Institute for Regenerative Medicine, Texas A&M Health Science Center, Temple, TX, 76502, USA.

Simi Gunaseelan
Department of Pharmaceutics, Ernest Mario School of Pharmacy, Rutgers University, 160Frelinghuysen Road, Piscataway, New Jersey 08854-0789, USA.

Gang Guo
State Key Laboratory of Biotherapy, West China Hospital, West China Medical School, Sichuan University, Chengdu, 610041, PR China.

Sean M. Harris
Center for Gene Therapy, Tulane University Medical School, New Orleans, LA, 70115, USA.

Bharat Joshi
Department of Cellular and Physiological Sciences, Life Sciences Institute, University of British Columbia, Vancouver, British Columbia, Canada.

Liliana D. Kojic
Department of Cellular and Physiological Sciences, Life Sciences Institute, University of British Columbia, Vancouver, British Columbia, Canada.

K. Sathish Kumar
Department of Chemical Engineering, SSN College of Engineering, Kalavakkam 603110, India.

Michael J. Leibowitz
Department of Molecular Genetics, Microbiology, and Immunology, Robert Wood Johnson Medical School, University of Medicine and Dentistry of New Jersey, Piscataway, New Jersey 08854, USA.
Cancer Institute of New Jersey, New Brunswick, New Jersey 08903-2681, USA.

Lara Leoni
Department of Bioengineering, University of Illinois at Chicago, USA.

Su Li
Department of Medicine, Tumor Hospital, Sun Yat-sen University, Guangzhou, China.

Zongjin Li
Molecular Imaging Program at Stanford (MIPS) and Bio-X Program, Department of Radiology, Stanford University, Stanford, CA 94305, USA.

Shuan Lin
Molecular Imaging Program at Stanford (MIPS) and Bio-X Program, Department of Radiology, Stanford University, Stanford, CA 94305, USA.

Ming-Zhu Liu
Department of Biochemistry and Molecular Biology, Shanghai Medical College, Fudan University, Shanghai, PR China.

Gordon J. Lutz
Drexel University College of Medicine, Department of Pharmacology and Physiology, Philadelphia, Pennsylvania 19102, USA.

Ivan R. Nabi
Department of Cellular and Physiological Sciences, Life Sciences Institute, University of British Columbia, Vancouver, British Columbia, Canada.

Hinyu Nedev
Lady Davis Research Institute, McGill University, Montreal, Quebec, Canada.

Agnieszka Paca
Institute of Biochemistry and Biophysics, Polish Academy of Sciences, Warsaw, Poland.

Manishkumar R. Patel
Molecular Imaging Program at Stanford (MIPS) and Bio-X Program, Department of Radiology, Stanford University, Stanford, CA 94305, USA.

Jacqueline Plaizier-Vercammen
Department of Pharmaceutical Technology and Physical Pharmacy, Faculty of Medicine and Pharmacy, Vrije Universiteit Brussel, Laarbeeklaan 103, B-1090 Brussels, Belgium.

Shahriar Pooyan
Department of Pharmaceutics, Ernest Mario School of Pharmacy, Rutgers University, 160Frelinghuysen Road, Piscataway, New Jersey 08854-0789, USA.

Darwin J. Prockop
Center for Gene Therapy, Tulane University Medical School, New Orleans, LA, 70115, USA.
Institute for Regenerative Medicine, Texas A&M Health Science Center, Temple, TX, 76502, USA.

Zhi Yong Qian
State Key Laboratory of Biotherapy, West China Hospital, West China Medical School, Sichuan University, Chengdu, 610041, PR China.

Arnold B. Rabson
Department of Molecular Genetics, Microbiology, and Immunology, Robert Wood Johnson Medical School, University of Medicine and Dentistry of New Jersey, Piscataway, New Jersey 08854, USA.
Cancer Institute of New Jersey, New Brunswick, New Jersey 08903-2681, USA.

Jiang Hong Rao
Molecular Imaging Program at Stanford (MIPS) and Bio-X Program, Department of Radiology, Stanford University, Stanford, CA 94305, USA.

H. Uri Saragovi
Lady Davis Research Institute, McGill University, Montreal, Quebec, Canada.

Guy Schoehn
Institute of Molecular and Structural Virology, FRE 2854 CNRS-UJF, Grenoble, France.

Rebecca C. Schray
Drexel University College of Medicine, Department of Pharmacology and Physiology, Philadelphia, Pennsylvania 19102, USA.

V. Selvaraj
Department of Chemical Engineering, Alagappa College of Technology, Anna University, Chennai 600025, India.

Sheikh Shafiq
New Drug Delivery System (NDDS), Zydus Cadila Research Centre, Ahemdabad, India.

Faiyaz Shakeel
Department of Pharmaceutics, Faculty of Pharmacy, Al-Arab Medical Sciences University, Benghazi-5341, Libya.

Shuai Shi
State Key Laboratory of Biotherapy, West China Hospital, West China Medical School, Sichuan University, Chengdu, 610041, PR China.

Gabriel A Silva
Departments of Bioengineering and Ophthalmology, and Neurosciences Program, University of California, San Diego, 9415 Campus Point Drive, La Jolla, California 92037-0946, USA.

Baljit Singh
Department of Veterinary Biomedical Sciences and Immunology Research Group, University of Saskatchewan, 52 Campus Drive, Saskatoon, SK, S7N 5B4, Canada.

Patrick J. Sinko
Department of Pharmaceutics, Ernest Mario School of Pharmacy, Rutgers University, 160Frelinghuysen Road, Piscataway, New Jersey 08854-0789, USA.
Cancer Institute of New Jersey, New Brunswick, New Jersey 08903-2681, USA.

Shashank R. Sirsi
Drexel University, Department of Biomedical Engineering, Philadelphia, Pennsylvania 19104, USA.

Stanley Stein
Department of Pharmaceutics, Ernest Mario School of Pharmacy, Rutgers University, 160Frelinghuysen Road, Piscataway, New Jersey 08854-0789, USA.
Cancer Institute of New Jersey, New Brunswick, New Jersey 08903-2681, USA.

Sarabjeet Singh Suri
Department of Veterinary Biomedical Sciences and Immunology Research Group, University of Saskatchewan, 52 Campus Drive, Saskatoon, SK, S7N 5B4, Canada.

Ewa Szolajska
Institute of Biochemistry and Biophysics, Polish Academy of Sciences, Warsaw, Poland.

Débora B. Vieira
Department of Biochemistry, Institute of Chemistry, University of São Paulo, CP 26077, CEP 05513-970, São Paulo, Brazil.

Li Wan
Department of Pharmaceutics, Ernest Mario School of Pharmacy, Rutgers University, 160 Frelinghuysen Road, Piscataway, New Jersey 08854-0789, USA.

Anxun Wang
Department of Oral and Maxillofacial Surgery, First Affiliated Hospital, Sun Yat-sen University, Guangzhou, China.

Yu Quan Wei
State Key Laboratory of Biotherapy, West China Hospital, West China Medical School, Sichuan University, Chengdu, 610041, PR China.

Jason H. Williams
Drexel University College of Medicine, Department of Pharmacology and Physiology, Philadelphia, Pennsylvania 19102, USA.

Sam M. Wiseman
Department of Surgery, St. Paul's Hospital, University of British Columbia, Vancouver, British Columbia, Canada.

Mandolin J. Whitney
Center for Gene Therapy, Tulane University Medical School, New Orleans, LA, 70115, USA.

Joseph C. Wu
Molecular Imaging Program at Stanford (MIPS) and Bio-X Program, Department of Radiology, Stanford University, Stanford, CA 94305, USA.
Department of Bioengineering, Stanford University, Stanford, CA 94305, USA.

Hai-Long Xie
Institute of Cancer Research, South China University, Hengyang, PR China.

Xiaoyan Xie
Molecular Imaging Program at Stanford (MIPS) and Bio-X Program, Department of Radiology, Stanford University, Stanford, CA 94305, USA.

Iftach Yacoby
Department of Molecular Microbiology and Biotechnology, The George S. Wise Faculty of Life Sciences, Tel-Aviv University, Ramat Aviv 69978, Israel.

Jing Liang Yang
State Key Laboratory of Biotherapy, West China Hospital, West China Medical School, Sichuan University, Chengdu, 610041, PR China.

Yao-Hung Yang
Molecular Imaging Program at Stanford (MIPS) and Bio-X Program, Department of Radiology, Stanford University, Stanford, CA 94305, USA.

Suzanne Zeitouni
Center for Gene Therapy, Tulane University Medical School, New Orleans, LA, 70115, USA.
Institute for Regenerative Medicine, Texas A&M Health Science Center, Temple, TX, 76502, USA.

Xi-Liang Zha
Department of Biochemistry and Molecular Biology, Shanghai Medical College, Fudan University, Shanghai, PR China.

Xiaoping Zhang
Department of Pharmaceutics, Ernest Mario School of Pharmacy, Rutgers University, 160 Frelinghuysen Road, Piscataway, New Jersey 08854-0789, USA.

Yan Zhang
Molecular Imaging Program at Stanford (MIPS) and Bio-X Program, Department of Radiology, Stanford University, Stanford, CA 94305, USA.

Xiu Ling Zheng
State Key Laboratory of Biotherapy, West China Hospital, West China Medical School, Sichuan University, Chengdu, 610041, PR China.

Monika Zochowska
Institute of Biochemistry and Biophysics, Polish Academy of Sciences, Warsaw, Poland.

List of Abbreviations

% F	Percent relative bioavailability
2'OMe	2'O-Methyl
5-Fu	5-Fluorouracil
7-Add	7-aminoactinomycin
AD	Adenovirus
AD	Alzheimer's disease
AFP	Alpha-1-fetoprotein
AIDS	Acquired immunodeficiency syndrome
AIIMS	All India Institute of Medical Sciences
AIM	Adipo-inductive media
AmB	Amphotericin B
AMF/PGI	Autocrine motility factor/phosphoglucose isomerase
ANOVA	Analysis of variance
Apaf	Apoptotic protease activating factor
API	Active pharmaceutical ingredient
ApoE	Apolipoprotein E
AR	Analytic reagent
ATCC	American type culture collection
AUC	Area under the concentration-time curve
$AUC_{0\rightarrow t}$	Area under curve from time 0 to t
$AUC_{0\rightarrow \omega}$	Area under curve from time 0 to infinitive
BA	Benzoic acid
BBB	Blood brain barrier
BCA	Bicinchoninic acid
BLM	Bleomycin
BSA	Bovine serum albumin
Cav1	Caveolin-1
CBB	Coomassie brilliant blue
CCM	Complete culture medium
CFU	Colony-forming unit
CG	Colloidal gold
CGC	Critical gelation concentration
C_{max}	Peak or maximum plasma concentration
CMC	Carboxymethylcellulose
CNS	Central nervous systems

COX-2	Cyclo-oxygenase-2
CPP	Cell penetrating peptide
CPT	Camptothecin
Ct-b	Cholera toxin b-subunit
CXB	Celecoxib
DAB	Diaminobenzidine
DB	Dodecahedron base
Dd	Dodecahedron
DDSs	Drug delivery systems
DDW	Double-distilled water
DHP	Dihexadecylphosphate
DIC	Differential interference contrast
DLS	Dynamic light scattering technique
DMD	Duchenne muscular dystrophy
DMEM	Dulbecco's modified eagle medium
DMF	N,N-dimethylformamide
DMSO	Dimethyl sulfoxide
DODAB	Dioctadecyldimethylammonium bromide
Dox	Doxorubicin
DSC	Differential scanning calorimeter
ECM	Extracellular matrix
EDC	1-Ethyl-3- (3-dimethylaminopropyl) carbodiimide
EDTA	Ethylene diamine tetra-acectic acid
EGF	Epidermal growth factor
EGFR	Epidermal growth factor receptor
EM	Electron microscopy
EMEM	Eagle's minimal essential medium
EPR	Enhanced permeability and retention
ERAD	Edoplasmic reticulum-associated degradation
ERK	Extracellular regulated kinases
ES	Embryonic stem
ESI-MS	Electrospray ionization mass spectra
ESOs	Exon skipping oligonucleotides
FAK	Focal adhesion kinase
FBS	Fetal bovine serum
FBS	Fetal calf serum
FCS	Foetal calf serum
FK	Phenylalanine-Lysine
Flk1	Fetal liver kinase-1

FTIR	Fourier transform Infra-red
GSH	Glutathione
HAART	Highly active antiretroviral therapy
HCPT	Hydroxycamptothecin
HCT	Human colon tumor
H-E	Hematoxylin-Eosin
HER2	Human epidermal growth factor receptor-2
HF	Hydrogen fluoride
HIV	Human immunodeficiency virus
HK	Honokiol
hMSCs	Human MSCs
HPLC	High-performance liquid chromatography
HPLC-UV	High performance liquid chromatography with UV detector
HPV	Human papillomavirus
HRP	Horseradish peroxidase
HSCs	Hematopoietic stem cells
HT29	Human colon adenocarcinoma grade II cell line
i.p.	Intraperitoneal
i.t.	Intratumoral
i.v.	Intravenous
ICAM-1	Intercellular adhesion molecule-1
IGP	Isotonic glucose phosphate buffer
IR	Inhibition rate
JC	John Cunningham virus
KOH	Potassium hydroxide
LbL	Layer-by-layer approach
LCGT	Lower critical gelation temperature
mAbs	Monoclonal antibodies
MALDI-TOF	Matrix-assisted laser desorption ionization time-of-flight
MEMS	Micro electro mechanical systems
MFI	Mean fluorescence intensity
mMSCs	Mouse MSCs
mMSCs	Murine MSCs
MOI	Multiplicity of infection
MP	Methylparaben
MP	Methylparahydroxybenzoate
MRI	Magnetic resonance imaging
MSCs	Multipotent mesenchymal stromal cells
MST	Median survival time

MTT	Methyl thiazolyl tetrazolium
MTX	Methotrexate
mβCD	Methyl-β-cyclodextrin
Ncam	Neural cell adhesion molecule
NCEs	New chemical entities
NG	Nanogold
NSCs	Neural stem cells
PACA	Polyalkylcyanoacrylates
PBLG	Poly(γ-benzyl L-glutamate)
PBS	Phosphate buffered saline
PDI	Polydisperse index
PEBBLE	Probes encapsulated by biologically localized embedding
PEG	Poly(ethylene glycol)
PEG-PBLG	Poly(ethylene glycol)-poly(γ-benzyl-L-glutamate)
PEG-PCL-PEG, PECE	Poly(ethylene glycol)-poly(ε-caprolactone)-poly(ethylene glycol)
PEI	Poly(ethylene imine)
PET	Polyethylene terephthalate
PET	Preservative efficacy test
PET-PLA	Polyethylene terephthalate-polylactic acid copolymer
Ph. Eur.	European pharmacopoeia
PI	Propidium iodide
PK	Pharmacokinetic
PLA	Polylactic acid
PLGA	Polylactic/glycolic acid
PMO	Phosphorodiamidate morpholino
PP	Propylparaben
PP	Propylparahydroxybenzoate
PTX	Paclitaxel
QD	Quantum dots
R.I.CK	Retro-inverso-D-cysteine-lysine)-Tat9
RES	Reticuloendothelial system
RF	Retardation factor
RGD	Arg-Gly-Asp
RI	Retro-inverso
rpm	Revolution per minute
RT-PCR	Reverse-transcription polymerase chain reaction
s.c.	subcutaneous
s.d.	Standard deviation

SA	Sorbic acid
SC	Stratum corneum
SEM	Scanning electron microscopy
siRNA	Short interfering
SLNs	Solid lipid nanoparticles
SMOs	Splice modulating oligonucleotides
SQV	Saquinavir
ssDNA	Single-stranded DNA
sulfo-NHS	N-hydroxysulfosuccinimide
SV40	Simian virus serotype 40
TA	Tibialis anterior
TAR	Trans-activation responsive element
TDT	Tumor doubling time
TEA	Triethanolamine
TH	Tyrosine hydroxylase
TLC	Thin layer chromatography
T_{max}	Time to reach peak plasma concentration
Topo I	Topoisomerase I
TV	Tumor volume
UCGT	Upper critical gelation temperature
USP	United States Pharmacopoeia
VB_{12}	Vitamin B_{12}
V_d	Distribution volume
VEGF	Vascular endothelial growth factor
VLP	Virus like particle
γ-BLG NCA	γ-benzyl L-glutamate N-carboxyanhydride

Contents

Chapter 1

Nanotechnology-based Drug Delivery Systems

Sarabjeet Singh Suri, Hicham Fenniri, and Baljit Singh

INTRODUCTION

Nanoparticles hold tremendous potential as an effective drug delivery system. In this review we discussed recent developments in nanotechnology for drug delivery. To overcome the problems of gene and drug delivery, nanotechnology has gained interest in recent years. Nanosystems with different compositions and biological properties have been extensively investigated for drug and gene delivery applications. To achieve efficient drug delivery it is important to understand the interactions of nanomaterials with the biological environment, targeting cell-surface receptors, drug release, multiple drug administration, stability of therapeutic agents, and molecular mechanisms of cell signaling involved in pathobiology of the disease under consideration. Several anti-cancer drugs including paclitaxel, doxorubicin, 5-fluorouracil, and dexamethasone have been successfully formulated using nanomaterials. Quantom dots, chitosan, polylactic/glycolic acid (PLGA), and PLGA-based nanoparticles have also been used for *in vitro* RNAi delivery. Brain cancer is one of the most difficult malignancies to detect and treat mainly because of the difficulty in getting imaging and therapeutic agents past the blood-brain barrier and into the brain. Anti-cancer drugs such as loperamide and doxorubicin bound to nanomaterials have been shown to cross the intact blood-brain barrier and released at therapeutic concentrations in the brain. The use of nanomaterials including peptide-based nanotubes to target the vascular endothelial growth factor (VEGF) receptor and cell adhesion molecules like integrins, cadherins, and selectins, is a new approach to control disease progression.

Nanoparticles used as drug delivery vehicles are generally <100 nm in at least one dimension, and consist of different biodegradable materials such as natural or synthetic polymers, lipids, or metals. Nanoparticles are taken up by cells more efficiently than larger micromolecules and therefore, could be used as effective transport and delivery systems. For therapeutic applications, drugs can either be integrated in the matrix of the particle or attached to the particle surface. A drug targeting system should be able to control the fate of a drug entering the biological environment. Nanosystems with different compositions and biological properties have been extensively investigated for drug and gene delivery applications (Brannon-Peppase and Blanchette, 2004; Pison et al., 2006; Schatzlein, 2005; Stylios et al., 2005; Yokoyama, 2005). An effective approach for achieving efficient drug delivery would be to rationally develop nanosystems based on the understanding of their interactions with the biological environment, target cell population, target cell-surface receptors (Groneberg et al., 2006), changes in cell receptors that occur with progression of disease, mechanism and site of drug action, drug retention, multiple drug administration, molecular mechanisms, and pathobiology of the disease under consideration. It is also important to understand the barriers to drug such as stability of therapeutic agents in the living cell environment. Reduced drug efficacy could be due to instability of drug inside the cell, unavailability due to multiple targeting or chemical properties of delivering molecules, alterations in genetic makeup of cell-surface receptors, over-expression of efflux pumps, changes in signaling pathways with the progression of disease, or drug degradation. For instance, excessive DNA methylation with the progression of cancer (Grady, 2005) causes failure of several anti-neoplastic agents like doxorubicin and cisplatin. Better understanding of the mechanism of uptake, intracellular trafficking, retention, and protection from degradation inside a cell are required for enhancing efficacy of the encapsulated therapeutic agent.

In this chapter we will discuss the drug delivery aspects of nanomedicine, the molecular mechanisms underlying the interactions of nanoparticles with cell-surface receptors, biological responses, and cell signaling, and the research needed for the widespread application of nanodelivery systems in medicine.

MATERIALS AND METHODS

Design of Nanotechnology-based Drug Delivery Systems

Nanoparticles can be used in targeted drug delivery at the site of disease to improve the uptake of poorly soluble drugs (Kipp, 2004; Ould-Ouali et al., 2005), the targeting of drugs to a specific site, and drug bioavailability. A schematic comparison of untargeted and targeted drug delivery systems is shown in Figure 1. Several anti-cancer drugs including paclitaxel (Fonseca et al., 2002; Koziara et al., 2006), doxorubicin (Yoo et al., 2000), 5-fluorouracil (Bhadra et al., 2003), and dexamethasone (Panyam and Labhasetwar, 2004) have been successfully formulated using nanomaterials. The PLGA and polylactic acid (PLA) based nanoparticles have been formulated to encapsulate dexamethasone, a glucocorticoid with an intracellular site of action. Dexamethasone is a chemotherapeutic agent that has anti-proliferative and anti-inflammatory effects. The drug binds to the cytoplasmic receptors and the subsequent drug-receptor complex is transported to the nucleus resulting in the expression of certain genes that control cell proliferation (Panyam and Labhasetwar, 2004). These drug-loaded nanoparticles formulations that release higher doses of drug for prolonged period of time completely inhibited proliferation of vascular smooth muscle cells.

Colloidal drug delivery modalities such as liposomes, micelles, or nanoparticles have been intensively investigated for their use in cancer therapy. The effectiveness of drug delivery systems can be attributed to their small size, reduced drug toxicity, controlled time release of the drug and modification of drug pharmacokinetics, and biological distribution. Too often, chemotherapy fails to cure cancer because some tumor cells develop resistance to multiple anti-cancer drugs. In most cases, resistance develops when cancer cells begin expressing a protein, known as p-glycoprotein that is capable of pumping anti-cancer drugs out of a cell as quickly as they cross through the cell's outer membrane. New research shows that nanoparticles may be able to get anti-cancer drugs into cells without triggering the p-glycoprotein pump (Koziara et al., 2004, 2006). The researchers studied *in vivo* efficacy of paclitaxel loaded nanoparticles in paclitaxel-resistant human colorectal tumors. Paclitaxel entrapped in emulsifying wax nanoparticles was shown to overcome drug resistance in a human colon adenocarcinoma cell line (HCT-15). The insolubility problems encountered with paclitaxel can be overcome by conjugating this drug with albumin. Paclitaxel bound to biocompatible proteins like albumin (Abraxane) is an injectable nano-suspension approved for the treatment of breast cancer. The solvent Cremophor-EL used in previous formulations of paclitaxel causes acute hypersensitivity reactions. To reduce the risk of allergic reactions when receiving paclitaxel, patients must undergo pre-medication using steroids and anti-histamines and be given the drug using slow infusions lasting a few hours. Binding paclitaxel to albumin resulted in delivery of higher dose of drug in short period of time. Because it is solvent-free, solvent-related toxicities are also eliminated. In Phase III clinical trial, the response rate of Abraxane was about twice than that of the solvent-containing drug Taxol.

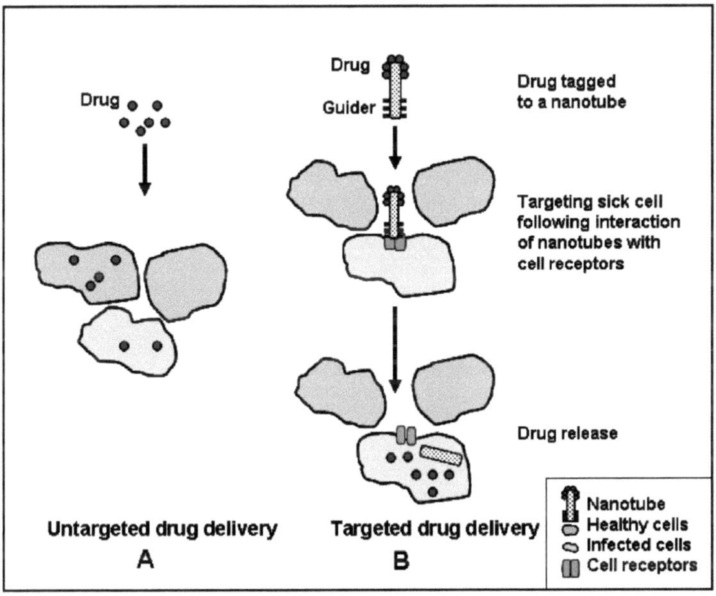

Figure 1. Untargeted and targeted drug delivery systems.

Nanoparticle-Mediated Delivery of siRNA

Short interfering RNA (siRNA) is emerging as a robust method of controlling gene expression with a large number of applications. Translation of nucleic acid-based therapy to clinical studies will require significant advances in the delivery system. Quantum dots (QD) have been used to monitor RNAi delivery (Chen et al., 2005). The PLGA and PLA based nanoparticles have also been used for *in vitro* RNAi delivery (Shinde et al., 2007). Although there has been some success in the delivery of siRNA using various nanomaterials, tracking their delivery, and monitoring their transfection efficiency is difficult without a suitable tracking agent or marker. Designing an efficient and self-tracking transfection agent for RNA interference is a big challenge. Recently, Tan et al. (2007) synthesized chitosan nanoparticles encapsulated with quantum dots and used such nanomaterial to deliver human epidermal growth factor receptor-2 (HER2/neu) siRNA. Such a novel nano carrier helped in monitoring the siRNA by the presence of fluorescent QDs in the chitosan nanoparticles. Targeted delivery of HER2 siRNA to HER2-overexpressing SKBR3 breast cancer cells has been specific with chitosan/quantum dot nanoparticles surface labeled with HER2 antibody targeting the HER2 receptors on SKBR3 cells (Tan et al., 2007).

Labeling of nanoparticles with a fluorescent marker, such as Cy-5, helps in visualizing uptake and accumulation of nanotubes using a fluorescent microscope. Recently, Howard et al. (2006) used such nanoparticles conjugated with siRNA specific to the BCR/ABL-1 junction sequence and found 90% reduced expression of BCR/ABL-1 leukemia fusion protein in K562 (Ph(+)) cells. Effective *in vivo* RNA interference was also achieved in bronchiolar epithelial cells of transgenic EGFP mice after nasal administration of chitosan/siRNA formulations. These findings highlight the potential application of this novel chitosan-based system in RNA-mediated therapy of systemic and mucosal disease.

Cancer

Targeting Cancer Cells with Nanoparticles

Cancer is one of the most challenging diseases today, and brain cancer is one of the most difficult malignancies to detect and treat mainly because of the difficulty in getting imaging and therapeutic agents across the blood-brain barrier and into the brain. Many investigators have found that nanoparticles hold promise for ferrying such agents into the brain (Costantino et al., 2005; Kreuter et al., 2002; Sumner and Kopelman, 2005). Apolipoprotein E was suggested to mediate drug transport across the blood-brain barrier (Michaelis et al., 2006). Loperamide, which does not cross the blood-brain barrier but exerts antinociceptive effects after direct injection into the brain, was loaded into human serum albumin nanoparticles and linked to apolipoprotein E. Mice treated intravenously with this complex induced antinociceptive effects in the tail-flick test. The efficacy of this drug delivery system of course depends upon the recognition of lipoprotein receptors. Kopelman and colleagues designed probes encapsulated by biologically localized embedding (PEBBLE) to carry a variety of unique agents on their surface and to perform multiple functions (Sumner and Kopelman, 2005). One target molecule immobilized on the surface could guide the PEBBLE to a tumor. Another agent could be used to help visualize the target using magnetic resonance imaging, while a third agent attached to the PEBBLE could deliver a destructive dose of drug or toxin to nearby cancer cells. All three functions can be combined in a single tiny polymer sphere to make a potent weapon against cancer. Another anti-cancer drug, doxorubicin, bound to polysorbate-coated nanoparticles is able to cross the intact blood-brain barrier and be released at therapeutic concentrations in the brain (Steiniger et al., 2004). Smart superparamagnetic iron oxide particle conjugates can be used to target and locate brain tumors earlier and more accurately than reported methods

(Zhang et al., 2004). It is known that folic acid combined with polyethylene glycol can further enhance the targeting and intracellular uptake of the nanoparticles. Therefore, nanomaterial holds tremendous potential as a carrier for drugs to target cancer cells.

Targeting Angiogenesis with Nanoparticles

Robust angiogenesis underlies aggressive growth of tumors. Therefore, one of the mechanisms to inhibit angiogenesis is to starve tumor cells. Angiogenesis is regulated through a complex set of mediators and recent evidence shows that integrin $\alpha v\beta 3$ and VEGFs play important regulator roles. Therefore, selective targeting of $\alpha v\beta 3$ integrin and VEGFs is a novel anti-angiogenesis strategy for treating a wide variety of solid tumors. One approach is to coat nanoparticles with peptides that bind specifically to the $\alpha v\beta 3$ integrin and the VEGF receptor (Li et al., 2004). The synthetic peptide bearing Arg-Gly-Asp (RGD) sequence is known to specifically bind to the $\alpha v\beta 3$ integrin expressed on endothelial cells in the angiogenic blood vessels, which can potentially inhibit the tumor growth and proliferation. Following hydrophobic modifications, glycol chitosan is capable of forming self-aggregated nanotube and has been used as a carrier for the RGD peptide, labeled with fluoresein isothiocyanate (FITC-GRGDS) (Park et al., 2004). These nanotubes loaded with FITC-GRGDS might be useful for monitoring or destroying the angiogenic tissue/blood vessels surrounding the tumor tissue. Our research group has been studying biological responses of RGDSK self-assembling rosette nanotubes (RGDSK-RNT). These rosette nanotubes are a novel class of nanotubes that are biologically inspired and naturally water soluble upon synthesis (Fenniri et al., 2001, 2002). These nanotubes are formed from guanine-cytosine motif as building blocks. However, one of the novel properties of the RNT is the ability to accept a variety of functional groups at the G/C motif which imparts functional versatility to the nanotubes for specific medical or biological applications. Therefore, the RNTs can be potentially modified to target a variety of therapeutic molecules *in vivo* to treat cancer and inflammatory diseases.

Nanosystems in Inflammation

Targeting Macrophages to Control Inflammation

The potential of macrophages for rapid recognition and clearance of foreign particles has provided a rational approach to macrophage-specific targeting with nanoparticles. Macrophages' ability to secrete a multitude of inflammatory mediators allows them to regulate inflammation in many diseases. Therefore, macrophages are potential pharmaceutical targets in many human and animal diseases. Although macrophages are capable of killing most of the microbes, many microorganisms (*Toxoplasma gondii*, *Leishmania* sp., *Mycobacterium tuberculosis* and *Listeria monocytogenes*) have developed potential ability to resist phagocytosis activity of macrophages. These pathogens subvert a macrophage's molecular machinery designed to kill them and come to reside in modified lysosomes. Therefore, nanoparticles-mediated delivery of antimicrobial agent(s) into pathogen-containing intracellular vacuoles in macrophages could be useful to eliminate cellular reservoirs (Gaspar et al., 1992; Zhang et al., 2007). This system can be used to achieve therapeutic drug concentrations in the vacuoles of infected macrophages and reduction in side effects associated with the drug administration and the release of pro-inflammatory cytokines. Polyalkylcyanoacrylates (PACA) nanoparticles have been used as a carrier for targeting anti-leishmanial drugs into macrophages. This nanomaterial did not induce interleukin-1 release by macrophages (Balland et al., 1996). Therefore, similarly designed nanosytems could be very useful in targeting macrophage infections in chronic diseases.

The anti-fungal and anti-leishmanial agent amphotericin B (AmB) has been complexed with lipids-based nanotubes to develop a less toxic formulation of AmB. Gupta and Viyas (2007) formulated AmB in trilaurin-based nanosize lipid particles (emulsomes) stabilized by soya phosphatidylcholine as a new intravenous drug delivery system for macrophage targeting. Nanocarrier-mediated delivery of macrophage toxins has proved to be a powerful approach in getting rid of unwanted macrophages in gene therapy and other clinically relevant situations such as autoimmune blood disorders, T cell-mediated autoimmune diabetes, rheumatoid arthritis, spinal cord injury, sciatic nerve injury, and restenosis after angioplasty. Alternatively, nanoparticles with macrophage-lethal properties can also be exploited. Exploiting a variety of macrophage cell receptors as therapeutic targets may prove a better strategy for antigen delivery and targeting with particulate nanocarriers.

Targeting Inflammatory Molecules

In the past two decades, many cell adhesion molecules have been discovered. Cell adhesion molecules are glycoproteins found on the cell surface that act as receptors for cell-to-cell and cell-to-extracellular matrix adhesion (Hynes, 2002; Hynes and Zhao, 2000). These cell adhesion molecules are divided into four classes called integrins, cadherins, selectins, and the immunoglobulin superfamily. These molecules are required for the efficient migration of inflammatory cells such as neutrophils and monocytes into inflamed organs and generation of host response to infections. There is, however, considerable evidence that excessive migration of neutrophils in inflamed lungs leads to exaggerated tissue damage and mortality. Therefore, a major effort is underway to fine tune the migration of neutrophils into inflamed organs. Recent advancements of the understanding of the cell adhesion molecules has impacted the design and development of drugs (i.e., peptide, proteins) for the potential treatment of cancer, heart, and autoimmune diseases (Chen et al., 2005; Gupta et al., 2005; Schiffelers et al., 2003). These molecules have important roles in diseases such as cancer (Christofori, 2003; Haass et al., 2005), thrombosis (Andrews and Berndt, 2004; Pancioli and Brott, 2004), and autoimmune diseases such as type-1 diabetes (Anderson and Siahaan, 2003; Shimaoka and Springer, 2004; Yusuf-Makagiansar et al., 2002). The RGD peptides have been used to target integrins $\alpha v\beta 3$ and $\alpha v\beta 5$, and peptides derived from the intercellular adhesion molecule-1 (ICAM-1) have been used to target the $\alpha v\beta 2$ integrin. Peptides derived from $\alpha v\beta 2$ can target ICAM-1 expressing cells. Cyclic RGD peptides have been conjugated to paclitaxel (PTX-RGD) and doxorubicin (Dox-RGD4C) for improving the specific delivery of these drugs to tumor cells. Mice bearing human breast carcinoma cells (i.e., MDA-MB-435) survived the disease when treated with Dox-RGD4C, while all the untreated control mice died because of the disease (Arap et al., 1998). This conjugate targets $\alpha v\beta 3$ and $\alpha v\beta 5$ integrins on the tumor vasculature during angiogenesis.

Extracellular regulated kinases (ERK) may regulate apoptosis and cell survival at multiple points that include increasing p53 and BAX action, increasing caspase-3 and caspase-8 activities, decreasing Akt activity, and increasing expression of TNF-α (Zhuang and Schnellmann, 2006). Our research group is investigating the interaction of RGD-RNT to αvβ3 integrins, following cell signaling through P38 kinases and its function in human lung epithelial cells, and bovine and equine neutrophil migration. Cyclo(1,12)PenITDGEATDSGC peptide (cLABL peptide), derived from the I-domain of the α subunit of leukocyte function-associated factor-1 (LFA-1) is known to bind ICAM-1. cLABL peptide has been conjugated with methotrexate (MTX) to give MTX-cLABL conjugate (Dunehoo et al., 2006). Because ICAM-1 is upregulated during tissue inflammation and several different cancers, this conjugate may be useful for directing drugs to inflammatory and tumor cells. The anti-inflammatory activity of MTX is due to the suppression of production of anti-inflammatory cytokines such as (interleukin-6) IL-6 and (interleukin-8) IL-8. Thus, the activity of MTX-cLABL conjugate was compared to MTX in suppressing the production of these cytokines in human coronary artery endothelial cells stimulated with TNF-α. The MTX-cLABL is more selective in suppressing the production of IL-6 than IL-8, which is opposite to MTX. The PLGA nanoparticles coated with cLABL peptides have also been shown to upregulate ICAM-1 (Zhang and Berkland, 2006). More detailed information on the mechanism(s) of internalization and intracellular trafficking of cell adhesion molecules is required to be exploited for delivering drug molecules to a specific cell type or for diagnosis of cancer and other diseases (heart and autoimmune diseases).

CONCLUSION

It appears that nano drug delivery systems hold great potential to overcome some of the barriers to efficient targeting of cells and molecules in inflammation and cancer. There also is an exciting possibility to overcome problems of drug resistance in target cells and facilitating movement of drugs across barriers such as those in the brain. The challenge, however, remains the precise characterization of molecular targets and to ensure that these molecules are expressed only in the targeted organs to prevent effects on healthy tissues. Secondly, it is important to understand the fate of the drugs once delivered to the nucleus and other sensitive cells organelles. Furthermore, because nanosystems increase efficiency of drug delivery, the doses may need recalibration. Nevertheless, the future remains exciting and wide open.

KEYWORDS

- **Apolipoprotein E**
- **p-Glycoprotein**
- **Polyalkylcyanoacrylates nanoparticles**
- **Vascular endothelial growth factor**

AUTHORS' CONTRIBUTIONS

Both the authors contributed equally in the preparation of this review chapter.

COMPETING INTERESTS

The author(s) declare that they have no competing interests.

Chapter 2

Novel Multi-component Nanopharmaceuticals for Anti-HIV Effects

Li Wan, Xiaoping Zhang, Simi Gunaseelan, Shahriar Pooyan, Olivia Debrah, Michael J. Leibowitz, Arnold B. Rabson, Stanley Stein, and Patrick J. Sinko

INTRODUCTION

Current anti-acquired immunodeficiency syndrome (AIDS) therapeutic agents and treatment regimens can provide a dramatically improved quality of life for human immunodeficiency virus (HIV)–positive people, many of whom have no detectable viral load for prolonged periods of time. Despite this, curing AIDS remains an elusive goal, partially due to the occurrence of drug resistance. Since the development of resistance is linked to, among other things, fluctuating drug levels, our long-term goal has been to develop nanotechnology-based drug delivery systems that can improve therapy by more precisely controlling drug concentrations in target cells. The theme of the current study is to investigate the value of combining AIDS drugs and modifiers of cellular uptake into macromolecular conjugates having novel pharmacological properties.

Bioconjugates were prepared from different combinations of the approved drug, saquinavir (SQV), the antiviral agent, R.I.CK-Tat9, the polymeric carrier, poly(ethylene) glycol, and the cell uptake enhancer, biotin. Anti-HIV activities were measured in MT-2 cells, an HTLV-1-transformed human lymphoid cell line, infected with HIV-1 strain Vbu 3, while parallel studies were performed in uninfected cells to determine cellular toxicity. For example, R.I.CK-Tat9 was 60 times more potent than L-Tat9 while the addition of biotin resulted in a prodrug that was 2,850 times more potent than L-Tat9. Flow cytometry and confocal microscopy studies suggest that variations in intracellular uptake and intracellular localization, as well as synergistic inhibitory effects of SQV and Tat peptides, contributed to the unexpected, and substantial differences in antiviral activity.

Our results demonstrate that highly potent nanoscale multi-drug conjugates with low non-specific toxicity can be produced by combining moieties with anti-HIV agents for different targets onto macromolecules having improved delivery properties.

Most current anti-AIDS drugs target two key enzymes in the HIV-1 replication cycle, reverse transcriptase, and protease. While the remarkable efficacy of protease and reverse transcriptase inhibitor combinations for the treatment of HIV-1 infection has been clearly established *in vitro* and in the clinic, not even a single AIDS patient has ever been cured. Accordingly, new anti-HIV drug candidates having alternate mechanisms of action are under investigation. For example, ALX40-4C (Doranz et al., 1997; O'Brien et al., 1996) blocks viral coreceptor CXCR4 and TAK-779 (Baba et al.,

1999) blocks coreceptor CCR5. The T-20 (Kilby et al., 1998; Wild et al., 1994) and T-1249 (Bangsberg et al., 2000; Castagna et al., 2005; Lazzarin et al., 2003) inhibit virus-cell fusion by binding to the viral envelope glycoprotein gp-41. Tat antagonists (Choudhury et al., 1998; Hamy et al., 1998) interrupt viral transcription. The NCp7 inhibitors (Turpin et al., 1999) hamper viral assembly and budding. To date, combination pharmacotherapy remains the most effective strategy for reducing viral loads in HIV-infected patients. However, given the variety of new chemical entities under development, combination therapies hold even greater future promise.

A major impediment to successful anti-HIV-1 therapy is the emergence of drug resistant strains harboring mutations in genes encoding these viral enzymes (Larder et al., 1995). Factors that are known or expected to contribute to the failure of highly active antiretroviral therapy (HAART) include pre-existing resistance (Opravil et al., 2002), low and fluctuating drug concentrations due to poor drug absorption or patient non-compliance (Bangsberg et al., 2000; Nieuwkerk et al., 2001; Paterson et al., 2000), and the presence of viral reservoirs and sanctuary sites (Schrager and D'Souza, 1998). Other mechanisms of resistance are becoming increasingly recognized in AIDS therapy. For example, drug-induced biopharmaceutical "resistance" (i.e., multi-drug resistance), an established concept in cancer pharmacotherapy (Cole et al., 1992; Goldie and Coldman, 1984), occurs when the upregulation of cell efflux transporter activity results in lower cellular exposure and decreased drug efficacy. Therefore, the ability to control blood and cellular drug concentrations is critical for managing the emergence of classical viral and multi-drug resistance.

Recent successes with HIV peptide fusion inhibitors such as T20 (e.g., enfuvirtide and fuzeon) (Lazzarin et al., 2003) suggest that small anti-HIV peptides can provide clinical utility complementing the antiviral activity of reverse transcriptase or protease inhibitors. However, many of these peptide drugs are poorly absorbed or are rapidly cleared from the body. The HIV-1 encodes a small non-structural protein, Tat (*trans*-activator of transcription), which is essential for transcriptional activation of virally encoded genes. Viruses with deletion of the Tat-function are non-viable (Jeang et al., 1999). Efficient replication and gene expression of HIV-1 requires a specific interaction of the Tat viral protein with the *trans*-activation responsive element (TAR), a highly stable stem-loop RNA structure (Kaushik et al., 2002). The interaction with TAR is mediated by a 9-amino acid basic domain (RKKRRQRRR, residues 49–57) of the Tat protein (Figure 1). This domain is essential for TAR RNA binding *in vivo* and is sufficient for TAR recognition *in vitro* (Madore and Cullen, 1993). A Tat-derived basic arginine-rich peptide alone binds TAR RNA with high affinity *in vitro* (Choudhury et al., 1998). A peptidyl compound, N-acetyl- RKKRRQRRR-(biotin)-NH_2, containing the 9-amino acid sequence of Tat protein basic domain, was shown to inhibit both Tat-TAR interaction *in vitro* and HIV-1 replication in cell culture (Choudhury et al., 1998). In addition to the TAR RNA interaction, the basic domain in Tat has at least three other functional properties. It constitutes a nuclear/nucleolar localization signal (Hauber et al., 1989; Ruben et al., 1989). The basic Tat peptide is also a prototypic cell penetrating peptide that can bring a cargo molecule across the plasma membrane. This was originally discovered when it was observed that Tat protein could freely enter cells (Frankel and Pabo, 1988). Small Tat peptides derived from the basic domain have also been shown to inhibit HIV replication in cultured T-cells by interacting with the HIV CXCR4 co-receptor present on the surface of T cells, thereby blocking infection by T-tropic HIV-1 strains (Ghezzi et al., 2000; Lohr et al., 2003; Xiao et al., 2000). These peptides may also have translational effects (Choudhury et al., 1999).

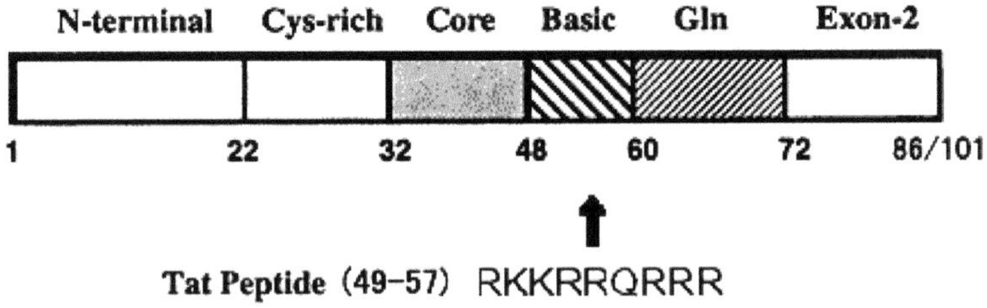

Figure 1. Schematic representation of Tat peptide, the basic domain in the viral Tat protein containing residue 49–57.

Therefore, we have been investigating Tat peptides as therapeutic agents (Choudhury et al., 1998, 1999). Considering the pleiotrophic effects of Tat domain peptides, it is not clear whether the delivery of these peptides to extracellular or intracellular targets or both is important for their antiviral effect. Furthermore, since these Tat peptides have cell penetrating activity (Zhang et al., 2004), they can also potentially be used to enhance the cellular uptake of an appended drug (Nori et al., 2003). However, Tat peptides have certain disadvantages, such as high systemic clearance due to *in vivo* degradation, non-specific binding to other biological components, and rapid renal clearance due to their low molecular weight and positive charges (Lee and Pardridge, 2001). A variety of different strategies have improved biopharmaceutical properties of peptide drugs. In our studies, we have utilized retro-inverso (RI) peptides and macromolecular PEG conjugates to overcome the many biopharmaceutical challenges faced by Tat peptides. The R.I.CK (retro-inverso-D-cysteine-lysine)-Tat9, N-acetyl- RKKRRQRRR -NH_2, consists of D-amino acids assembled in the reverse order of the natural L-amino acid Tat9 peptide, N-acetyl-RKKRRQRRR-NH_2. Thus, R.I.CK-Tat9 has a similar shape and charge distribution to the natural L-amino acid peptide but is more stable to proteases and retains pharmacological activity (Wang, 1997). The PEGylation has been shown to be one of the most successful techniques for improving the pharmacokinetic and pharmacodynamic properties of peptide drugs by increasing stability and reducing renal clearance and protein binding (Harris and Chess, 2003).

The second agent used in this study, SQV was the first HIV-protease inhibitor approved by the US Food and Drug Administration. Its structure mimics the phenylalanine-proline cleavage sequence at positions 167 and 168 of the HIV gag-pol polyprotein (Debouck, 1992). Thus, SQV prevents cleavage of gag and gag-pol protein precursors by HIV protease in acutely and chronically infected cells, arresting maturation and blocking nascent virions from becoming infectious (Roberts et al., 1990). However, therapeutic use of SQV suffers from problems of low absorptive and high secretory permeability, bioconversion to inactive metabolites, and poor solubility (Aungst, 1999; Sinko et al., 2004). The oral bioavailability of SQV in clinical formulations is low and/or variable with limited penetration into the lymphatic and central nervous systems (CNS) (Flexner, 1998; Sawchuk and Yang, 1999). While its low and variable bioavailability is primarily attributed to metabolism by cytochrome P-450 3A, recent results published by our group (Williams et al., 2002) and others (Jones et al., 2001) suggest that multiple membrane transporters may also contribute significantly to the delivery problems of SQV.

We showed that the activity of SQV prodrug conjugates was reduced when SQV was conjugated to $PEG_{3.4\,K}$, compared to the maximal achievable antiviral efficacy (Gunaseelan et al., 2004). But activity was restored by the addition of R.I.CK-Tat9 to the conjugate (EC_{50} = 15 nM). However, the mechanism of enhancement for the SQV-$PEG_{3.4\,k}$-R.I.CK-Tat9 conjugates was not clearly established since, in addition to targeting intracellular TAR, Tat possesses cell penetrating properties (Nori et al., 2003; Zhang et al., 2004) that may promote conjugate uptake into the cell and/or it may exert anti-HIV-1 activity by means of cell surface binding to CXCR4 receptors (Ghezzi et al., 2000; Lohr et al., 2003; Xiao et al., 2000). In the current study, the preclinical *in vitro* effectiveness of a small peptidic Tat antagonist, R.I.CK-Tat9, alone or in combination with SQV on multifunctional poly(ethylene glycol) (PEG)-based bioconjugates is demonstrated. Furthermore, the mechanism of enhanced activity of the SQV-$PEG_{3.4\,k}$-R.I.CK-Tat9 conjugates was addressed by flow cytometry and confocal microscopy. The current results suggest that the increased anti-HIV activity of SQV-$PEG_{3.4\,k}$-R.I.CK-Tat9 is due to the enhanced intracellular uptake and synergistic inhibitory effects of SQV on HIV protease and Tat peptides on both CXCR4 co-receptor interaction and/or HIV-1 transcriptional activation.

MATERIALS AND METHODS

Synthesis of R.I.CK-Tat9 and SQV Conjugates

The R.I.CK-Tat9 and its derivatives, compounds 1–3 (Figure 2) were synthesized manually on a MBHA Rink amide resin (Novabiochem, La Jolla, CA) via Fmoc chemistry in the presence of coupling activating reagents, BOP (benzotriazol-1-yl-oxytris(dimethylamino)phosphonium hexafluorophosphate), and HOBt (N-hydroxy-benzotriazole) (Sigma-Aldrich, St. Louis, MO). The ε-Dde (1-(4,4-dimethyl-2,6-dioxocyclohex-1-ylidene)ethyl) protecting group (in the N-terminal lysine residue) was selectively removed using 2% hydrazine in DMF (dimethylformamide) and reacted to attach the appended groups biotin-NHS or carboxyfluorescein-NHS (Sigma-Aldrich, St. Louis, MO) on solid support. The peptides were then acetylated, cleaved, and purified on a Vydac C_{18} column (10 μm, 2.2 × 25 cm, Vydac, Hesperia, CA) with detection at 220 nm; fluorescence of labeled peptides was detected at 535 nm (emission) and 485 nm (excitation). The purified products were lyophilized and confirmed by electrospray ionization mass spectra (ESI-MS).

In the synthesis of R.I.CK-Tat9-PEG bioconjugates (Figure 3), R.I.CK(fluorescein)-Tat9 was conjugated to mPEG-MAL by the reaction of the thiol group of R.I.CK(fluorescein)-Tat9 with the maleimide group on mPEG-MAL, which formed a stable thioether bond between PEG and R.I.CK(fluorescein)-Tat9. The eight amino groups of $PEG_{10\,k}$-$(NH_2)_8$ (MW 10 kDa, 8-arm branched, Nektar Therapeutics, Huntsville,

AL) were first activated with 3-fold molar excess of the heterobifunctional cross-linker, N-maleimidobutyryloxysuccinimide ester (GMBS) (Pierce Biotechnology, Rockford, IL), in DMF to form a maleimide activated PEG. The reaction was stirred overnight at room temperature. The product was precipitated with cold ether and dried under vacuum to yield the solid PEGylated product. The GMBS linker essentially converts a primary amino group to a maleimide group that can react with a thiol group to form a stable thioether bond. This activated intermediate seven was reacted with a 3-fold molar excess of 1, 2, and 3, respectively, with coupling reagents HOBt (4-fold molar excess) and BOP (3-fold molar excess) in DMF. The DIEA (diisopropylethylamine, 1% v/v) was added to adjust to neutral pH. For control, the eight amino groups of 8-arm PEG amine were reacted with carboxyfluorescein-NHS in the presence of 1% DIEA in DMF to yield 11 $PEG_{10\,k}$-(fluorescein)$_8$ lacking Tat peptides. The products were recrystallized from cold ether and dried under vacuum overnight. These bioconjugates were purified using size-exclusion chromatography using a Sephacryl S-100 column (Amersham, Piscataway, NJ) in 0.1 M PBS, pH 7.4, with detection at 220 nm. For 10, fluorescence was detected at 535 nm (emission) and 485 nm (excitation). The formation of the bioconjugates was confirmed by MALDI-TOF mass spectrometry and the concentrations of bioconjugates were determined by amino acid analysis.

In the synthesis of the SQV conjugates (Figure 4), the active hydroxyl function of SQV (extracted from Inverase, Roche) was esterified with Fmoc-Cys(S-Trt)-COOH using DIPC (1,3-diisopropylcarbodiimide)/DMAP (4-(dimethylamino)pyridine) as coupling reagent. The SQV-Cys ester was obtained with 82% yield after Fmoc removal with piperidine, followed by TFA(trifluoroacetic acid)-deprotection of the Trt (trityl) group. The esterification of the hydroxyl of SQV after silica gel purification was confirmed by ESI-MS and 1H and 13C NMR. The ESI-MS (m/z): 774.5 $(M + H)^+$; 796.5 $(M + Na)^+$. The PEGylation was carried out using $PEG_{3.4\,k}$-NHS in the presence of DIEA/DCM. This product was purified using gel permeation chromatography (Sephadex LH-20 column in DMF, 239 nm) resulting in 70 % yield. The formation of above was confirmed by MALDI-TOF (m/z (%) 3837.6) and ^1H and ^{13}C NMR. The thiol group of the cysteine in PEGylated form of SQV-Cys-ester was then activated with 2,2'-dithiodipyridine. Addition of one to the activated PEGylated form of SQV-Cys-ester gave with 65% yield after gel permeation purification. Mass spectrometry of these products demonstrated peaks at the expected molecular weights using MALDI-TOF (m/z (%) 5447.6.

Release Kinetics of R.I.CK-Tat9 by Cleavage of Thioether Bond

The stability of fluorescein-labeled $PEG_{10\,k}$-(R.I.CK-Tat9)8 bioconjugates was investigated in PBS (pH 7.4) and rabbit plasma, at 37°C. The stability of the bioconjugates was also investigated in PBS (pH 7.4) at 37°C by treating them with 5 μM glutathione (GSH) (Sigma-Aldrich, St. Louis, MO), a physiologically relevant reducing reagent that is responsible for intracellular reductive environment inside cells. Initially, different concentrations (0.01–10.0 μM) of R.I.CK (fluorescein)-Tat9 were dissolved separately in PBS (pH 7.4) and in plasma and their fluorescence measured by Tecan fluorescence microplate reader (excitation at 485 nm, emission at 535 nm) to obtain calibration curves in PBS (pH 7.4) and in plasma. Thereafter, the bioconjugate solutions were incubated separately in PBS (pH 7.4) and in spiked rabbit plasma at 37°C, along with GSH treated bioconjugates in PBS (pH 7.4) at 37°C. Aliquots were withdrawn at different time points and centrifuged at 14,000 × g for 90 min with a Microcon™ filter (molecular weight cut-off= 10,000 Da) (Amicon Inc., Beverly, MA). The drug moiety cleaved from the bioconjugate during the incubation passes through the filter whereas the drug moiety that remains linked to the PEG carrier is retained. (Note that a PEG polymer of 3,400 Da behaves as a > 10,000 Da peptide on ultrafiltration.) The retentates resulting from the different incubation time points were withdrawn and subjected to fluorescence detection. Each measurement was done in duplicate. The concentrations of the bioconjugates were determined from a fluorescence calibration curve that was established in the same media. The rate constant (k) was obtained from the linear plot of ln (bioconjugate)t versus incubation time, t (hr), where (bioconjugate)t = concentration of bioconjugate at different incubation time, t, (Figure 5). The half-life ($t_{1/2}$) of the cleavage of thioether bond from the bioconjugates was calculated from the relation $t_{1/2} = 0.693/k$ where k is the slope of the linear plot.

Release Kinetics of SQV by Cleavage of Ester Bond

A fluorogenic protease inhibition assay was used to measure the hydrolysis kinetics of SQV-Cys ester which was the common intermediate for all the synthesized R.I.CK-Tat9-SQV bioconjugates. The chemical stability of this ester was determined in PBS at pH 7.4 and in spiked plasma both measured at 37°C as reported earlier (Gunaseelan et al., 2004).

Antiviral Assays

The *in vitro* anti-HIV activity of PEG conjugates was determined by a MTT-based HIV-1 susceptibility assay reported previously (Gunaseelan et al., 2004) using MT-2 cells, an HTLV-1-transformed human T-cell leukemia cell line, infected with the HIV-1 strain LAV-Vbu3. The cytotoxicity of the conjugates was evaluated in parallel. The MT-2 cells were grown in RPMI 1640 DM (Dutch modification) medium supplemented with 20% fetal bovine serum (FBS), 1% w/v pen-strep, and 1% w/v L-glutamine and maintained at 37°C in 5% CO_2 in an incubator. The cultured MT-2 cells were diluted to 2×10^5 cells/ml and infected at a multiplicity of infection (MOI) of 0.01 (1 viral particle per 100 cells), causing the death of 90% of the cells 5 days later. The tested conjugates were diluted with RPMI 1640 medium and were added to the cultured MT-2 cells after viral infection. Each conjugate was tested in triplicate for its antiviral activity. Cell viability was measured by the colorimetric MTT test at 540 nm, which is directly proportional to the number of living cells. The conjugate EC_{50} and LC_{50} values were determined from the curves of the percentage of viral cell killing and cytotoxicity against compound concentration (Table 1, Figure 6).

Confocal Microscopy

The MT2 cells were treated with fluorescein-labeled R.I.CK-Tat9 or its conjugates for 24 hr. Where indicated, a fluid phase endocytosis marker, tetramethylrhodamine-Dextran/10 kDa (Invitrogen/Molecular Probe), was used at 0.25 mg/ml in co-incubation with a fluorescein-labeled compound. All images were taken of live cells on a Leica

TCS SP2 Spectral Confocal Microscope using the XYZ mode and 0.25 micrometer per section. The fluorescence wavelength windows for different dyes were well separated to ensure no breach-through from one dye to another.

Flow Cytometry

The MT-2 cells were grown to 2 days post-confluency and aliquots of 2×10^6 cells were washed briefly and incubated in 96-well microplates with 1 μM $PEG_{10\ K}$, R.I.CK(fluorescein)-Tat9, $PEG_{3.4\ K}$-R.I.CK(fluorescein)-Tat9, and $PEG_{10\ K}$-(R.I.CK(fluorescein)-Tat9)$_8$ bioconjugate for 24 hr. Trypan blue staining was used for quenching of cell surface bound fluorochrome emission. After the 24 hr incubation with tested conjugates, the medium was immediately removed from the wells. Part of the cells were washed and resuspended in 0.02 M sodium acetate buffer (pH 5.8). The remaining cells were suspended in sodium acetate buffer containing 0.2 mg/ml trypan blue. After 20s, the cells were washed twice and resuspended in the sodium acetate buffer. The total cell associated fluorescence was then analyzed by flow cytometry using a Coulter EPICS PROFILE equipped with a 25 mW argon laser. For each analysis, 10,000–20,000 events were accumulated. The total cell associated fluorescence was the cell associated fluorescence of cells without quenching by trypan blue. The intracellular fluorescence was the cell associated fluorescence of cells quenched by trypan blue. The cell surface bound fluorescence is the difference between the total cell associated fluorescence and the intracellular fluorescence.

DISCUSSION

While recent advances in anti-AIDS therapeutics have resulted in the introduction of more potent drugs, a cure for HIV infection remains an elusive goal. Many factors contribute to the inability of current therapeutic regimens to cure HIV infection. However, central to the problem is the variability of drug concentrations in the blood and target tissues resulting from poor patient adherence to complicated regimens, the inability of these potent agents to selectively target infected tissues, and the poor penetration or retention of drugs in reservoir and sanctuary sites. It is becoming more obvious that better drug delivery and targeting technologies are required to increase total body persistence, target cell exposure and retention of these potent therapeutic agents. In the current study, we have produced and tested the first of a series of nanoscale drug delivery vehicles in order to better target HIV infected cells and possibly to provide novel modes of action.

The present report describes the design, synthesis, and initial characterization of a series of PEG-based bioconjugates in order to achieve maximum therapeutic payload of Tat peptide, to explore multi-drug delivery on one bioconjugate and to determine the potential role of Tat in the cellular uptake and HIV inhibition by the conjugates. These bioconjugates were designed (i) to carry multiple copies of the R.I.CK-Tat9 drug linked by stable thioether bonds to 8-arm poly(ethylene) glycol (PEG), (ii) to carry multiple drugs such as SQV for combination therapy, (iii) to have an extended biological and chemical half-life, (iv) to selectively release appended drug molecules inside the cell because of the differential in reducing capacity between blood and the internal cell environment and finally, (v) to enhance cellular uptake of the drug and bioconjugate through the use of uptake enhancing moieties like biotin attached to the R.I.CK-Tat9. These modifications were designed to increase the therapeutic peptide's bioavailability, biodistribution, and delivery into HIV sanctuary sites of both the therapeutic Tat peptide and appended drugs, exemplified here by SQV.

The current study is aimed at improving the therapeutic potential of a Tat-antagonistic compound R.I.CK-Tat9. It is an analog of the 9-amino acid sequence of the TAR-binding basic domain of Tat protein in which the direction (polarity) of the amino acid sequence is reversed and the chirality of each amino acid residue is inverted from L to D. The RI analog peptides are expected to have shapes and charge distributions of their side chains similar to the natural L-amino acid peptides, but are highly resistant to proteolysis (Chorev and Goodman, 1995; Fromme et al., 2003). Furthermore, Wender et. al. found that the L-, D-, and R.I. forms of Tat9 showed similar cellular uptake in serum-free medium, while in the presence of serum the D-form was modestly more active and the R.I. form much more active than the L-form, indicating the likely role of proteolysis in limiting the activity of natural peptides (Wender et al., 2000). The current results show that R.I.CK-Tat9 had a 60-fold higher anti-HIV activity than L-Tat9, consistent with the enhanced stability and/or increased intracellular availability of R.I.CK-Tat9.

Choudhury et al. showed that Tat9-C(biotin) with S-biotinylation of the cysteine residue was taken up 30-fold more efficiently by Jurkat cells than was unbiotinylated Tat9-C (3% vs. 0.1%, respectively) (Choudhury et al., 1998). This was attributed to increased hydrophobic interactions with the plasma membrane (Chen et al., 1995) and it was hypothesized that biotinylation would result in enhanced inhibiton of transactivating activity by the biotinylated compound. The current results confirm this hypothesis since the biotinylated RI-Tat9 was 47 times more potent than the RI-Tat9 and was approximately as potent as SQV in inhibiting HIV-1.

The central hypothesis of the current study is that improved delivery would result in an enhancement in the pharmacological properties of Tat inhibitors, in particular R.I.CK-Tat9. Thus, it was anticipated that PEGylation of R.I.CK-Tat9 would enhance the pharmacological properties *in vivo* for more effective delivery. The PEG residues were chosen to avoid *in vivo* binding of R.I.CK-Tat9 to plasma proteins and rapid elimination from the blood (Foroutan and Watson, 1999). Thus, PEGylation provides a way to increase the stability and body persistence of the R.I.CK-Tat9, which could result higher *in vivo* activity. However, the PEG conjugates reduced the antiviral activity of R.I.CK-Tat9 or R.I.CK(biotin)-Tat9 in cell culture experiments (Table 1). The thioether bonds, used in the linkage between R.I.CK-Tat9 or R.I.CK(biotin)-Tat9 and PEG were very stable, insuring that Tat was not released from the conjugate. These results suggest the quantitatively more important antiviral effect of R.I.CK-Tat9 depends upon its release from PEG, presumably reflecting a requirement for entry into infected cells.

An oligocationic peptide compound (ALX40-4C), designed to mimic the basic domain of the HIV-1 Tat (O'Brien et al., 1996), was also found to interfere with viral entry through the inhibition of the chemokine receptor CXCR4 on the host cell membrane (Doranz et al., 1997). The blocking of viral entry resulted in a more potent response than the inhibition of transactivation by that compound (O'Brien et al., 1996). To delineate whether the antiviral mechanism of the R.I.CK-Tat9 conjugates is by inhibition of transactivation or by blocking of cell surface co-receptor, R.I.CK-Tat9 was labeled with the fluorescence tag carboxyfluorescein-NHS and conjugated to $PEG_{3.4\,K}$ and $PEG_{10\,K}$ for stability and uptake mechanism studies of the final conjugates. Flow cytometry showed 93.8%, 53.6%, and 19.0% of total cell-associated R.I.CK(fluorescein)-Tat9, $PEG_{3.4\,K}$-R.I.CK(fluorescein)-Tat9, and $PEG_{10\,K}$-(R.I.CK(fluorescein)-Tat9)$_8$, respectively, were within the cells. In contrast, the control fluorescein labelled PEG lacking the Tat peptide, $PEG_{10\,K}$-(fluorescein)$_8$, showed little cell association by flow cytometry and no cell surface binding by fluorescence microscopy (data not shown). The confocal microscopy studies showed that cells incubated with 1μM R.I.CK(fluorescein)-Tat9 or $PEG_{3.4\,K}$-R.I.CK(fluorescein)-Tat9 showed significant higher intracellular fluorescence, while cells incubated with $PEG_{10\,K}$- (R.I.CK(fluorescein)-Tat9)$_8$ showed primarily cell surface-associated fluorescence. These results suggested that the observed anti-HIV activity of the uncleavable $PEG_{10\,K}$-(R.I.CK-Tat9)$_8$ conjugates is a result of the binding of the conjugate to cell surface CXCR4 receptor, which is consistent with observations of other groups (Doranz et al., 1997; O'Brien et al., 1996). However, the reduced potency of the conjugates relative to free R.I.CK-Tat9 suggests that this peptide may have more anti-HIV-1 activity at intracellular sites than at the cell surface. These results support the model that the most potent mechanism of action of this peptide agent is inhibition of the transcriptional effects of the viral Tat protein.

While expected to be a stronger binder to CXCR4, $PEG_{10\,K}$-(R.I.CK-Tat9)$_8$ is less promising than $PEG_{3.4\,K}$-R.I.CK-Tat9 in intracellular targeting. The intracellular space consists of two topological compartments—the cytosol/nucleus and all membrane-bound organelles including endosomes and lysosomes. The HIV-1 protease and reverse transcriptase, the cellular targets of the majority of current anti-HIV-1 drugs, are located in the cytosol, whereas the TAR region of all HIV-1 mRNA transcripts, the cellular target of both conjugates and their released R.I.CK-Tat9, is located in the nucleus. Compared to $PEG_{3.4\,K}$-R.I.CK-Tat9, less $PEG_{10\,K}$-(R.I.CK-Tat9)$_8$ is internalized. Significant portions of both internalized conjugates are within endosomes. Unless they escape, endosome-confined conjugates and their drug-carrying derivatives cannot reach these cellular targets. At present, there is some evidence in the literature for the endosomal escape of Tat peptide-conjugates or fusion proteins. We recently discovered a possible pH-dependent endosomal escape mechanism that could operate at the mildly acidic pH of 6.5 of early endosomes (to be published). Once they escape from endosomes, both conjugates and their released R.I.CK-Tat9 must enter the nucleus in order to meet their TAR target. The cytosol and the nucleus are continuous through nuclear pores, which have a functional diameter of about 40 nm. This pore size roughly equals the effective size of a linear PEG molecule of 20 kDa (Caliceti and Veronese, 2003), implying that the 25 kDa $PEG_{10\,K}$-(R.I.CK-Tat9)$_8$ might not be able to enter the nucleus while the 5 kDa $PEG_{3.4\,K}$-R.I.CK-Tat9 might.

In this study, we used uninfected MT2 cells that are transformed $CD4^+$ T cells, which are capable of supporting HIV-1 replication. Depending on a particular anti-HIV-1 agent tested and the MOI used, MT2 cells can serve as a useful model for HIV-1 infected or uninfected T cells *in vivo*. Critical to current HAART regimens is that both infected and uninfected T cells should be adequately loaded with anti-HIV-1 drugs at all times. In the infected cells, the drugs prevent the production of mature, infectious viruses. In the uninfected cells, the drugs play a prophylactic role, ensuring abortive infection, or replication whenever infection occurs. Constant new HIV-1 infection must take place as both HIV-1 and virus-replicating T cells have short *in vivo* half-life yet the virus keeps evolving and cessation of HAART inevitably leads to viral load rebounding. We now know that during all stages of HIV disease $CD4^+$ T cell depletion occurs predominantly in the gut (Brenchley et al., 2004).

Certain aspects of the performance of PEG conjugates (e.g., plasma persistence and protein binding) can only be studied *in vivo* and are not addressed in the current study. The known *in vivo* advantages of PEGylation of various pharmacophores indicates the potential that PEG-based bioconjugates could display useful therapeutic properties of increased plasma half-life (Davis et al., 1981), lower cytotoxicity (Conover et al., 1997), and reduced protein binding, which could outweigh the observed reduction in efficacy seen in this study for some PEGylated drugs. This will require further future study in *in vivo* models and is beyond the scope of the current studies.

Multiple-drug cocktail regimens have been associated with the recent successes in improving the quality of life of patients with AIDS. However, delivery of drugs to the bloodstream rather than too many of the known sites of high viral replication may not insure that the maximal therapeutic effect will be obtained. A potential first step in achieving this maximal effect is to better control the exposure of infected cells to multiple therapeutic agents. In this proof-of-principle study, the prototypical protease inhibitor, SQV, was conjugated to $PEG_{3.4\,K}$ and $PEG_{3.4\,K}$-R.I.CK-Tat9. The conjugation of PEG to SQV yielded a much less active prodrug conjugate SQV-Cys- $PEG_{3.4\,K}$ with EC_{50} at 900 nM. The 60-fold lower activity of the conjugate compared to the parent drug could be due to the slow cleavage of the ester bond and/or low cell uptake of the conjugate. However, the addition of Tat to SQV-Cys-$PEG_{3.4\,K}$ resulted in a conjugate with an EC_{50} of 0.015μM, the same *in vitro* potency as the free SQV. The increased activity of SQV-$PEG_{3.4\,K}$-R.I.CK-Tat9 may be attributable to a variety of factors including the enhanced intracellular uptake by the bifunctional conjugates containing both Tat peptide and SQV, the synergistic effects of SQV on HIV protease and Tat peptides on both HIV Tat-TAR binding and/or on cell surface receptor CXCR4. All of these results suggest that higher anti-HIV activity was attained mainly due to the enhanced intracellular uptake of SQV-$PEG_{3.4\,K}$-R.I.CK-Tat9 resulting in improved delivery of SQV. However, the synergistic effects of SQV on HIV protease and Tat peptides on both HIV TAR and/or CXCR4 are likely to contribute.

RESULTS

Synthesis of R.I.CK-Tat9 and SQV Conjugates

A series of R.I.CK-Tat9 and SQV bioconjugates was synthesized and characterized. The peptides, L-Tat9, R.I.CK-Tat9, R.I.CK(biotin)-Tat9, and R.I.CK(ε-carboxyfluorescein)-Tat9 (Figure 2) were synthesized, purified, and their structures were confirmed by electrospray ionization mass spectrometry (ESI-MS). For R.I.CK-Tat9

PEG bioconjugates, the thiol group of the cysteine residue at the N-terminus of R.I.CK-Tat9 or its derivatives was linked to the maleimide group on mPEG-MAL (Figure 3A) or amino groups of branched 8-arm $PEG_{10\,K}$-$(NH_2)_8$ through a stable thioether bond using a heterobifunctional cross-linker N-maleimidobutyryloxysuccinimide ester (GMBS) (Figure 3B). As a control, the eight amino groups of 8-arm PEG amine were reacted with carboxyfluorescein-NHS and yielded $PEG_{10\,K}$-(ε-carboxyfluorescein)$_8$ lacking Tat peptides. These bioconjugates were purified using size-exclusion chromatography on a Sephacryl S-100 column. The formation of each bioconjugate was confirmed by MALDI-TOF mass spectrometry and the concentration of each bioconjugates was determined by quantitative amino acid analysis. The overall design for all SQV conjugates was to link the various components using covalent bonds that varied in their stability properties (Figure 4). A biodegradable ester bond was made between the hydroxyl group of SQV and the carboxyl group of Cys. The esterification of the hydroxyl of SQV was confirmed by ESI-MS and ^{1}H and ^{13}C NMR. The thiol group of Cys was used to attach R.I.CK-Tat9 and its derivatives via a reducible disulfide bond, while the amino group of Cys was used to attach $PEG_{3.4\,k}$ via a more stable amide bond. The thiol group of the cysteine in PEGylated form of SQV-Cys-ester was activated with 2,2'-dithiodipyridine. Then, disulfide bond formation resulted from addition of R.I.CK-Tat9 to the activated PEGylated form of SQV (SQV-Cys($PEG_{3.4\,k}$)(TP)), giving SQV-Cys($PEG_{3.4\,k}$)(R.I.CK-Tat9), in 65% yield after gel permeation purification. Mass spectrometry using MALDI-TOF of these products demonstrated peaks at the expected molecular weights.

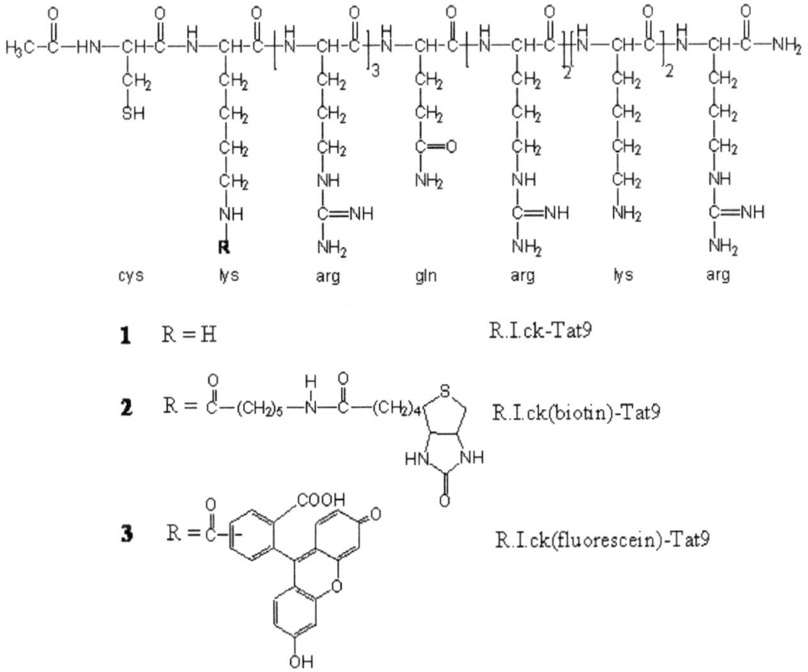

Figure 2. Schematic representation of R.I.CK-Tat9 and its derivatives.

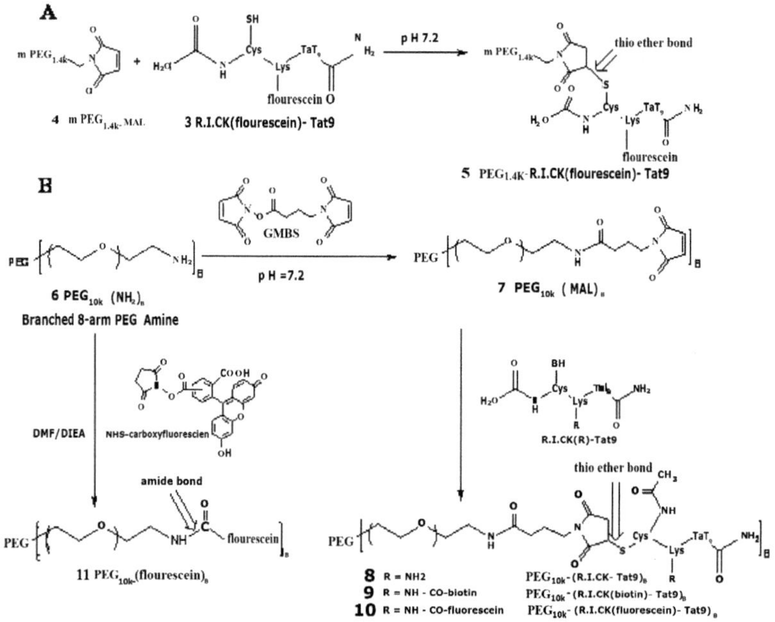

Figure 3. Synthetic scheme of Tat-PEG bioconjugates with single (3A) or multiple copies (3B) of R.I.CK-Tat9 and fluorescein-labeled control PEG lacking Tat peptides.

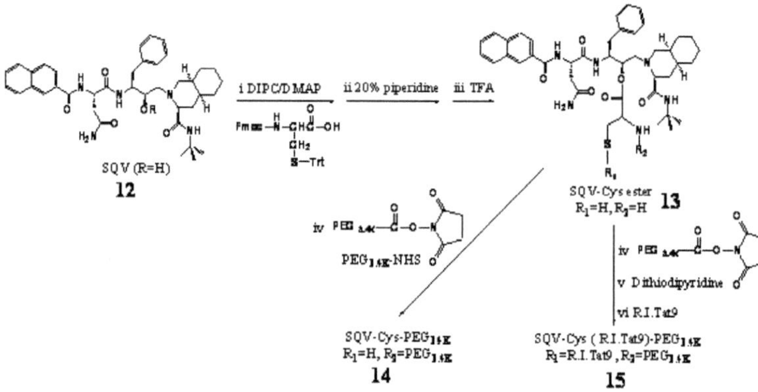

Figure 4. Synthetic scheme of Tat-SQV bioconjugates (i) 3 equivalents Fmoc-Cys(S-Trt)-COOH in CH_2Cl_2 with DIPC/DMAP; (ii) 20% piperidine in CH_2Cl_2 ; (iii) TFA/CH_2Cl_2 (1:1); (iv) 2 equivalents Fmoc-$PEG_{3.4\,K}$-NHS in CH_2Cl_2 with DIEA; (v) 2 equivalents 2,2′-Dithiodipyridine in DMSO; (vi) 2 equivalents. R.I.CK-Tat9 in DMSO.

Stability Studies

The stability of the covalent linkages attaching pharmacophores to the conjugates was determined. The R.I.CK-Tat9 was linked to $PEG_{10\,k}$ using a relatively stable thioether bond. The stability of this bond was assessed by incubating $PEG_{10\,K}$-(R.I.CK(fluorescein)-Tat9)$_8$ bioconjugates in PBS (pH 7.4), spiked plasma or PBS (pH 7.4) with 5 μM reduced GSH at 37°C. Aliquots were withdrawn at different time points and centrifuged at 14,000 × g for 90 min with a 10 kDa cut-off Microcon™ filter. The conjugated R.I.CK(fluorescein)-Tat9 was retained in the filter as retentates and separated from the cleaved free R.I.CK(fluorescein)-Tat9 that passed through the filter. Thereafter, the fluorescence of conjugated R.I.CK(fluorescein)-Tat9 was measured using a Tecan fluorescence microplate reader with an excitation wavelength at 485 nm and an emission wavelength at 535 nm. This method was used rather than measuring fluorescence in the flow-through, since the concentration of cleaved R.I.CK(fluorescein)-Tat9 could not be quantified due to high degree of adsorption caused by its positive charges (unpublished data). The calibration curves of fluorescein-labeled R.I.CK-Tat9 in PBS (pH 7.4) and in plasma were linear with correlation coefficients of 0.9993 and 0.9997, respectively. The concentration of the bioconjugates decreased with time (Figure 5). Plots of ln ((bioconjugate)t) against incubation time (t) were linear within the concentration range studied indicating that cleavage occurs by a first order process (Figure 5). The PEG_{10k}-((R.I.CK(fluorescein)-Tat9)$_8$ bioconjugate showed a longer half-life ($t_{1/2}$= 50.6 hr) in PBS (pH 7.4) than in plasma ($t_{1/2}$ of 24.4 hr). The half-life of this bioconjugate decreased significantly from 50.6 to 10.5 hr in the presence of 5 μM GSH in PBS (pH 7.4).

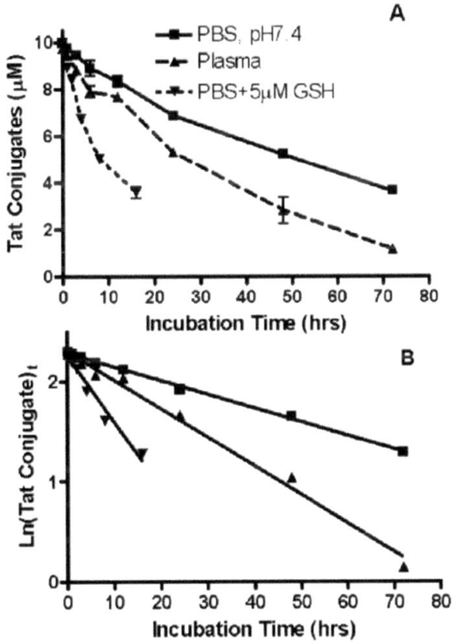

Figure 5. Panel A: Release of R.I.CK(fluorescein)-Tat9 from PEG_{10k}-((R.I.CK(fluorescein)-Tat9)$_8$ in PBS (pH 7.4) (■), in plasma (▲), or PBS (pH 7.4) with 5μM GSH (▼) at 37°C respectively, using fluorescence detection at excitation wavelength 485 nm and emission wavelength 535 nm. The concentrations of the bioconjugates were determined from fluorescence calibration curves that were established in the same media. All measurements were done in duplicates. Panel B: Plot of ln(bioconjugate)t versus incubation time (t) of the PEG- (R.I.CK(fluorescein)-Tat9)$_8$ in PBS (pH 7.4) (■), in plasma (▲) or PBS (pH 7.4) with 5 μM GSH (▼) at 37°C respectively. The rate constant (k) is the slope of this linear plot. The half-lives ($t_{1/2}$) for the thioether bond cleavage were calculated using the relation $t_{1/2}$ = 0.693/k.

The SQV was linked to R.I.CK-Tat9 through a SQV-Cys ester bond. The stability of the ester was evaluated in PBS at pH 7.4 and in spiked plasma, measured at 37°C using a recently developed fluorogenic protease assay for free SQV (Gunaseelan et al., 2004). The release of active SQV was observed with half-lives of 14 hr and 0.9 hr in PBS at pH 7.4 and in spiked plasma, respectively (Gunaseelan et al., 2004).

Biological Activity

The anti-HIV activity of each bioconjugate derived from R.I.CK-Tat9 and SQV was evaluated *in vitro* in HIV-infected MT-2 cells (Figure 6) utilizing an established antiviral assay (Gunaseelan et al., 2004). The L-form of Tat9 showed weak anti-HIV activity (EC_{50} = 51.3 μM) while the RI form of Tat peptide showed much stronger anti-HIV activity (EC_{50} = 0.85 μM). Biotin appended to the R.I.CK-Tat9 peptide greatly enhanced the activity of the peptide (EC_{50} = 0.018 μM), possibly due to the increased cellular uptake (~30-fold) conferred by biotin (Chen et al., 1995). The conjugation with a 10 kDa branched PEG might be expected to enhance the stability of the peptide by protecting it from attack by peptidases, even though the unnatural D-amino acids in the R.I. peptides may already confer ample protease-resistance. We found that R.I.CK-Tat9 is released from $PEG_{10\,k\text{-}(}$R.I.CK-Tat9$)_8$ conjugates very slowly ($t_{1/2}$ = 50.6 hr) and that most of the fluorescence labeled PEG10k-(R.I.CK-Tat9$)_8$ conjugate remained bound to the MT-2 cell surface rather than being internalized (Figures 7 and 8). Thus, the PEG conjugates of R.I.CK-Tat9 and R.I.CK(biotin)-Tat9 both displayed similar antiviral activity with EC_{50} of 1.47 μM and 1.5 μM, respectively, which was weaker than that of the non-PEGylated forms (Figure 6 and Table 1). This result suggests that the intracellular inhibitory effect of Tat peptide may be quantitatively more important than the extracellular blocking of HIV infection previously described for Tat-based peptides, although targeting cell surface receptors might still be an important secondary mechanism of viral inhibition by either biotinylated or non-biotinylated peptides.

The activity of SQV in drug conjugates compared to the maximal achievable antiviral efficacy of free SQV (EC_{50} = 15 nM) was reduced with addition of $PEG_{3.4\,k}$ alone (EC_{50} = 900 nM), but restored with the addition of R.I.CK-Tat9 to the SQV-$PEG_{3.4\,k}$ conjugate (EC_{50} = 0.015 μM), the same *in vitro* potency as free SQV.

The cytotoxicities of the R.I.CK-Tat9 and SQV bioconjugates were measured by incubating non-infected MT-2 cells in the presence of different concentrations of the bioconjugates for 5 days at 37°C. The cytotoxicity (LC_{50}) of all the tested bioconjugates was in the low micromolar range (12.5–46.8 μM). The L-form of Tat9 showed the poorest therapeutic index with essentially equivalent EC_{50} and LC_{50}. In contrast, a number of the multi-component bioconjugate molecules such as R.I.CK(biotin)-Tat9 and SQV-$PEG_{3.4\,k}$-R.I.CK-Tat9 exhibited very favorable therapeutic indices of 2600 and 833, respectively. The ratios of LC_{50}/EC_{50} (i.e., *in vitro* therapeutic index) are shown in Table 1.

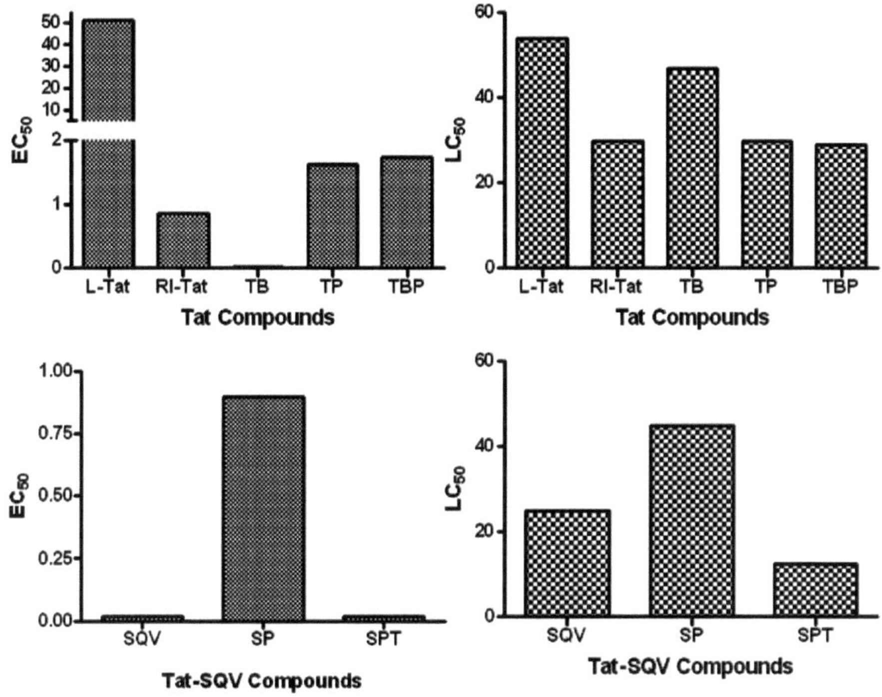

Figure 6. Representative data from MTT assays showing the anti-HIV activity (EC_{50}) of Tat and SQV compounds using MT-2 cells infected with HIV-1 strain Vbu 3 at 0.01 MOI. Cytotoxiciy (LC50) was determined usjng uninfected cells. (TB: R.I.CK(biotin)-Tat9, TP: PEG_{10k}-(R.I.CK-Tat9)$_8$, TBP: PEG_{10K}-(R.I.CK(biotin)-Tat9)$_8$, SQV: saquinavir, SP: SQV-Cys- $PEG_{3.4K}$, SPT: SQV- $PEG_{3.4K}$-R.I.CK-Tat9)

Table 1. Anti-HIV activity (EC_{50}) and cytotoxicity(LC_{50}) data of R.I.CK-Tat9 based bioconjugates in MT-2 cell culture infected with HIV-1 strain LAV-Vbu3 (MOI of 0.01).

Compound	Number	EC_{50} (μM)	R^b	LC_{50} (μM)	Therapeutic Index (LC_{50}/EC_{50})
L-Tat9	-	51.3	-	53.8	1
R.I.CK-Tat9	1	0.85	-	29.8	35
R.I.CK(biotin)-Tat9	2	0.018	0.02	46.8	2600
PEG_{10K}-(R.I.CK-Tat9)$_8$	8	1.47	1.7	29.1	20
PEG_{10K}-(R.I.CK (biotin)-Tat9)$_8$	9	1.50	1.8	29.7	20
SQV($MeSO_3H$) (control)	12	0.015	-	25	1667
SQV-Cys-$PEG_{3.4K}$	14	0.90	60	4.5	50
SQV-Cys(R.I.CK-Tat9)-$PEG_{3.4K}$	15	0.015	1	12.5	833

Flow Cytometry and Confocal Microscopy

Flow cytometry (Figure 7) showed that MT2 cells incubated with fluorescein-labeled control PEG lacking Tat peptides had a low fluorescence and no cell-associated fluorescence by fluorescence microscopy (data not shown), indicating PEG did not bind or enter the cells. In contrast, cells incubated with 1 μM (concentrations of conjugates containing Tat9 are indicated in Tat9 equivalents) R.I.CK(fluorescein)-Tat9, $PEG_{3.4\ k}$-R.I.CK(fluorescein)-Tat9, or $PEG_{10\ k}$- (R.I.CK(fluorescein)-$Tat9)_8$ had significant amounts of total cell-associated fluorescence, with cells incubated with $PEG_{3.4\ k}$-R.I.CK(fluorescein)-Tat9 and $PEG_{10\ k}$- (R.I.CK(fluorescein)-$Tat9)_8$ having twice as much fluorescence as cells incubated with R.I.CK(fluorescein)-Tat9. When the cell surface-bound fluorescence was quenched with trypan blue, 93.8% of the total cell-associated fluorescence was intracellular in cells incubated with R.I.CK(fluorescein)-Tat9, 53.6% of total in cells incubated with $PEG_{3.4\ k}$-R.I.CK(fluorescein)-Tat9, and only 19% in cells incubated with $PEG_{10\ k}$- ((R.I.CK(fluorescein)-$Tat9)_8$. Since it is known that arginine-rich peptides bind to CXCR4, this suggests that multivalent Tat9 binding to CXCR4 on the cell surface impedes conjugate internalization.

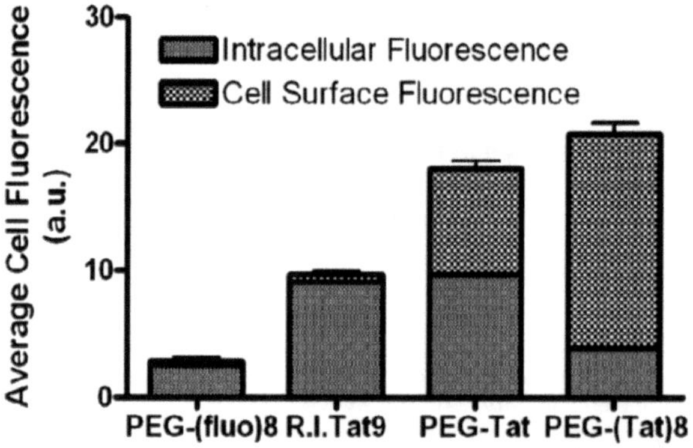

Figure 7. Quantitative data from flow cytometry showing the intracellular fluorescence and cell surface bound fluorescence of fluorescein-labeled $PEG_{10\ K}$ (PEG-$(fluo)_8$), R.I.CK-Tat9 (R.I. Tat9), $PEG_{3.4\ K}$-R.I.CK-Tat9 (PEG-Tat), and $PEG_{10\ K}$-(R.I.CK-$Tat9)_8$ (PEG-$(Tat)_8$) after 24 hr incubation with MT-2 cells at 37°C for 24 hr. The total cell associated fluorescence was quantified by flow cytometry. The intracellular fluorescence was measured after the cell surface-bound fluorescence was quenched by 0.2 mg/ml trypan blue at pH 5.8. The cell surface bound fluorescence is the difference between the total cell associated fluorescence and the intracellular fluorescence.

Confocal microscopy studies (Figure 8) showed that in cells incubated with 1 μM R.I.CK(fluorescein)-Tat9 or $PEG_{3.4\ k}$-R.I.CK(fluorescein)-Tat9, there was significantly higher fluorescence intracellularly than on the cell surface. On the other hand, cells incubated with $PEG_{10\ k}$- (R.I.CK(fluorescein)-$Tat9)_8$ showed primarily cell surface bound fluorescence. Note that in Figure 8, only a middle section of the cells is presented for each compound and the nucleus-cytosol boundaries of some cells can be discerned in the DIC (differential interference contrast) images. This result is consistent with the results from flow cytometry.

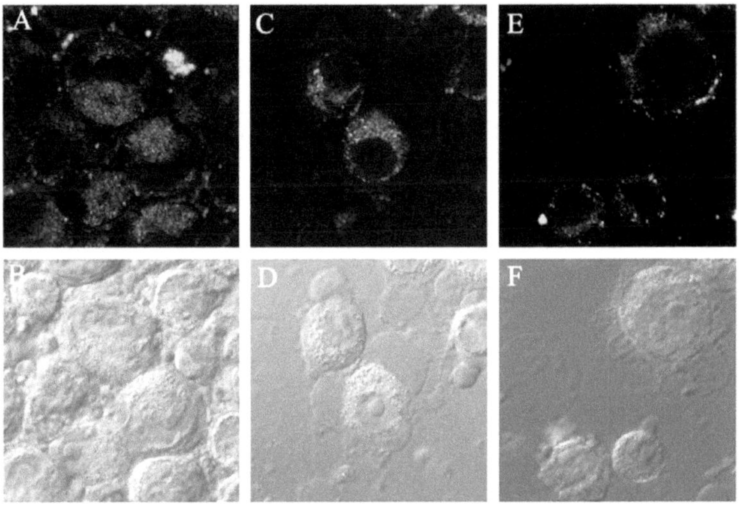

Figure 8. Confocal microscopic images of suspended MT-2 cells incubated with R.I.CK(fluorescein)-Tat9 (A, B), $PEG_{3.4\,k}$-R.I.CK(fluorescein)-Tat9 (C, D) and $PEG_{10\,K}$- (R.I.CK(fluorescein)-Tat9)$_8$ (E, F) for 24 hr (all 1μM relative to Tat9). (A, C, and E show fluorescence images while B, D, and F are light images generated by differential interference contrast (DIC) of the same fields. All focal planes are through the middle of the cells. A and C show bright intracellular fluorescence, while E shows primarily cell surface bound fluorescence.

Since the targets of both SQV (HIV-1 protease) and one of the Tat targets (HIV-1 mRNA TAR region) are in the cytosol/nucleus compartment and since flow cytometry and the confocal data shown in Figure 8 do not distinguish between the cytosol/nucleus and endosome compartments for the intracellular fluorescence, we incubated cells with either R.I.CK(fluorescein)-Tat9 or $PEG_{3.4\,k}$-R.I.CK(fluorescein)-Tat9 and a fluid phase endocytosis marker, tetramethylrhodamine-labeled dextran (10 kDa). The results (Figure 9) showed that at a relatively high concentration (7μM) R.I.CK(fluorescein)-Tat9 or $PEG_{3.4\,k}$-R.I.CK(fluorescein)-Tat9 (green) were mainly co-localized with the fluid phase endocytosis marker rhodamine-dextran (red) in punctate dots (orange/yellow in the merged panels, Figures 9D, H), suggesting predominant endosomal location. Only in cells incubated with R.I.CK(fluorescein)-Tat9, was there some faint green fluorescence that was not co-localized with the fluid phase endocytosis marker (arrows in Figure 9D), suggesting some cytosolic location.

Overall, the confocal data are consistent with the conclusion from flow cytometry analysis that the majority of R.I.CK-Tat9 is within cells, the majority of $PEG_{10\,k}$-(R.I.CK-Tat9)$_8$ is on the cell surface, and $PEG_{3.4\,k}$-R.I.CK-Tat9 is roughly equally distributed between cell surface and intracellular locales. The confocal data further suggest that after exposure to 1μM conjugate, intracellular R.I.CK-Tat9, and $PEG_{3.4\,k}$-R.I.CK-Tat9 are all predominantly within endosomes. Since the cytosol/nucleus compartment accounts for the vast majority of cellular volume, any R.I.CK-Tat9 and $PEG_{3.4\,k}$-R.I.CK-Tat9 molecules that escaped from endosome, or entered cytosol directly from outside cell, would be diluted. As a result, the detection of cytosolic fluorescence is not sensitive and we cannot rule out the presence in cytosol/nucleus compartment of a fraction of total intracellular R.I.CK-Tat9 and PEG$_{3.4\,k}$-R.I.CK-Tat9. Therefore, the potent anti-HIV-1 activity of SQV-PEG$_{3.4\,k}$-R.I.CK-Tat9 due to addition of the R.I.CK-Tat9 moiety could be attributable to a variety of factors including the inhibitory effect of Tat9 peptide on viral interaction with co-receptor CXCR4 and/or on HIV-1 transcriptional activation, either of which might be synergistic with SQV inhibition of HIV protease.

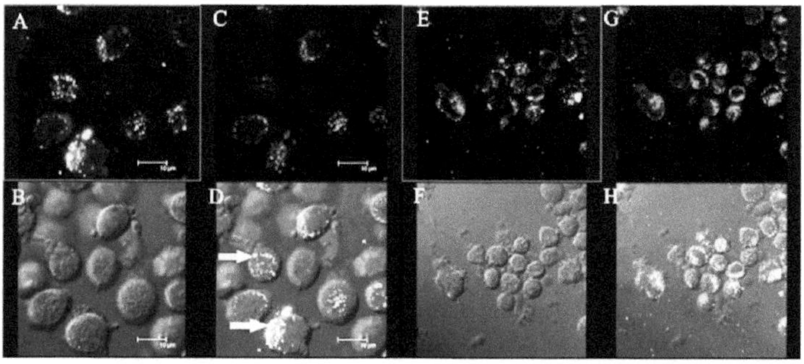

Figure 9. Confocal microscopic images of suspended MT2 cells incubated with R.I.CK(fluorescein)-Tat9 (A-D) or PEG$_{3.4K}$-R.I.CK(fluorescein)-Tat9 (E-H) in the presence of endocytosis marker rhodamine-dextran at 37°C for 24 hr. A and E show fluorescein fluorescence (green), B and F are DIC images, C and G show rhodamine-dextran (red), and D and H show overlaying of the green and red images. Colocalization of two dyes (orange-yellow in the overlay images) implies endosomal uptake of PEG$_{3.4K}$-R.I.CK-Tat9. Cells incubated with R.I.CK(fluorescein)-Tat9 showed some faint green fluorescence that was not co-localized with the fluid phase endocytosis marker (arrows in Figure 9D), suggesting some cytosolic localization.

CONCLUSION

In the current study, the preclinical *in vitro* effectiveness of a small peptidic Tat antagonist, R.I.CK-Tat9, alone or with SQV using PEG-based bioconjugates was demonstrated. While the PEG-linkage alone did not potentiate the activity of R.I.CK-Tat9, the addition of SQV to R.I.CK-Tat9-PEG bioconjugates significantly enhanced the anti-retroviral activity to the level comparable to free SQV. These bifunctional conjugates were more potent than the PEG conjugates with R.I.CK-Tat9 or SQV alone. These results demonstrate that the macromolecular bioconjugates could deliver drugs to multiple targets, bringing drug delivery systems down to the molecular level. Since *in vitro* studies of anti-HIV activity do not account for factors that would enhance *in vivo* potency (e.g., increased body persistence and decreased binding), it is quite possible that the advantages of SQV-PEG$_{3.4\,K}$R.I.CK-Tat9 conjugates over the parent drugs could become evident by *in vivo* testing. In addition, all of the bioconjugates demonstrated low cytotoxicity.

The modular approach for producing a targeted nanopharmaceutical delivery system that we have taken allows for appending different drug combinations or combinations of drugs and cellular uptake enhancing agents in order to maximize the therapeutic effect. Therefore PEG bioconjugates could constitute a powerful delivery system for either single drug administration or combination therapy. However, further mechanistic studies are needed to optimize the structure (e.g., size, shape, and other features) of the PEG bioconjugates. Additional studies are needed to assess the potential *in vivo* benefits (long half-life, lower clearance rate) of these conjugates.

KEYWORDS

- **Acquired immunodeficiency syndrome**
- **Glutathione**
- **Human immunodeficiency virus**
- **Saquinavir**
- ***trans*-Activation responsive**

AUTHORS' CONTRIBUTIONS

Li Wan: Performed synthetic and quality control chemistry, stability, flow cytometry, confocal microscopy studies, interpretation of results, and participated in drafting the manuscript. Xiaoping Zhang: Performed confocal microscopy and participated in study and conjugate design and drafting the manuscript. Simi Gunaseelan: Performed synthetic and quality control chemistry and participated in drafting the manuscript. Shahriar Pooyan: Performed synthetic and quality control chemistry. Olivia Debrah: Performed HIV and general toxicity studies. Michael J Leibowitz: Participated in study and conjugate design and critically reviewing manuscript. Arnold B. Rabson: Participated in study design and supervised HIV and toxicity studies and critically reviewing manuscript. Stanley Stein: Participated in conjugate and study design and interpretation of results. Patrick J. Sinko: Participated in conjugate and study design and interpretation of results and drafting the manuscript.

ACKNOWLEDGMENTS

This work was supported by Grants AI 33789 and 51214 from National Institutes of Health. The following reagent was obtained through the NIH AIDS Research and Reference Reagent Program, Division of AIDS, NIAID, NIH: HIV-1HXB2 KIIA Protease, cat# 4375 from Drs. David Davis, Stephen Stahl, Paul Wingfield, and Joshua Kaufmann. The authors thank Dr. H.-C. Lin for assistance in development of the antiviral assays.

COMPETING INTERESTS

The author(s) declare that they have no competing interests.

Chapter 3

Hydroxycamptothecin-loaded Nanoparticles to Enhance Drug Delivery

Anxun Wang and Su Li

INTRODUCTION

Hydroxycamptothecin (HCPT) has been shown to have activity against a broad spectrum of cancers. In order to enhance its tissue-specific delivery and anti-cancer activity, we prepared HCPT-loaded nanoparticles made from poly(ethylene glycol)-poly(γ-benzyl-L-glutamate) (PEG-PBLG), and then studied their release characteristics, pharmacokinetic characteristics, and anti-cancer effects. The PEG-PBLG nanoparticles incorporating HCPT were prepared by a dialysis method. Scanning electron microscopy (SEM) was used to observe the shape and diameter of the nanoparticles. The HCPT release characteristics *in vitro* were evaluated by ultraviolet spectrophotometry. A high-performance liquid chromatography (HPLC) detection method for determining HCPT in rabbit plasma was established. The pharmacokinetic parameters of HCPT/PEG-PBLG nanoparticles were compared with those of HCPT.

The HCPT-loaded nanoparticles had a core-shell spherical structure, with a core diameter of 200 nm and a shell thickness of 30 nm. Drug-loading capacity and drug encapsulation were 7.5 and 56.8%, respectively. The HCPT release profile was biphasic, with an initial abrupt release, followed by sustained release. The terminal elimination half-lives ($t_{1/2\beta}$) of HCPT and HCPT-loaded nanoparticles were 4.5 and 10.1 hr, respectively. Peak concentrations (Cmax) of HCPT and HCPT-loaded nanoparticles were 2627.8 and 1513.5 μg/l, respectively. The apparent volumes of distribution of the HCPT and HCPT-loaded nanoparticles were 7.3 and 20.0 l, respectively. Compared with a blank control group, Lovo cell xenografts, or Tca8113 cell xenografts in HCPT or HCPT-loaded nanoparticle treated groups grew more slowly and the tumor doubling times were increased. The tumor inhibition effect in the HCPT-loaded nanosphere-treated group was significantly higher than that of the HCPT-treated group ($p < 0.01$). Tumor inhibition in the control group by PEG-PBLG nanoparticles was not observed ($p > 0.05$).

Compared to the HCPT- and control-treated groups, the HCPT-loaded nanoparticle-treated group showed a more sustained release, a longer circulation time, increased delivery to tissue, and an enhanced anti-cancer effect. The HCPT-loaded nanoparticles appear to change the pharmacokinetic behavior of HCPT *in vivo*.

In recent years, microspheres, liposomes, and biodegradable polymers have been used in site-specific drug delivery systems (Mainardes and Silvam, 2004; Wang et al., 2007; Zentner et al., 2001). Hydrophilic-hydrophobic diblock copolymers exhibit amphiphilic behavior and form micelles with core-shell architecture. The hydrophobic block forms the inner core, which acts as a drug incorporation site, especially for the hydrophobic drugs. The hydrophilic block forms the hydrated outer shell, which plays a role in preventing uptake by the reticuloendothelial system (RES) (Jeong et al., 2004; Zentner et al., 2001). The predominant characteristics of these copolymers that have been reported include solubilization of hydrophobic drugs, sustained release, selective targeting, and lower interactions with the RES (Dong et al., 2004; Jeong et al., 2004; Zentner et al., 2001). Nanoparticles made from poly(γ-benzyl L-glutamate) (PBLG) and poly(ethylene oxide) (PEG) are hydrophilic-hydrophobic diblock copolymers which have these predominant characteristics (Jeong et al., 1999; Li et al., 2004). Thus, this PEG-PBLG copolymeric carrier may serve as an appropriate vehicle for drug delivery (Jeong et al., 1999; Li et al., 2004).

The anti-cancer activity of camptothecin (CPT) and its natural and synthetic analogs has been shown in a broad spectrum of cancers, including leukemias and cancers of the liver, stomach, breast, and colon (Ding et al., 2002, 2004; Zhou et al., 2001). Among natural CPTs, 10-HCPT has been shown to be more active and less toxic (Ding et al., 2002; Ping et al., 2006; Zhou et al., 2001) however, natural HCPT is in a lactone form and is water-insoluble. One way to improve the solubility of HCPT is to change the lactone form to the carboxylate form by adding NaOH. However, this leads to less activity and more unwanted toxicity (Sanchez et al., 2003; Zhang et al., 1998). At the same time, HCPT has a short half-life *in vivo* and poor biodistribution (Li et al., 1996).

To improve the solubility of CPT analogs, the lactone form of the analogs was incorporated into liposomes or nanoparticles (Machida et al., 2000; Onishi and Machida, 2003; Williams et al., 2003). These delivery systems show favorable pharmacokinetics and biodistribution (Machida et al., 2000; Onishi and Machida, 2003; Williams et al., 2003). In the present study, we prepared HCPT-loaded PEG-PBLG nanoparticles and investigated the *in vitro* release, pharmacokinetics, and anti-cancer effect. Our results showed that HCPT-loaded nanoparticles changed the pharmacokinetic behavior of HCPT *in vivo*. The HCPT-loaded nanoparticles had a more sustained release, a longer circulation time, increased delivery to tissue, and an enhanced anti-cancer effect.

MATERIALS AND METHODS

The PEG-PBLG block copolymers were prepared by polymerization of γ-benzyl L-glutamate N-carboxyanhydride (γ-BLG NCA) initiated with mono amine-terminated PEG in a methylene dichloride solution by the method described previously (Li et al., 2004). The HCPT (lactone form) powder (>98.5% purity) and HCPT liquid injection were obtained from Huangshi Lishizhen Pharmaceutical Co. (Hubei, China). All other reagents were of analytical grade. Human colon cancer cells (Lovo cell line) or oral squamous carcinoma cells (Tca8113 cell line) were grown in RPMI 1640 (GIBCO, USA) with 10% fetal calf serum (GIBCO), 100 units/ml penicillin G, and 100 μg/ml streptomycin at 37°C in 5% CO2. New Zealand rabbits (2–3 kg) and SPF BALB/c nude mice, 6–8 weeks of age (20–30 g) were purchased from the Animal Center of Sun Yat-sen University. Animal experiments were performed with the permission of the Animal Ethical Commission of Sun Yat-sen University.

Preparation and Identification of HCPT-loaded Nanoparticles

The HCPT-loaded PEG-PBLG nanoparticles were prepared by dialysis, as described previously (Li et al., 2004). Briefly, PEG-PBLG diblock copolymer and HCPT (1:1 W/W) were dissolved in N,N-dimethylformamide (DMF), then dialyzed using a dialysis bag (molecular cut-off 3500 g/mol; Spectrum Medical Industries, Inc., Houston, TX) against double-distilled water for 24 hr. The solution inside the dialysis bag was centrifuged and supernatant (nanoparticles) was filtered through a 0.45 μm filter. A 640 UV spectrophotometer (Beckman) was used to identify the HCPT-loaded PEG-PBLG nanoparticles at the wavelengths, 200–400 nm. The morphology of nanoparticles was observed using a scanning electron microscope (SEM, HITACHI-600; Japan).

Drug-loading Capacity and Drug Encapsulation

The HCPT-loaded PEG-PBLG nanoparticles were added into the dialysis bag, which was placed in DMF. The solution outside the dialysis bag was stirred at 37°C for 3 hr and then the drug concentration was measured using a UV spectrophotometer at 326 nm. Absorbency of the solution (A) was used to calculate the drug-loading capacity and drug encapsulation according to the following formulae: drug loading capacity $= M_{HCPT}/M_{HCPT/PEG\text{-}PBLG}$ and drug encapsulation $= M_{HCPT}/M_{drug\ devoted}$, where M_{HCPT} was the drug content of the detected solution ($M_{HCPT} = D_{HCPT} \times V$, $D_{HCPT} = A_{sample}/A_{standard}) \times D_{standard}$, D: concentration, V: volume), $M_{HCPT/PEG\text{-}PBLG}$ was the quantity of the detected solution of HCPT/PEG-PBLG nanoparticles, and M_{drug} devoted was the initial quantity of HCPT

In Vitro Release

The HCPT-loaded nanoparticles were added to a dialysis bag and then introduced into a vial with PBS at different pHs (6.86 and 9.18). The medium was stirred at 94 ± 4 revolutions/min at 37°C. At the indicated time intervals (observed until 96 hr), the medium was removed and replaced with fresh PBS. The absorbency of samples of these replaced media was detected by an UV spectrophotometer at 326 nm. The released HCPT in these replaced media at different time intervals was calculated from the standard curve, which was set up in the same way. Then, the release curve of HCPT-loaded nanoparticles was described.

Pharmacokinetic Study of HCPT-loaded Nanoparticles in Rabbit Plasma

Six New Zealand rabbits were randomized into two groups. After 12 hr of fasting, a bolus of the sample, equivalent to 12 mg/kg of HCPT or HCPT-loaded nanoparticles, was injected intravenously into each rabbit. Blood samples were withdrawn from the aural vein at the indicated time intervals. After centrifugation, the plasma supernatant was added to acetic acid (pH 3) to produce the lactone form of HCPT. Then, cold methanol-acetonitrile (1:1, v/v) was used to precipitate proteins. After centrifuging at 10,000 r/min for 5 min at 4°C, 50 μl of the supernatant were injected into the HPLC, HP1100; Agilent) to determine the lactone concentration. The analytical column used was Hypersil C18 (5 μm, ID 4.6 mm × 300 mm). The mobile phase was 0.075 mol/l ammonium acetate buffer (pH 6.4)/acetonitrile (78:22 (v:v)). The column was eluted at a flow rate of 1.0 ml/min at room temperature; and the effluent was monitored spectrofluorometrically with an excitation wavelength of 269 nm and an emission wavelength of 550 nm. The concentrations of HCPT were calculated based on the standard curve, which was set up using standard HCPT solution, and the pharmacokinetic parameters of HCPT distribution were estimated using 3p87 programs, or calculated with open two-compartment models.

Tumor Inhibition Effect of HCPT-loaded Nanoparticles *In Vivo*

The xenograft model of colon cancer was established subcutaneously in the right flank of BALB/c nude mice. After xenografts about 5 mm in diameter formed (day 3), the mice were randomly assigned to 4 groups (n = 8) as follows: control, PEG-PBLG, HCPT, and HCPT/PEG-PBLG. Then HCPT or HCPT/PEG-PBLG, 3 mg/kg, was intraperitoneally injected daily for 7 times. In the control group, the same volume of PBS or PEG-PBLG was injected intraperitoneally. Mice were sacrificed on day 21. Tumor size was measured by calipers (length and width) every 3 days. The tumor volume ($V = 1/2$ length $\times$ width^2) was calculated and the tumor growth curve was generated ($y = A e^{kt}$). The tumor doubling time ($T = \ln 2/K$, k: growth rate) and inhibition rate on day 21 were calculated. The inhibition rate was calculated as follows: (1-the volume change of experiment group/the volume change of control group) $\times$ 100%. The establishment, grouping, and treatment protocol of the Tca8113 cell xenograft (oral squamous cell carcinoma) was similar to the Lovo cell xenograft, except for the following differences: (1) treatment began on day 8, (2) the drug was injected every 2 days for 8 times (16 days), and (3) the mice were sacrificed on day 34. The anti-tumor activity was evaluated as described above.

DISCUSSION

Drug-loaded nanoparticles made from natural and synthetic macromolecular materials that are biocompatible and biodegradable have been used for controlling the release of drugs and changing pharmacokinetics and the targets of drug action (Mainardes and Silvam, 2004; Zentner et al., 2001). Nanoparticles have been used to load anti-cancer drugs to enhance their anti-cancer effect and decrease their toxicity (Onishi and Machida, 2003; Williams et al., 2003), especially for water-insoluble drugs. Nanoparticles made from PEG and PBLG, which are biocompatible and biodegradable macromolecule materials, have been used to load drugs (Jeong et al., 1999; Li et al., 2004). In this study, HCPT-loaded PEG-PBLG nanoparticles were prepared by dialysis, and the drug loading capacity was 7.5%, which was obviously higher than that of HCPT-loaded polybutylcyanoacrylate nanoparticles (1.22%) prepared by the adsorption-enwrapping method (Zhang and Lu, 1997).

Like many other copolymer nanoparticles (Jeong et al., 1999; Li et al., 2004), the shape of HCPT-loaded nanoparticles was mostly spherical or ellipsoid. Close observation of SEM photographs revealed grayish and bright white profiles in the copolymer nanoparticles, which indicated that they are of the core shell type. The grayish center portion, which was 200 nm in diameter, was assigned to the core of the hydrophobic PBLG, and the bright white ring, which was 30 nm in thickness, was assigned to the shell of the hydrophilic PEG. Studies have revealed that nanoparticles are not easily phagocytized by phagocytes when the thickness of the PEG layer is 10 nm for every

100 nm thickness of micelles (Zhang et al., 2007). Thus, the size of the nanoparticles was suitable to avoid uptake by the RES.

Numerous data have shown that the release of drugs from nanoparticles is biphasic, with abrupt and sustained release components (Sanchez et al., 2003). Abrupt release includes release of the drug adsorbed at the surface of the nanoparticles or diffused from the polymer matrix. Abrupt release enables the drug to quickly reach effective blood concentrations. Sustained release is the release of the drug that was enwrapped inside the nanoparticles and occurs when the nanoparticles biodegrade, or diffuse from the polymer matrix. Sustained release is advantageous to maintain effective blood concentrations of the drug. In this study, the release profile of the HCPT-loaded nanoparticles also consisted of an abrupt release and a sustained release. The HCPT-loaded nanoparticles also showed a quick release pattern in the alkaline condition *in vitro*. This may be related to the fact that the lactone form of HCPT converts to the carboxylate form in the alkaline condition and becomes water-soluble.

The HCPT is an inhibitor of topoisomerase I (Topo I). Other researchers have revealed that only the lactone form of HCPT can form a stable compound with Topo I and DNA, which may be responsible for its anti-cancer effect (Zhou et al., 2001). The carboxylate form of HCPT has a low anti-cancer effect, high toxicity, and poor stability. Previous pharmacokinetic studies with HCPT have indicated that HCPT has a short half-life, a poor affinity for tissue, and a higher combination rate with plasma protein (Li et al., 1996; Zhang et al., 1998). In this study, we found the same results. Therefore, to improve the anti-cancer effect and decrease the toxicity of HCPT, many researchers have investigated a new preparation of HCPT (Machida et al., 2000; Williams et al., 2003; Zhang and Lu, 1997). Williams et al. (2003) prepared SN-38- (an active compound of irinotecan) loaded phospholipid-PEG nanoparticles by the solvent-evaporation method, which enhanced the lactone ring stability in the presence of human serum albumin and prolonged the existence of the active drug (lactone form) and the half-life *in vivo*. The HCPT-loaded nanoparticles prepared by Zhang (Zhang and Lu, 1997) were targeted to the liver and had a sustained release effect. In our study, the pharmacokinetic parameters of HCPT changed after it was enveloped in the PEG-PBLG nanoparticles. Compared with HCPT, the pharmacokinetic parameters for the HCPT/PEG-PBLG nanoparticles had the following changes: (1) the terminal elimination half-life increased, (2) the peak concentration decreased, and (3) the apparent volume of distribution increased. These results indicate that the HCPT-loaded nanoparticles have the following characteristics: (1) sustained release, (2) prolonged half-life, and (3) increased affinity to tissue. Therefore, they have the properties of an ideal new preparation of HCPT. The studies of Li et al. (2004) and Jeong et al. (1999) have also shown that 5-fluorouracil- or adriamycin-loaded PEG-PBLG nanoparticles have similar pharmacokinetic characteristics.

The HCPT has known clinical efficacy against a variety of solid tumors in humans (Ding et al., 2002; Zhou et al., 2001). In this study, free HCPT inhibited the xenograft growths of colon cancer and oral squamous cell carcinoma, and prolonged the tumor doubling times. These findings were also demonstrated in our previous studies (Ding et al., 2002; Wang et al., 2005). Compared with free HCPT, HCPT-loaded nanoparticles had a higher inhibitory effect on colon cancer and oral squamous cell carcinoma.

Williams et al. (2003) reported a similar result; after treatment with SN-38-loaded phospholipd-PEG, the anti-cancer effect against HT-29 colon xenografts was higher compared to CPT-11. The higher anti-cancer effect of HCPT-loaded nanoparticles may be due to one or more of the following reasons. First, the HCPT-loaded nanoparticles have sustained release, a prolonged half-life, and increase the apparent volume of distribution. These characteristics may increase the exposure time of the drug to tumor tissues. Second, the HCPT-loaded nanoparticles stabilize the lactone form of HCPT, which inhibits the activity of Topo I. The longer the period of stabilization, the stronger the anti-cancer effect. Third, tumor tissue has an abundant blood supply and tumor cells exhibit higher phagocytotic ability. Together, these characteristics would make nanoparticles more likely to enter the tumor cells and would improve the anti-cancer effect.

RESULTS

Characteristics of HCPT-loaded Nanoparticles

In this study, HCPT-loaded PBLG/PEG nanoparticles were prepared using dialysis. After analysis by UV spectrophotometey, we found that the solution of HCPT in a standard sample, or the simple mixture of a solution of HCPT and PBLG/PEG, had high absorbency in the wavelength range, 326–368 nm (Figures 1A, B). However, the absorbency of the solution of HCPT-loaded PBLG/PEG nanoparticles was greatly decreased (Figure 1C), representing the formation of HCPT-loaded PEG-PBLG nanoparticles. On the basis of absorbency at 326 nm, the drug-loading capacity and drug encapsulation of HCPT-loaded nanoparticles were 7.5 and 56.8%, respectively.

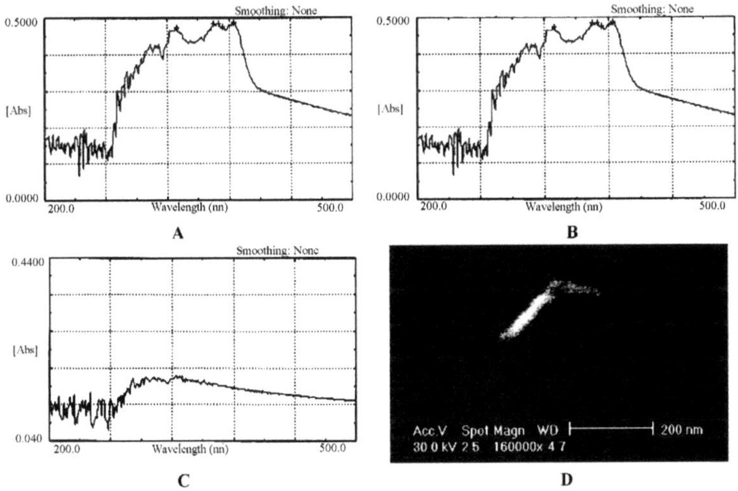

Figure 1. Characteristics of HCPT-loaded nanoparticles. (A-C): UV spectrum of HCPT detected by ultraviolet spectrophotometry. At wavelengths of 326 and 368 nm, both the HCPT standard sample (A) and the mixture of HCPT and PBLG/PEG (B) had high absorbency, but the absorbency of HCPT-loaded PBLG/PEG nanoparticles (C) was greatly decreased. (D) The morphology of HCPT-loaded nanoparticles was found under scanning electron microscopy (x 160,000) to be a core-shell structure, spherical or elliptical, with a smooth surface. The hydrophobic central core was a grayish area, approximately 200 nm in diameter. The hydrophilic shell was a bright white ring, approximately 30 nm thick.

The morphology of HCPT-loaded nanoparticles (Figure 1D) was found to be a core-shell structure that was spherical or elliptical, with a smooth surface. The hydrophobic central core, the grayish area inside the bright white ring, was approximately 200 nm in diameter. The hydrophilic shell, the bright white ring, was approximately 30 nm in thickness.

Abrupt-sustained Release of HCPT-loaded Nanoparticles

The standard curve of a HCPT solution was derived from the following equation: y = 10.7 x + 0.0056 (r = 0.9999). The HCPT release from PEG-PBLG nanoparticles at pHs 6.86 and 9.18 *in vitro* is shown on Figure 2. The HCPT release profile was biphasic, with an initial abrupt release, followed by sustained release. Abrupt release occurred at 2 hr, and 1/3 of the loaded HCPT was released by that time. Then, the release of HCPT entered sustained release following initial abrupt release. After 96 hr, 3/5 of the loaded HCPT was still enveloped in the nanoparticles. In this release study, HCPT-loaded nanoparticles showed a quicker release pattern in the more alkaline condition.

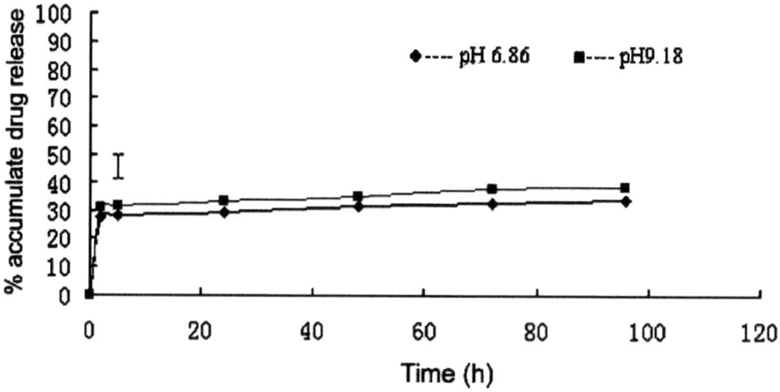

Figure 2. Release characteristics of HCPT from PEG-PBLG nanoparticles *in vitro* in different buffers. The HCPT release profile was biphasic with an initial abrupt release, followed by sustained release. The abrupt release occurred at 2 hr and 1/3 of the loaded-HCPT was released during this period. Then, the HCPT entered the sustained release; after 96 hr, 3/5 of the loaded-HCPT was still enwrapped in the nanoparticles. In this release study, HCPT-loaded nanoparticles also showed a quick release pattern in the alkaline condition.

Pharmacokinetic Characteristics of HCPT-loaded Nanoparticles

The standard curve for HCPT in rabbit plasma was derived from the following equation: y = 2.75 x +2.90 ($\gamma > 0.9999$), where Y is the concentration (μg/l) and X is the peak height. The limit of determination was 2 μg/l. The mean plasma concentrations over time for the free HCPT and the HCPT-loaded nanoparticles are illustrated in Figure 3. The HCPT release profile from HCPT-loaded nanoparticles was biphasic with an initial abrupt release, followed by sustained release. Abrupt release occurred at 1 hr and the peak concentration was 1,513.5 μg/l. During the sustained release, the plasma concentration was between 7.4–84.7 μg/l. As shown in Table 1, the pharmacokinetics of HCPT changed after it was loaded into PEG-PBLG nanoparticles. The terminal elimination half-life was longer, the peak concentration decreased, and the apparent volume of distribution increased.

Table 1. The pharmacokinetic parameters of HCPT or HCPT-loaded nanoparticles after IV administration at a single dose of 12 mg/kg in rabbit.

	$t_{1/2}$ (h)	C_{max} (μg/L)	T_{max} (h)	V_d (L)	AUC (μg · h/L)
HCPT	4.5	2627.8	0	7.3	2459.0
HCPT/PEG-PBLG	10.1	1513.5	1	20	2175.9

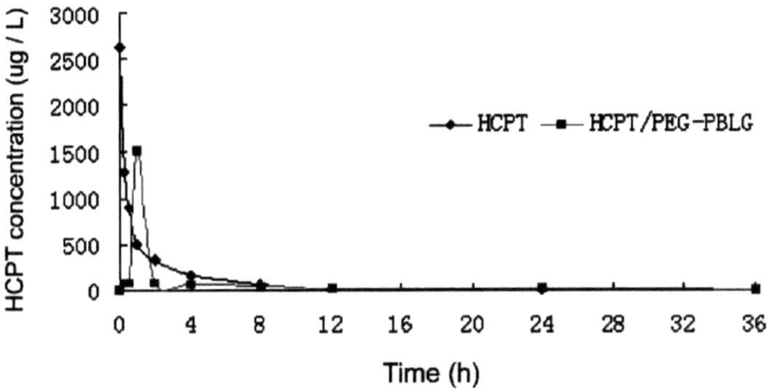

Figure 3. The mean plasma concentration of HCPT after IV administration of HCPT or HCPT/PEG-PBLG nanospheres at a single dose of 12 mg/kg. The HCPT release profile from HCPT-loaded nanoparticles showed a biphasic with an initial abrupt release, followed by a sustained release. The abrupt release occurred at 1 hr and the peak concentration was 1513.5 μg/l. The release then became sustained, with a plasma concentration between 84.7 and 7.4 μg/l.

Tumor Inhibition Effect of HCPT-loaded Nanoparticles *In Vivo*

Tumor-associated swellings were visible in all the mice. As demonstrated by the tumor growth curve of Lovo (Figure 4A) and Tca8113 cell xenografts (Figure 4B), xenograft growth was fast in the blank and PEG-PBLG control groups, but significantly depressed in the HCPT-or HCPT/PEG-PBLG-treated groups. As shown in Table 2, tumor doubling time lengthened with treatment. The inhibition rate for HCPT alone was between 60 and 70%, but was greater than 80% for the HCPT-loaded nanoparticles. The tumor volumes of the HCPT and HCPT-loaded nanoparticle-treated groups were significantly less than those of the blank and PEG-PBLG control groups ($P < 0.01$). There was also significantly more tumor inhibition in the HCPT-loaded nanoparticle treated group than in the HCPT treated group ($P < 0.01$). However, there was no significant difference in tumor inhibition between the two control groups ($P > 0.05$). No significant toxicity was observed in any of the groups.

Table 2. The anti-cancer effect of HCPT-loaded nanoparticles in the treatment of xenografts.

	Lovo cells xenograft			Tca8113 cells xenograft		
	TDT (d)	IR (%)	TV(cm^3)	TDT (d)	IR (%)	TV(cm^3)
Blank control	3.0	0	4.336 ± 0.485	3.5	0	3.888 ± 0.547
PEG-PBLG	2.9	0	4.206 ± 0.308*	3.6	0	3.944 ± 0.179*
HCPT	4.3	70.0%	1.299 ± 0.082#	4.5	59.8%	1.564 ± 0.286#
HCPT/PEG-PBLG	4.9	83.8%	0.701 ± 0.067#§	4.9	85.6%	0.559 ± 0.062 #§

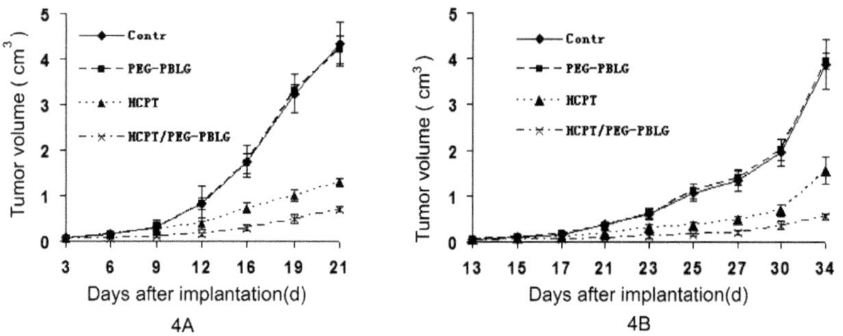

Figure 4. The tumor growth curve of Lovo cell xenografts (A) or Tca8113 cell xenografts (B). Xenografts grew quickly in the blank and PEG-PBLG control groups, but growth was significantly slowed in the HCPT- and HCPT/PEG-PBLG-treated groups.

CONCLUSION

From this research, we found that PEG-PBLG nanoparticles are useful for the solubilization and sustained release of HCPT. The HCPT-loaded PEG-PBLG nanoparticles improved the tissue-specific delivery and the anti-cancer effect of HCPT by changing the pharmacokinetic behavior of HCPT *in vivo.*

STATISTICAL ANALYSIS

In all cases, experiments were replicated in triplicate and data represent mean ± standard deviation (s.d.). Statistical analysis of the inhibitory effect on tumor growth was performed using one-way analysis of variance. The $P < 0.05$ denoted significance in all cases.

KEYWORDS

- **High-performance liquid chromatography**
- **Hydroxycamptothecin**
- **Reticuloendothelial system**
- **Scanning electron microscopy**

AUTHORS' CONTRIBUTIONS

Anxun Wang and Su Li were responsible for experimental design and completion of all laboratory work presented in this chapter. The manuscript was drafted by Anxun Wang. All authors approved and read the final manuscript.

ACKNOWLEDGMENTS

This work was supported by research grants from the Natural Science Foundation of Guangdong Province, No.021865, and the Science and Technique Project of Guangdong Province, No. 2004B30901002.

COMPETING INTERESTS

The authors declare that they have no competing interests.

Chapter 4

Targeted Drug-carrying Phage Nanomedicines

Hagit Bar, Iftach Yacoby, and Itai Benhar

INTRODUCTION

Systemic administration of chemotherapeutic agents, in addition to its anti-tumor benefits, results in indiscriminate drug distribution and severe toxicity. This shortcoming may be overcome by targeted drug-carrying platforms that ferry the drug to the tumor site while limiting exposure to non-target tissues and organs.

We present a new form of targeted anti-cancer therapy in the form of targeted drug-carrying phage nanoparticles. Our approach is based on genetically-modified and chemically manipulated filamentous bacteriophages. The genetic manipulation endows the phages with the ability to display a host-specificity-conferring ligand. The phages are loaded with a large payload of a cytotoxic drug by chemical conjugation. In the presented examples we used anti ErbB2 and anti ERGR antibodies as targeting moieties, the drug hygromycin conjugated to the phages by a covalent amide bond, or the drug doxorubicin conjugated to genetically-engineered cathepsin-B sites on the phage coat. We show that targeting of phage nanomedicines via specific antibodies to receptors on cancer cell membranes results in endocytosis, intracellular degradation, and drug release, resulting in growth inhibition of the target cells *in vitro* with a potentiation factor of >1,000 over the corresponding free drugs.

The results of the proof-of concept study presented here reveal important features regarding the potential of filamentous phages to serve as drug-delivery platform, on the affect of drug solubility or hydrophobicity on the target specificity of the platform and on the effect of drug release mechanism on the potency of the platform. These results define targeted drug-carrying filamentous phage nanoparticles as a unique type of antibody-drug conjugates.

Since the introduction of monoclonal antibodies (mAbs), and the initial clinical trials of antibody therapy in cancer patients, there has been progress in antibody-based therapeutics, particularly in oncology. The usage of naked mAbs has gradually evolved into drug immunoconjugates. In general drug immunoconjugates are composed of targeting entities (mainly mAbs) chemically conjugated to a cytotoxic drug. The outcome is improved drug efficacy with reduced systemic toxicity. To date, the most clinically-advanced forms of armed antibodies are antibody-isotope and antibody-drug conjugates (Carter and Merchant, 1997; Kreitman, 1999; Schrama, 2006). Key issues in designing and testing immunoconjugates include: (1) the nature of the target molecule, its abundance at the target, whether it is internalizing and at what rate, and its specificity to the target, cells or tissues. (2) the linkers used to attach the drug to the targeting moiety (Ulbrich and Subr, 2004), (3) the drug-carrying capacity of the carrier is also a key issue in its potency, thus conjugation schemes, such as the use of branched linkers were devised to maximize the drug payload per target site (King et al., 1999).

A second class of targeted drug delivery platforms are the drug-carrying nanomedicines, such as liposomes, nanoparticles, drug-loaded polymers, and dendrimers (Brannon-Peppas and Blanchette, 2004; Duncan, 2006; Ferrari, 2005; Luo and Prestwich, 2002; Medina et al., 2004). With a few exception such as targeted liposomes, and antibody-targeted polymeric carriers (Dziubla et al.,2008; Muro et al., 2006; Stephenson et al., 2004; Torchilin, 2006), nanomedicines do not utilize a targeting moiety to gain target specificity. Rather, they rely on the "enhanced permeability and retention" (EPR) effect that results from the rapid deployment of blood vessels within rapidly growing tumors resulting in blood vessels in the tumor being irregular in shape, dilated, leaky, or defective. As a result, large drug-carrying platforms may gain selective access to the tumor while their exit at non-target sites is limited (Iyer et al., 2006; Luo and Prestwich, 2002; Maeda et al., 2000). While the immunoconjugates are limited in drug-carrying capacity, usually less than 10 drug molecules per targeting moiety (Chari, 1998), nanomedicines by nature deliver a much larger payload to the target cells. Recently, a novel approach for combining antibody-mediated targeting to cell-surface receptors with a large drug-carrying payload was provided in the description of minicells; enucleated bacteria that are loaded with cytotoxic drugs and targeted using bi-specific antibodies (MacDiarmid et al., 2007).

Filamentous bacteriophages (phages) are the workhorse of antibody engineering and are gaining increasing importance in nanobiotechnology (Nam et al., 2006; Petty et al., 2007; Sarikaya et al., 2003; Souza et al., 2006; Sweeney et al., 2006). Phage-mediated gene delivery into mammalian cells was developed following studies that identified "internalizing phages" from libraries of phage-displayed antibodies or peptides. (Becerril et al., 1999; Gao et al., 2003; Kassner et al., 1999; Larocca and Baird, 2001; Larocca et al., 2001; Poul and Marks, 1999; Poul et al., 2000; Urbanelli et al., 2001). Recently, an efficient integrated phage/virus system was developed where tumor targeting and molecular-genetic imaging were merged into an integrated platform (Hajitou et al., 2006, 2007).

Recently we exploited the potential of phages for targeted delivery by applying them as anti-bacterial nanomedicines. The phages were genetically engineered to display a target-cell specificity-conferring molecule, up to five targeting molecules/phage if displayed on all copies of the phage g3p coat protein. The targeted phages were chemically conjugated, via a cleavable bond to a large payload of an antibiotic, with a maximal loading capacity of more than 10,000 drug molecules/phage (Yacoby et al., 2006). The anti-bacterial system was based on drug release at (and not within) the target site. Here we present an evaluation of targeted phage nanomedicines to be applied against cancer cells, with target-mediated internalization followed by intracellular drug release. We show that the growth of target cells can be specifically inhibited when the drug is conjugated either be a covalent bond or through an engineered cathepsin-B cleavage site to the phage coat. Due to the modular nature of the platform, this new class of targeted, drug-carrying viral particles may enable a wide range of applications in biology and medicine.

MATERIALS AND METHODS

Cell Lines

Cell lines used were the human breast carcinoma cell lines SKBR3 and MDA-MB231, the human epidermoid carcinoma A431 cell line, and the human kidney HEK293 cell line. Cells were maintained in Dulbecco's modified Eagle medium (DMEM) containing 10% foetal calf serum (FCS), unless mentioned otherwise.

All the chemicals used were of analytical grade and were purchased from Sigma (Israel). Unless stated otherwise, reactions were carried out at room temperature (about 22°C).

Linking Phages to the Targeting Antibodies

Phage fUSE5-ZZ that can be complexed with IgGs was recently described (Yacoby et al., 2006). Briefly, this is a derivative of the filamentous phage vector fUSE5 (Smith Lab Phage Display Vectors) that was engineered to display the IgG Fc-binding ZZ domain on all copies of the g3p minor coat protein. Filamentous phages were routinely propagated in DH5-αF' cells using standard phage techniques as described (Enshell-Seijffers et al., 2001). Phages were usually recovered from overnight 1 l cultures of carrying bacteria. The bacteria were removed by centrifugation and the phage-containing supernatant was filtered through a 0.22 μm filter. The phages were precipitated by addition of 20% (w/v) polyethylene glycol 8000 PEG/2.5 M NaCl followed by centrifugation as described (Enshell-Seijffers et al., 2001). The phage pellet was suspended in sterile miliQ double-distilled water (DDW) at a concentration of 10^{13} pfu/ml and stored at 4°C.

To form a complex with targeting antibodies, 10^{12} phage in 1 ml PBS were mixed with 1.6 μg of the IgG: chFRP5 (Mazor et al., 2007), Herceptin® (trastuzumab, Genentech, USA), Erbitux® (cetuximab, ImClone, USA) or control normal human IgG (Sigma, Israel). The phage-IgG mixtures were left for at least 1 hr at room temperature. This phage to IgG ration yields occupancy of about 50% of the available ZZ sites on the phage (Yacoby et al., 2006).

Construction of Phage fUSE5-ZZ-(g8p)DFK

The fUSE5-ZZ was further modified to display the lysosomal cysteine protease cathepsin-B cleavable DFK tri-peptide (Dubowchik and Firestone, 1998) on all copies of the g8p major coat protein. The DFK tri-peptide was inserted into the N-terminal region of g8p by two subsequent steps. First, fUSE5-ZZ DNA was amplified by PCR using primers P8-DFK/R-FOR (5'-CTGACTTTARGGGTCCTGCAGAAGCGGCCTTT-GACTCCC-3') with M13g3BamHI-REV (5'-TATTCACAAACGAATGGATCC 3') and in a second reaction using primers P8-DFK/R-REV (CAGGACCCRTAAAGT-CAGCGAAAGACAGCATCGGAACG-3') with P5-BsrGI-FOR (5'-TCGTCAG-GGCAAGCCTTATTC-3'). Second, the resulting DNA fragments were assembled using primers P5-BsrGI-FOR and M13g3BamHI-REV. The assembled PCR product was purified, digested with restriction enzymes BsrGI and BamHI, and cloned into a similarly digested fUSE5-ZZ phage vector. The resulting phage was named fUSE5-ZZ-(p8)DFK. The g8p major coat protein of fUSE5-ZZ-(p8)DFK contains an amino terminal aspartate for drug conjugation by ECD chemistry to its carboxyl residue followed by the cathepsin-B cleavage site phenylalanine-Lysine (FK). In addition, it contains mutations that eliminated almost all of the naturally occurring free carboxyl groups on g8p that may be susceptible to EDC conjugation.

Drug Conjugation to Phages by the EDC Chemistry

The phage major coat protein g8p contains 3 carboxylic amino acid (glu2; Asp4; asp5) that can be conjugated by application of (1-Ethyl-3-(3-dimethylaminopropyl) carbodiimide (EDC) chemistry, a rapid reaction performed at mild acidic pH (4.5–5.5) (Staros et al., 1986). All the conjugations were done within a total volume of 1 ml of 0.1 M Na-citrate buffer; pH = 5, 0.75 M NaCl, 2.5×10^{-6} mol of the aminoglycoside, 5×10^{12} and phages that were already complexed with the targeting IgG. The reaction was initiated by the addition of 2.5×10^{-6} mol of EDC, which was repeated two more times at time intervals of 30 min. Reactions were carried out at room temperature (~22°C) with gentle stirring in 2 ml Eppendorf tubes for a total of 2 hr. The targeted drug-carrying phage nanoparticles were separated from the reactants by two successive dialysis steps of 16 hr each against 1,000 volumes of sterile 0.3 M NaCl.

Quantifying Linked Doxorubicin Molecules/Phage by Cathepsin-B Cleavage in a Cell-Free System

The 2×10^{12} doxorubicin-conjugated fUSE5-ZZ-(g8p)DFK phages were suspended within 300 μl cathepsin-B reaction buffer as described (Dubowchik and Firestone, 1998). Next, 7 units of cathepsin-B (Sigma, Israel) were added for 24 hr at 37°. The phages were precipitated with PEG/NaCl and the supernatant was analyzed by reverse-phase HPLC and MALDI-TOF MS. For the HPLC analysis, a reverse phase C-18 column was used on a Waters machine with a gradient 0–100% of acetonitrile in the mobile phase, at 1 ml/min flow rate. Under these conditions, the doxorubicin containing peak at 480 nm was eluted 24–25 min after sample injection.

Evaluation of Target Cell Binding by Whole-Cell ELISA

Unless stated otherwise, all secondary antibodies, HRP-conjugated or fluorescent were from Jackson Immunoresearch Laboratories (USA). Evaluation of the binding ability of fUSE5-ZZ phages complexed with chFRP5 or trastuzumab to SKBR3 cells was done by whole-cell ELISA (Mazor et al., 2007). Following trypsinization, cells were washed once with 2% FCS, in PBS (incubation buffer, pH 7.4). In each experiment approximately 106 cells were divided into individual immunotubes (Nunc, Sweden). To confirm the specificity, phages (10^{10} and 10^{11} phage/ml) were added to the cell tubes for 1.5 hr at 4°C. After washing ×2 with incubation buffer, HRP-conjugated rabbit anti M13 antibodies (GE healthcare, USA, 1/5,000 dilution) were added to the immunotubes for 1 hr at 4°C. Detection of cell bound phage was performed by addition of 0.5 ml of the chromogenic HRP substrate TMB (Dako, USA) to each tube and color development was terminated with 0.25 ml of 1 M H_2SO_4. Finally, the tubes were centrifuged for 10 min at 4,000 rpm and color intensity of supernatants was measured at 450 nm.

Analysis of Phage Internalization Using Confocal Microscopy

Internalization of IgG-complexed phages into SKBR3 and A431 cells was studied using confocal microscopy as follows: Cells were grown on 24 mm cover slips in DMEM supplemented with 10% FCS essentially as described (Mazor et al., 2007). Subsequently, the medium was replaced by 450 μl DMEM without FCS into which 5 × 108 phages were added in 50 μl. After 3 hr incubation at 37°C, the cells were gently washed ×3 with PBS and 100 μl of 1 μg/ml of membrane labeling CM-Dil (Molecular probes, USA) were added following incubation for 5 min at 37°C and 15 min at 4°C. Next, the cells were washed × 3 with PBS and fixed by 30 min incubation with 500 μl of 4% formaldehyde followed by washing with 1 ml PBS. To ensure efficient cell permeability, cells were washed with 250 μl of 0.2% triton × 100 in PBS, after which cells were blocked with 90% FCS in PBS containing 0.05% Tween 20 (Sigma, Israel) for 30 min. The blocking solution was aspirated and monoclonal mouse anti-M13 (1/100 dilution; GE healthcare, USA) was added for 1 hr incubation following × 2 washes with 2% BSA in PBS. Subsequently, cells were incubated with 1:100 diluted FITC conjugated goat anti-mouse IgG for 1 hr at room temperature. Finally, the cells were gently washed × 3 with PBS and images were acquired using a LSM 510 laser scanning confocal microscope (Vontz 3403B).

Cell Viability Assay

The *in-vitro* cell-killing activity of hygromycin carrying fUSE5-ZZ-chFRP5 or doxorubicin carrying fUSE5-ZZ-(g8p)DFK-trastuzumab and fUSE5-ZZ-(g8p)DFK-cetuximab antibody complexed phage nanoparticles was measured by an MTT assay. Human breast carcinoma A431, SKBR3 target cells, or HEK293 control cells were seeded in 96-well plates at a density of 10^4 cells/well in DMEM supplemented with 10% FCS. Targeted drug-carrying phage nano-particles and relevant control phages were added to samples in 100 μl containing 5×10^{11} phages and serial 3-fold dilutions thereof and the cells were incubated at 37°C in 5% CO_2 atmosphere. Forty-eight hours later, the media was replaced by phage-free media (100 μl per well) containing 5 mg/ml MTT reagent (Thiazolyl Blue Tetrazoliam Bromide, Sigma, Israel, dissolved in PBS) and the cells were incubated for another 4 hr MTT-formazan crystals were dissolved by the addition of 20% SDS, 50% DMF, pH 4.7 (100 μl per well) and incubation for 16 hr at 37°C in 5% CO_2 atmosphere. Absorbance at 570 nm was determined on a microtiter plate reader. Identical concentrations and combinations were tested in four separate wells per assay and the assay was performed at least three times. The results were expressed as percentage of living cells in comparison to the untreated controls that were processed simultaneously using the following equation: (A570 of treated sample/A_{570} of untreated sample) ×100.

DISCUSSION

This study presents targeted, drug-carrying filamentous bacteriophages (phages) as a drug delivery platform for targeting cancer cells. Our phages represent a modular targeted drug-carrying platform of nanometric dimensions (particle diameter 8 nm, length of a few hundred nm) where targeting moieties, conjugated drugs and drug release mechanisms may be exchanged at will. Specifically, we have generated engineered phages that carried either the drug hygromycin covalently linked to the phage coat, or the drug doxorubicin linked through a cathepsin-B cleavable peptide that was engineered into the major coat protein of the phage. As targeting moieties we used three IgG antibodies; trastuzumab; and chFRP5 that target ErbB2 and cetuximab that target the EGFR. When target cells were treated with the targeted drug-carrying phages, selective cell killing could be demonstrated with a potentiation factor of up to several thousand over the free drug.

In our study we used EGFR and ErbB2 as targets; both are very well characterized in the field of targeted anti-cancer therapy. In fact, two of the three antibodies we used as targeting moieties are used clinically to treat cancer patients (trastuzumab and cetuximab). All three antibodies we used were shown before to facilitate the delivery of cytotoxic payloads to target cells and tumor models (Austin et al., 2005; Kobayashi et al., 2002; Mazor et al., 2007; von Minckwitz et al., 2005; Wels et al., 1992; Yip et al., 2007) In addition, antibody-displaying filamentous phages have been shown to undergo internalization into target cells, which laid the foundation for proposing to use such "internalizing phages" as gene delivery vehicles (Becerril et al., 1999; Hajitou et al., 2006, 2007; Liu et al., 2007; Nielsen and Marks, 2000; Poul et al., 2000).

The drug-carrying capacity of the platform is a key issue in its potency. With antibody-drug conjugates, the amount of cytotoxic drug that can be conjugated to the antibody is usually limited by the conjugation chemistry that, if pushed to the upper limit, may reduce its capacity to bind antigen. As a result, such conjugates carry no more than eight drug molecules per mAb (Chari, 1998). Recently more elaborate drug conjugation schemes, such as the use of dendrimers and branched linkers to increase carrying capacity were devised to maximize the drug payload per targeting molecule that binds a target site (King et al., 2002; Wu and Senter, 2005; Wu et al., 2006). Our phages carry as much as 104 drug molecules/phage which maximizes the intracellular drug load upon internalization of the platform into the target cells.

Considering the linkers used to attach the drug to the targeting moiety, an ideal linker should be stable in the serum and readily degraded within the intracellular milieu. Some examples from the field of antibody-drug conjugates are acid-labile linkers and enzyme-cleavable linkers (Ulbrich and Subr, 2004). We chose to evaluate two approaches; direct covalent conjugation of the drug to the carrier and conjugation of the drug through an engineered cathepsin-B cleavage site. Our results (Figure 5) show that both approaches are viable, but the results may vary with different drugs and/or targeting antibodies. Phages that were used to deliver covalently linked hygromycin to ErbB2 expressing cells (chFRP5 IgG as the targeting moiety, Figure 5A) could cause specific cell growth inhibition. When phages were used to deliver doxorubicin to either erbB2 expressing cells (trastuzumab as the targeting moiety, Figure 5C) or EGFR expressing cells (cetuximab as the targeting moiety, Figure 5D), phages to which the drug was linked covalently were inefficient in inhibiting cell growth, while phages that carried the cathepsin-B releasable drug were more efficient, suggesting that with this particular phage-drug combination, an engineered drug release mechanism is necessary to maximized potency. We could not link hygromycin to DFK-displaying phages, since we found that hygromycin with a single amino-acid adduct (as is the product of cathepsin-B release drug in our system) is inactive as a drug (data not shown).

Early antibody-drug conjugates were comprised of a mAb covalently linked to several molecules of a clinically used anti-cancer drug. The linker connecting the antibody and the drug was either non-cleavable or cleavable upon entry into the cell. In the early development phase of antibody-drug conjugates, it was believed that the tumor specificity of anti-cancer drugs could be improved merely by linking these drugs directly to antibodies via amide bonds (Chari, 1998). In most cases, the conjugates lacked cytotoxic potency and were less potent than the un-conjugated drugs (Endo et al., 1987). Only in the past few years the critical parameters for optimization have been identified and have begun to be addressed. These include low drug potency, inefficient drug release from the mAb and difficulties in releasing drugs in their active state (Wu and Senter, 2005). On the basis of this much research has been focused on designing new linker technology. The use of peptides which are susceptible to enzymatic cleavage, as conditionally stable linkers for drugs to mAbs. The peptides are designed for high serum stability and rapid enzymatic hydrolysis, once the mAb-drug conjugate is internalized into lysosomes of target cells, for example, cathepsin-B sensitive peptides. Cathepsin-B is a cysteine protease found in all mammalian cell lysosomes. The cathepsin-B cleavable di-peptide Phe-Lys was used for conjugating doxorubicin to BR96 mAb which were previously conjugated through a hydrazone labile linker (Dubowchik and Firestone, 1998). The resulting immunoconjugate showed levels of immunological specificity that had been unobtainable using the corresponding hydrazone-based conjugates.

The objective of the experiments described herein was a feasibility study of applying targeted drug delivery as an anti-cancer tool. The system was designed on three key components: (1) a targeting moiety, exemplified here by various monoclonal tumor specific antibodies complexed via the ZZ domain (Yacoby et al., 2007). (2) A high-capacity drug carrier, exemplified here by the filamentous phage, with its 3,000 copies of major coat protein, each amendable to drug conjugation. (3) A drug linked directly or through a labile linker that is subject to controlled release, exemplified here by hygromycin conjugate directly or by doxorubicin that was linked through a cleavable peptide expressed on all copies of phage major coat protein. In the case of covalently-linked hygromycin, we postulate that a partial non-selective release in the lysosomes post internalization would eventually lead to a specific killing of target cell. Several features led us to use hygromycin as the model drug: The first was the simplicity in which hygromycin can be conjugated to the phages through simple EDC chemistry. Hygromycin has two primary amino groups, one for phage conjugations and the other for drug or analyte conjugation (such as FITC as we have reported previously) (Yacoby et al., 2007). Another important feature at this stage is the high drug solubility in water. With this chemistry, a carrying capacity in excess of 10^4 drug molecules/phage was previously reported by us (Yacoby et al., 2007).

The second example was a controllable release mechanism that was genetically engineered into the phage major coat protein g8p (p8). We mutated the N-terminus of p8 to express a cathepsin-B cleavage peptide with the sequence of DFK (Dubowchik and Firestone, 1998). Aspartate (D) was added to the sequence FK for the creation of two options for chemical conjugation; through the α-amine or through the carboxyl side chain. In addition to this mutation, the native aspartic side chains were mutated to non carboxyl side chains (asp 11 (Figure 3A) was retained since it is buried within the phage coat and inaccessible to conjugation (Sidhu, 2001)). The native lys8 was mutated to glu7 in the newly mutated p8 and used as internal control for drug conjugation and to maintaining balanced number of charged residues that are important for phage solubilization. Indeed, from Figure 3C one may appreciate that there was partial release of doxorubicin upon cathepsin-B treatment, since doxorubicin molecules linked to glu7 were not released. Since two of the native carboxyl residues asp4 and asp5 were deleted it is important to note that by this genetic modification in the structure of the major coat protein-8 we have reduced the potential drug capacity by more than 60%.

Doxorubicin was used as a model drug; primary by two reasons; the first is its reporter properties, fluorescence as well as specific emission in the wavelength of 480 nm. This property was helpful for monitoring of drug release. The second is the relative tolerance for conjugation of linkers into the single primary amine located to the aminoglycoside ring tailored specifically for the solubilization of this highly hydrophobic drug. Doxorubicin was conjugated to phages through EDC chemistry, resulting with reddish solution. The releasing experiment with commercial cathepsin-B led to a complete release of all connected doxorubicin molecules. Each DFK phage release about ~3,500 doxorubicin molecules as we measured by a specific reading at 480 nm with a reference of a calibration curve of free doxorubicin. This results correlates with the maximal theoretical capacity of this phages. Using HPLC analysis, we found that the release was limited to the DFK phage only, while doxorubicin linked covalently to the wild-type phage coat was not released. Further MALDI-TOF MS analysis showed that the released moiety was doxorubicin with aspartate linked to it. Such adducts are common when labile linkers are used do deliver drugs, and in the case of doxorubicin, do not seem to inactivate it. This is similar to the released drug of the "non-cleavable" antibody-drug conjugates where upon degradation in the lysosomal compartment, the drug remains covalently linked to a single amino acid, either lysine for maytansinoid conjugates, or cysteine for auristatin conjugates (Doronina et al., 2006; Erickson et al., 2006; Kovtun and Goldmacher, 2007).

Internalization of the phages, unconjugated or armed with drug could be demonstrated by fluorescence confocal microscopy (Figure 2). The result of the target cell killing assays showed that the soluble drug hygromycin connected through a non cleavable stable amide bond, directly to phage coat carboxyl residues, could achieve impressive potency improvement, in factor of >1,000 over the free drug (Figure 5A) (5×10^{10} phages carrying 10^4 drug molecules/phage, carry 0.43 μg free drug, which inhibits cell growth as well as ~1 mg of free drug). This occurred although poor drug release within the cells could be expected.

The interpretation of the results of doxorubicin-carrying phages is more complex, since the goal of this system was a proof of new concept for the construction of cleavable linkers by genetic engineering instead of conventional organic chemical linkage. Our results show the DFK peptide to be specifically cleaved by cathepsin-B, specifically at the engineered site (Figure 3) and within the target cells. Further, doxorubicin-carrying DFK phages (Figures 3B, C, white bars) are more potent in comparison the phages that carry covalently-linked doxorubicin (Figures 3B, C, grey bars) even though the latter carry 10,000 drug molecules/phage while the former carry 3,500 drug molecules. Moreover, phages to which doxorubicin was covalently linked, although they were target-specific, inhibited cell growth less efficiently than non-specific, human IgG linked DFK phages, further demonstrating the contribution of the engineered drug-release mechanism to the potency of the platform. As for the limited specificity of doxorubicin-carrying DFK phages, we have already observed that coating phages with a high density of hydrophobic molecules limit the solubility of the phages (Yacoby et al., 2007) and cases them to become "sticky," that is, to bind non-specifically to bacteria and to cells (unpublished results). The results shown in Figures 5B, C suggest that this may also be the case with doxorubicin-carrying phages, since comparably levels of cell-killing could be observed when that phages were linked to the targeting antibodies, or to the irrelevant control, normal human IgG. Such non-specific killing could not be observed with hygromycin-armed phages (Figure 5A). Doxorubicin is known as a drug of which doses are limited by unwanted toxicity to non-tumor tissues (Albright et al., 2005). Doxorubicin and other anthracyclines are amphiphilic molecules known to interact with cell membranes (Gallois et al., 1998), which may cause non-specific binding. Large polymer-doxorubicin conjugates were reported as having limited solubility (Andersson et al., 2005), which may also affect target specificity. One may conclude that drug delivery platforms that carry the drug on the outside will be limited to highly water soluble drugs that do not bind non-discriminately to cells. However, a remedy to this limitation may be found in linking the hydrophobic drug to the phage through a solubility-enhancing linker, as we have recently reported (Yacoby et al., 2007). We have shown that the potency and the target specificity of anti-bacterial chloramphenicol-armed phages was substantially improved when this hydrophobic drug was linked to the phage coat through small hydrophilic molecules that served as solubility-enhancing linkers. On the other hand, phages that were directly armed with the hydrophobic drug chloramphenicol were less specific (Yacoby et al., 2007). An additional advantage of such an added hydrophilic coat is that it reduces both the immunogenicity and antigenicity of the drug-carrying phages upon injection into mice (unpublished data).

RESULTS

Binding Analysis with Monoclonal Antibodies Complexed Phage Nanoparticles Using Whole Cell ELISA

The comparative binding analysis was done by whole-cell ELISA as described in Materials and Methods. In order to assess the affect the binding abilities of the different targeting moieties the fUSE5-ZZ, phage vector that polyvalently displays the ZZ domain which enables the phages to form a stable complex with target-specific antibodies was used. The results of this assay are shown in Figure 1. As shown, the antibody-complexed phages exhibited cell specific binding which corresponded to the level of ErbB2 expression on the target cells, a weak binding to the control MDA-MB231 cell line (that expresses ErbB2 at a low level) was apparent and a much higher binding signal with ErbB2 overexpressing SKBR3 cell line indicating specific binding. No significant signal was obtained when control phages fUSE5-ZZ complexed with normal human IgG were used.

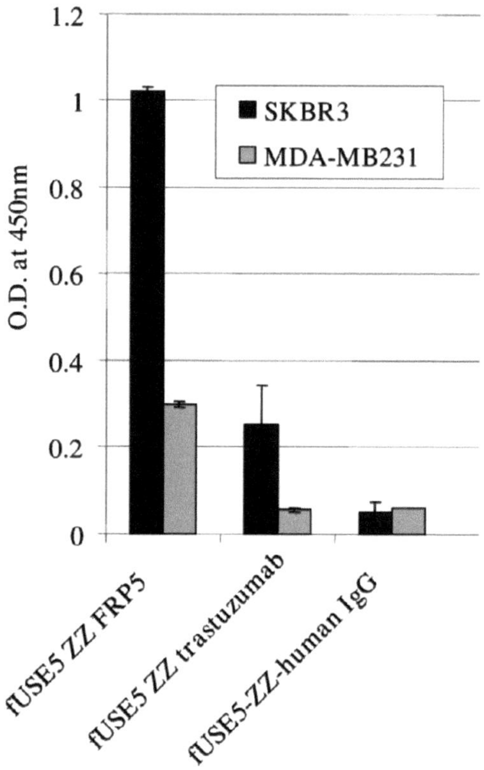

Figure 1. Comparative binding analysis of antibody displaying phages using whole cell ELISA. fUSE5-ZZ-chFRP5, fUSE5-ZZ-trastuzumab, and control phages fUSE5-ZZ-human IgG were added into wells that contain ErbB2 over-expressing SKBR3 cell line (black bars) or human mammary carcinoma MDA-MB231 cells as control cell line (gray bars) that express a low level of ErbB2. Binding was evaluated by the addition of HRP-conjugated rabbit anti M13 antibodies followed by addition chromogenic HRP substrate TMB. The results were plotted as absorbance at 450 nm. Data represent mean values ± SD of quadruplicate phage samples taking from one of three independent experiments.

Evaluation of Phage Internalization Using Confocal Microscopy

To function as a targeted drug-carrying platform, the antibody-complexed phages should be efficiently internalized into the target cells. To address this issue, we analyzed the capability of fUSE5-ZZ-chFRP5 complex to internalize into ErbB2 overexpressing human breast adenocarcinoma SKBR3 cells and human epidermoid carcinoma cell line A431 cells using confocal microscopy. A positive internalization signal is typically characterized by bright fluorescence vesicles within the cell cytoplasm together with a decrease in membranous fluorescence. As shown in Figure 2A, antibody-complexed fUSE5-ZZ-chFRP5 phages where internalized into both types of cells. The orange color dots that appeared within the cells are possibly the outcome of a combination between the red dyed membrane and the phage marked with green color generated by the secondary FITC conjugated antibody, which may suggest a lysosomal incorporation of the internalized phages.

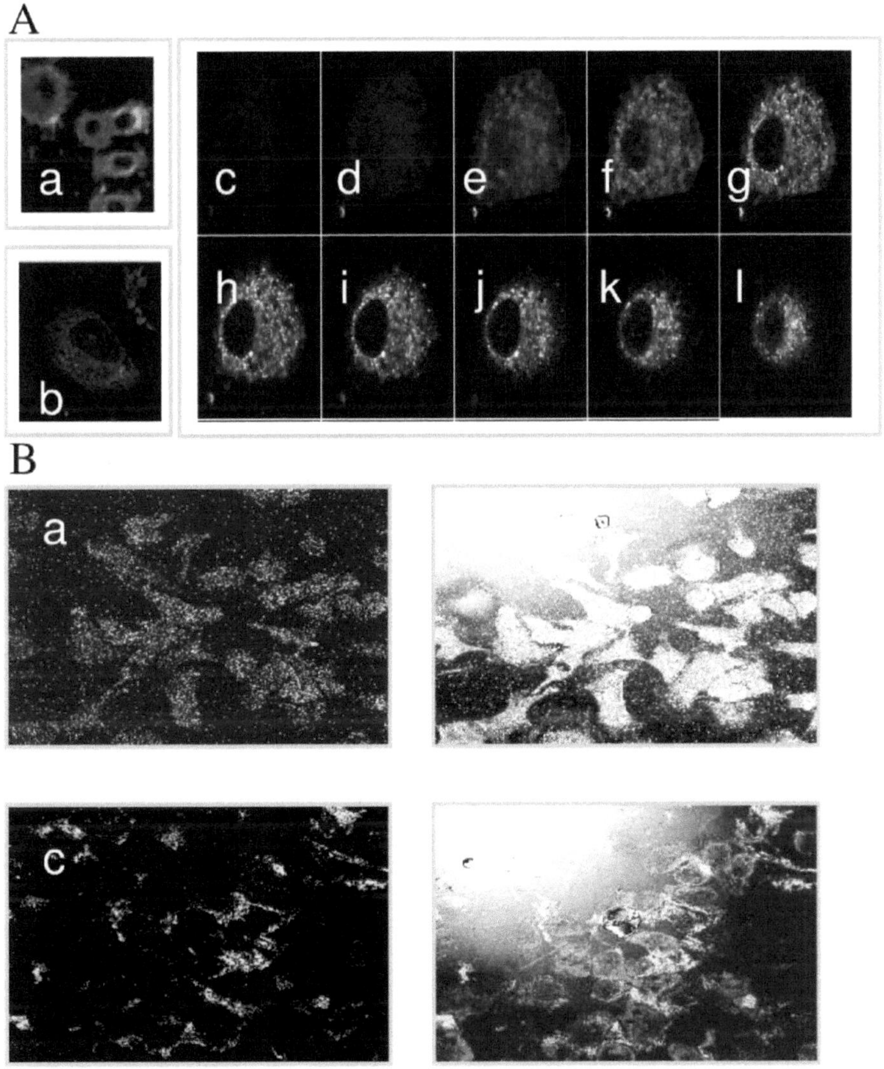

Figure 2. Evaluation of phage internalization into A431 and SKBR3 cells using confocal microscopy. (A) Immunofluorescence Staining: (a) control fUSE5-ZZ-human IgG phages (b), no phage, only antibodies (c-l) serial cuts of A431 cells that were treated with fUSE5-ZZ-chFRP5 phages. Membranes were labeled by using red fluorescent CM-Dil cell tracker (MoBiTec, Guttingen, Germany). Phages were detected by monoclonal mouse anti-M13 followed by incubation with FITC conjugated goat anti-mouse IgG (green fluorescence). (B) Evaluation of internalization of FITC labeled, drug conjugated phages into SKBR3 cells using confocal microscopy. (a) and (b) fUSE5-ZZ-chFRP5 phages, (c) and (d) control fUSE5-ZZ complexed with normal human IgG. As a reference, actin filaments with the cells were labeled by using red fluorescent dye Phalloidin (Sigma, Israel). Phages were labeled directly by FITC. Phages were added to the cells for 2 hr before analysis by confocal microscopy. Panels (a) and (c) show the green fluorescence of Fluorescein while in panels (b) and (d) the green fluorescence is overlaid on the red fluorescence.

Evaluation of Internalization of Drug Conjugated Phage Using Confocal Microscopy

The internalization of antibody-complexed phages following drug conjugation was evaluated also following drug conjugation. In this experiment, hygromycin conjugated fUSE5-ZZ complexed with chFRP5 was tested with SKBR3 cells. As opposed to detection with anti phage antibodies as shown in Figure 2A, here the visualization of hygromycin carrying phages was obtained by conjugating FITC to the phage through a free primary amine found in hygromycin, resulting in green fluorescent labeled fUSE5-ZZ-chFRP5 as previously described (Yacoby et al., 2007). The assay was done in different time points: 2, 12, 24 hr, in order to evaluate phage internalization rate. As shown in Figure 2B, hygromycin carrying phages were internalized into the cells, which could be observed 2 hr after adding phages to the cells. In fact, internalization seemed to be maximal when observed at 2 hr, and the fluorescent signal diminished during later time point (not shown). In contrast, hygromycin conjugated phages that were complexed with human IgG did not internalize. These results suggested that conjugating a large payload of drug to the phage coat does not seen to inhibit internalization of the antibody-complexed phages, probably occurring through receptor-mediated endocytosis.

Chemical Conjugation of Hygromycin and Doxorubicin to Phage Nanoparticles

Conjugation of the two drugs to the phage nanoparticles was done by using EDC chemistry, forming an amide bond between the exposed carboxyl side chains on the phage coat, mostly the ones exposed on g8p, and a free primary amine on the drugs. The drugs we used were hygromycin (an aminoglycoside antibiotics) or doxorubicin (an anthracycline antibiotic). Approximately 10,000 molecules of hygromycin were conjugated to each phage by using EDC chemistry as we recently described (Yacoby et al., 2007). The EDC reaction causes the formation of a covalent bond between the phage major coat protein, g8p and the drug which does not facilitates a controlled release form of the drug at the target site. However, as shown in Figure 2, the targeted phage nanoparticles are internalized into the cells possibly entering the lysosomal compartment where they are susceptible to digestion by lysosomal proteases. This led us to the assumption that lysosomal deconstruction of the phage may mediate drug release within the cell.

To obtain controlled release of the conjugated drug, fUSE5-ZZ-(g8p)DFK phage was designed. The fUSE5-ZZ-(g8p)DFK phages display the lysosomal cysteine protease cathepsin-B cleavage site on the phage major coat protein, g8p. In this phage almost all other carboxyl groups on g8p which were susceptible to EDC conjugation were eliminated by site-directed mutagenesis enabling the drug to be released mainly through cathepsin-B activity, a single carboxyl group was left as an internal control for the *in vitro* drug release experiments. The sequence of native g8p in comparison with the g8p coat protein of phage fUSE5-ZZ-DFK is shown in Figure 3A and the scheme of the doxorubicin-loaded phage is shown in Figure 3B.

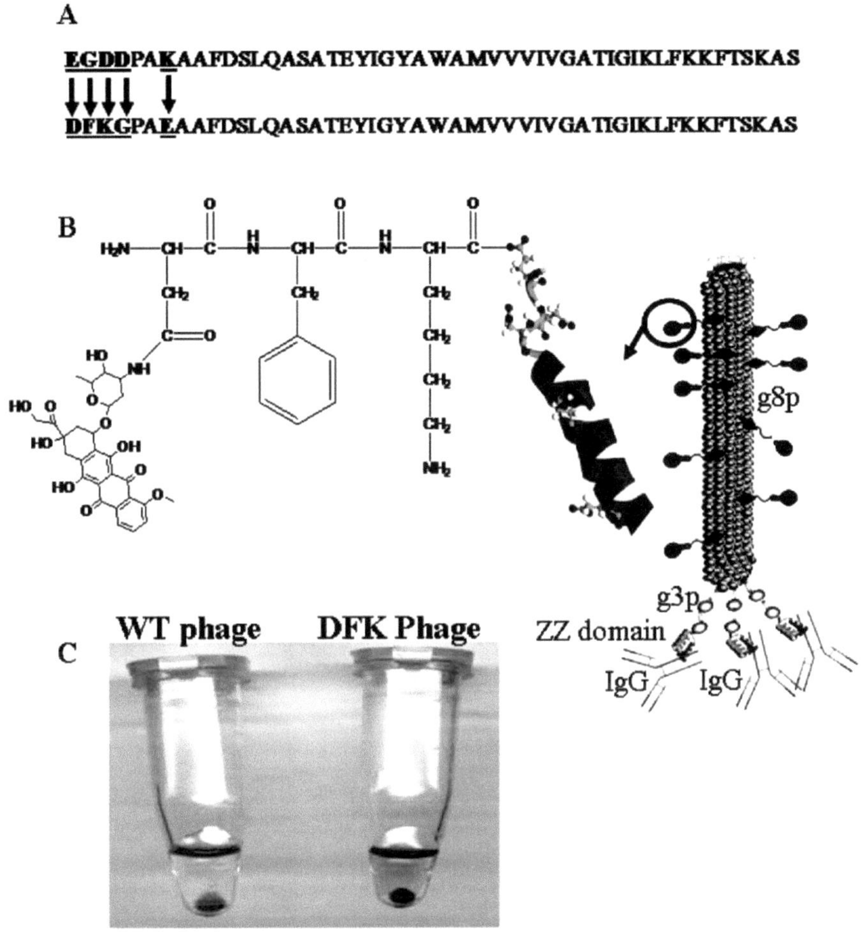

Figure 3. Controlled release of doxorubicin release from drug-carrying phages. (A) The sequence amino-acid sequence (single-letter code) of the g8p coat protein of fUSE5-ZZ-(p8)DFK phages (top) and native fUSE5 (bottom). The mutated residues are marked by black arrows. (B) Drawing (not to scale) of a single fUSE5-ZZ-(p8)DFK phage; In the phage scheme on the right, small turquoise spheres represent major coat protein g8p monomers. Purple spheres and sticks represent the five copies of minor coat protein g3p, which is fused to a 3-color helix representing the IgG binding ZZ domain. The Y shaped structure represents complexed IgG. An engineered g8p monomer is shown on the left. The helix represents a partial structure of a single major coat protein p8, conjugated through an amino terminal aspartate (D) of the sequence DFK carboxyl side chains a molecule of doxorubicin (red). (C) A Photograph of the cathepsin-B release experiment tubes, on the right, doxorubicin carrying fUSE5-ZZ-(p8)DFK phages that was incubated with cathepsin-B, followed by PEG/NaCl precipitation, a reddish soluble D-DOX (verified by HPLC and MS in Figure 5) is seen as well as a reddish pellet representing the drug conjugated through the internal glutamate residue. On the left is a tube containing fUSE5-ZZ phages that was incubated with cathepsin-B, followed by PEG/NaCl precipitation, the transparent colorless solution indicate no drug release.

In Vitro Release of Doxorubicin from fUSE5-ZZ(g8p)DFK Phages

Following doxorubicin conjugation to the phages we evaluated drug release mediated by the lysosomal hydrolase cathepsin-B. As shown in Figure 3C, drug release could be observed by the red color of the phage-free supernatant following PEG/NaCl precipitation of cathepsin-B-treated, doxorubicin conjugated fUSE5-ZZ(g8p)DFK phages. In contrast, no drug was released from similarly-treated, doxorubicin conjugated fUSE5-ZZ phages (that do not carry the DFK sequence).

The red supernatant that was recovered from the cathepsin-B-treated, doxorubicin conjugated fUSE5-ZZ(g8p)DFK phages was further analyzed by HPLC at the specific adsorption wavelength of doxorubicin (480 nm). As shown in Figure 4A, a specific peak corresponding to doxorubicin could be detected. Such a peak could not be observed when fUSE5-ZZ(g8p)DFK phages that do not carry doxorubicin were analyzed under identical conditions. In addition the MALDI-TOF MS analysis of this red supernatant revealed a specific peak corresponding the weight of aspartic acid-doxorubicin adduct, which is the N-terminal amino acid of the displayed DFK peptide Figure 4B.

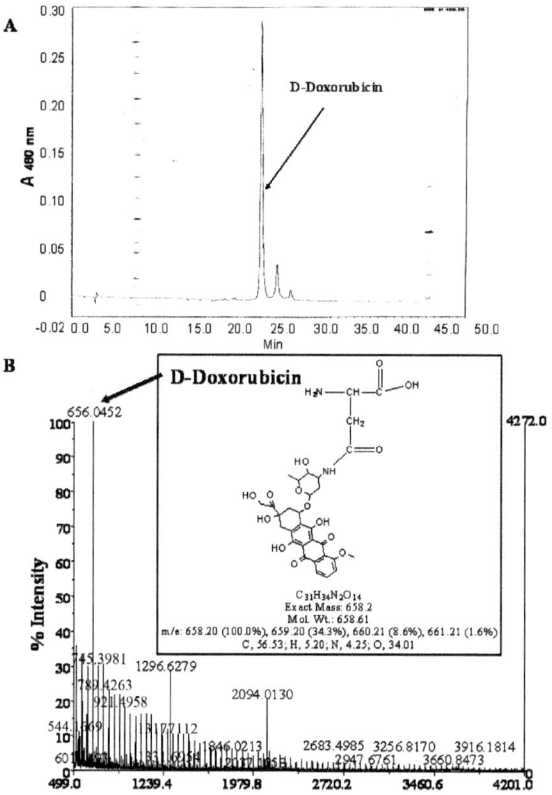

Figure 4. Analysis of the Cathepsin-B released material. (A) The crude cathepsin-B released material from re-suspended, PEG-precipitated, cathepsin-B treated, doxorubicin-carrying fUSE5-ZZ-(p8) DFK phages was analyzed using a gradient of acetonitrile in water on a Waters HPLC machine (RP; C-18 column) following the doxorubicin specific emission wavelength 480 nm. Cathepsin-B released material eluted at 24–25 min post injection. (B) The crude cathepsin-B released material was analyzed by MALDI TOF MS. The theoretical mass of the aspartate-doxorubicin (shown in the insert) was observed by the mass spectrometry analysis as a major peak 656.04 (marked by arrow) corresponding to the weight of aspartate-doxorubicin.

Specific Cytotoxicity of Targeted Hygromycin Conjugated Phages Towards Target Cells

Evaluation of the cell cytotoxicity of hygromycin carrying fUSE5-ZZ phages complexed with chFRP5 was done by *in vitro* cell-killing experiments. The ErbB2-expressing SKBR3 cells were incubated for 48 hr with 5×10^{11} of hygromycin carrying phages, and the relative number of viable cells in comparison with cells grown in the absence of the phage was determined using an enzymatic MTT assay. As shown in Figure 5A, hygromycin carrying fUSE5-ZZ-chFRP5 phages inhibited target cell growth by 50%, (Figure 5A treatment a), a > 1,000-fold improvement in hygromycin potency (in comparison to the free drug). No killing was observed when the cells were treated with, hygromycin conjugated fUSE5-ZZ-phages in complex with human IgG (non-targeted) (Figure 5A treatment b) or to targeted fUSE5-ZZ-chFRP5 that were not conjugated to the drug (Figure 5A treatment c). In contrast, the viability of HEK293 cells that were treated with the same dose of hygromycin carrying phages was not affected at all (Figure 5B).

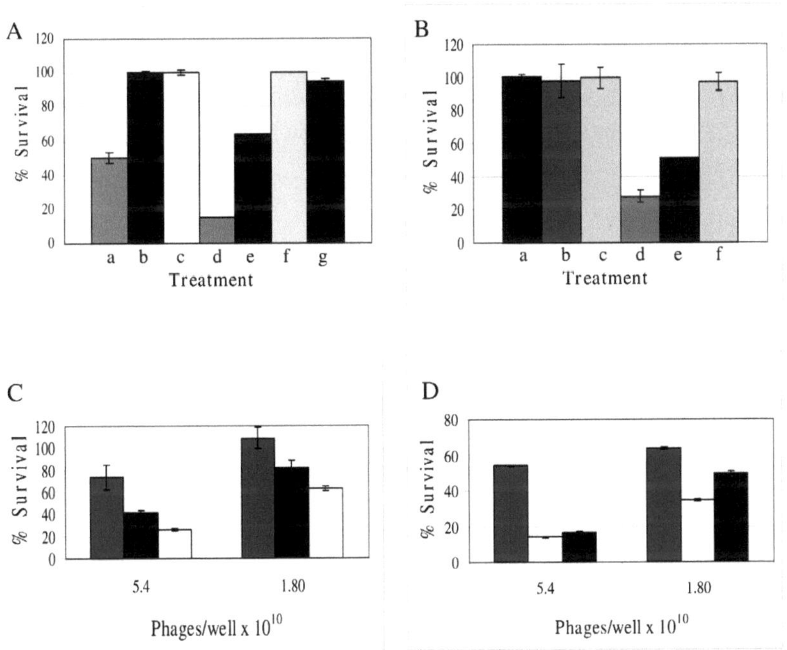

Figure 5. Toxicity analysis of targeted drug-carrying phages by *in vitro* cell-killing assays. (A) Hygromycin carrying phages on SKBR3 target cells SKBR3 cells were incubated with 5 x 10^{11} of hygromycin carrying fUSE5-ZZ-chFRP5 phages (a), hygromycin carrying fUSE5-ZZ-human IgG (b), hygromycin carrying fUSE5-ZZ-human IgG (c), 2 mg free hygromycin/well (d), 0.2 mg free hygromycin/well (e), 0.02 mg free hygromycin/well (f) 0.002 mg free hygromycin/well (g). (B) Hygromycin carrying phages on HEK293 non-target cells HEK293 cells were incubated with 5 x 10^{11} of hygromycin carrying fUSE5-ZZ-human IgG phages (a), hygromycin carrying fUSE5-ZZ-trastuzumab phages (b), hygromycin carrying fUSE5-ZZ-cetuximab phages (c), 1 mg/ml free hygromycin (d), 0.1 mg/ml free hygromycin (e), 0.01 mg/ml free hygromycin (f). (C) Trastuzumab-targeted, doxorubicin carrying phages on SKBR3 target cells SKBR cells were incubated with serial dilutions of doxorubicin

Figure 5. *(Caption Continued)*

carrying phages; grey bars, doxorubicin carrying fUSE5-ZZ-trastuzumab, black bars fUSE5-ZZ-(p8) DFK-human IgG, white bars, doxorubicin carrying fUSE5-ZZ-(p8)DFK-trastuzumab. (D) Cetuximab-targeted, doxorubicin carrying phages on A431 target cells A431 cells were incubated with serial dilutions of doxorubicin carrying phages; grey bars, doxorubicin carrying fUSE5-ZZ-cetuximab, black bars fUSE5-ZZ-(p8)DFK-human IgG white bars, doxorubicin carrying fUSE5-ZZ-(p8)DFK-cetuximab. The relative number of viable cells was determined using an enzymatic MTT assay and is indicated as the absorption at 570 nm. The results are expressed as percentage of living cells respect to untreated controls. Data represent mean values ± SD of three independent experiments.

Specific Cytotoxicity of Doxorubicin Conjugated fUSE5-ZZ(p8)DFK Phages Towards ErbB2-expressing Cells

Evaluation of the cell cytotoxicity of doxorubicin conjugated fUSE5-ZZ(p8)DFK in complex with the anti ErbB2 antibodies trastuzumab (Herceptin®) (Figure 5C) or anti EGFR cetuximab (Erbitux®) (Figure 5D) was done with *in vitro* cell-killing experiments with A431 and SKBR3 cells. Here the drug was designed to be released in a controlled manner. Doxorubicin was conjugated to the phage using the EDC chemistry, through the engineered DFK tri-peptide where the drugs release is mediated through the cathepsin-B activity in the endosomal-lysosomal compartments. As shown in Figures 5C, and 5D, doxorubicin carrying fUSE5-ZZ(g8p)DFK in complex with each of the targeting IgGs, but also with the non-targeting human IgG caused efficient killing of the target cells, in a dose-dependent manner. When doxorubicin was conjugated to fUSE5-ZZ phages in complex with trastuzumab (without the DFK sequence), growth inhibition was minimal.

CONCLUSION

To conclude, our study demonstrated a proof of principle of targeted, drug-carrying filamentous bacteriophage as anti-cancer agents. The issues of pharmacokinetics, biodistribution and immunogenicity and tumor penetration: these parameters are key issues in current phage therapy studies (Merril et al., 1996; Zou et al., 2004). Basically, phages are immunogenic on one hand, and upon intravenous injection are removed quickly by the reticuloendothelial system on the other. Attempts to modulate phage pharmacokinetics were based on isolating long-circulating mutants of phage lambda (Merril et al., 1996). But no such studies were done with the filamentous phages. We believe that chemical modification of the phage coat (as we do during drug conjugation) should modulate the pharmacokinetics, the biodistribution, and the immunogenicity in comparison to bare phages. Regarding tumor penetration, phages can not be regarded as huge complexes as may be evident from their molecular weight which is about 15 million Dalton. Due to their needle-like structure, they may very well penetrate into tumors, as may be suggested by the study where xenografts in nude mice were eradicated following IV injection of phages that delivered a therapeutic gene (Hajitou et al., 2006). We are currently comparing the immunogenicity, pharmacokinetics, and biodistribution of un-conjugated to drug-carrying phages in animal studies.

KEYWORDS

- **Anti-cancer therapy**
- **Chemotherapeutic agents**
- **Human breast carcinoma**
- **Potentiation factor**

AUTHORS' CONTRIBUTIONS

Hagit Bar designed and carried out experiments and analyzed the data; Iftach Yacoby designed and carried out experiments, participated in analyzing the data and in writing the manuscript. Itai Benhar designed the study and wrote the manuscript.

ACKNOWLEDGMENTS

This study was supported in part by a grant from the Israel Public Committee for Allocation of Estate Funds, Ministry of Justice, Israel, and by the Israel Cancer Association. Iftach Yacoby was supported by a Dan David Ph.D. scholarship for young scholars in future dimension.

Chapter 5

Artemisinin-derived Antimalarial Dry Suspensions for Pediatric Use

Magnus A. Atemnkeng, Katelijne De Cock,
and Jacqueline Plaizier-Vercammen

INTRODUCTION

Artemisinin-derivative formulations are now widely used to treat *P. falciparum* malaria. However, the dry powder suspensions developed for children are few and/or are of poor quality. In addition to the active compound, the presence of a suitable preservative in these medicines is essential. In this study, an evaluation of the preservative content and efficacy in some dry suspensions available on the Kenyan market was performed.

The UV spectrophotometry was used to identify the preservatives in each sample while high performance liquid chromatography with UV detector (HPLC-UV) was used for quantification. After reconstitution of the powders in water, the dissolution of the preservatives was followed for 7 days. Antimicrobial efficacy of the preservatives was assessed by conducting a preservative efficacy test (PET) following the European pharmacopoeia (Ph. Eur.) standards.

Four different preservatives were identified namely methylparahydroxybenzoate (MP), propylparahydroxybenzoate (PP), benzoic acid, and sorbic acid. The MP and PP were identified in Artesiane® (artemether 300 mg/100 ml), Alaxin® (dihydroartemisinin 160 mg/80 ml), andGvither® (artemether 300 mg/100 ml) respectively. Sorbic acid was present in Artenam® (artemether 180 mg/60 ml) while benzoic acid was identified in Santecxin® (dihydroartemisinin 160 mg/80 ml) and Artexin® (dihydroartemisinin 160 mg/80 ml) respectively. Cotecxin® (dihydroartemisinin 160 mg/80 ml) did not contain any of the above preservatives. After reconstitution in water, preservativesin 50% (3/6) of the products did not completely dissolve and the PET results revealed that only Artenam® and Gvither® met the requirements for antimicrobial efficacy. The other products did not conform.

These results show that pediatric antimalarial dry powder formulations on the market may contain ineffective or incorrect amounts of preservatives. This is a potential risk to the patient. Studies conducted on the dry powder suspensions should include the analysis of both the active ingredient and the preservative, including the efficacy of the latter.

The artemisinin-derivatives, artemether, artesunate, arteether, and dihydroartemisinin, are currently the most potent antimalarial medicines on the market. They are widely available in the different pharmaceutical dosage forms including tablets, injections, suppositories, and dry powders (Van der Meersch, 2005).

Since artemisinin and its derivatives are poorly water-soluble and are not very stable in solution, the preparations have to be formulated in the dry form for subsequent reconstitution into a wet suspension with water just before use. The dry powders for reconstitution are normally designed for children from 0–5 years of age, who are not able to swallow tablets. In the malaria endemic countries, living conditions are often poor, including scarce access to clean portable drinking water (Haines and Smith, 1997). As a result, microorganisms can easily thrive when the dry powder is reconstituted with poor quality water. In addition, children suffering from malaria, as well as AIDS or typhoid, have a weakened immunological system and are, therefore, more susceptible to other infections. Moreover, the drugs are packaged in multiple dose containers, making the preparation highly susceptible to contamination following frequent use. Hence, pharmaceutical preparations which need an aqueous vehicle such as syrups and powders for oral suspensions require safeguards from microbial contamination, which may affect product stability or infect the consumer. This is accomplished by the addition of antimicrobial agents in the formulation to destroy and inhibit the growth of those organisms that may contaminate the product during manufacture or use (European Pharmacopoeia IV, 2003).

The International Committee on Harmonization (ICH) guidelines (International Committee on Harmonization, 1992) requests that for submission of drug registration dossier on dry powders for oral suspensions, data should be provided for the content of the active pharmaceutical ingredient (API) as well as the type(s) and amount(s) of the preservative(s) used. In addition, the efficacy of the antimicrobial preservation should be demonstrated by challenging the reconstituted suspension in its final container with specified microorganisms. This implies that the preservative used in the dry powder must completely dissolve on addition of water to impart the preservation action.

Sources of this microbial contamination may include air and water, manufacturing equipment, manufacturing personnel and/or the consumer (Anger et al., 1996). Bacterial contamination of products through consumer use has resulted in presence of mixed and harmful microbial flora in the product (Wilson et al., 1971).

Major studies on antimalarial formulations are limited to the active ingredients without mention of the preservatives when studied in syrups and dry powders. In view of the biological role that this excipient plays towards the maintenance of the preparation and the recovery of the patient, there is a dire need for greater attention and awareness directed towards the importance of preservation in pediatric formulations.

Several chemical preservative agents exist and have been widely employed in the cosmetic, food, and pharmaceutical industries (Anger et al., 1996). For oral use, the choices of the preservatives are limited. These include benzoic acid (BA) C_6H_5COOH and sorbic acid (SA) C_5H_7COOH, which are generally effective to control mould and yeast growth, and the parahydroxybenzoic acid esters: methylparaben (MP) $C_6H_4(OH)COOCH_3$ and propylparaben (PP) $C_6H_4(OH)COOC_3H_7$, which are most commonly used to control bacterial growth due to their broad antimicrobial spectrum with good stability and non-volatility (The Japanese standards of cosmetic ingredients-with commentary, 1984). The MP and PP are usually used in combination as they possess a synergistic activity when used together. However, overuse of preservatives may cause allergic reactions hence, they should be shown not to be cytotoxic or sensitizing (Klocker et al., 2004; Soni et al., 2001).

Recently, the artemisinin-derivative drugs have become a major target for counterfeiters. Fake and substandard versions of original brands have previously been reported in Southeast Asia (Lon et al., 2006; Newton et al., 2003) and now in Africa (Atemnkeng et al., 2007). The substandard copies were present in all dosage forms but most especially in the tablets and dry powders. In the latter, quality analysis should also be performed on the preservatives. No report has been published on efficacy of preservatives in artemisinin-like antimalarial drugs.

Thus, the aim of this study was (1) to identify the commonly used antimicrobial agents in the artemisinin-containing dry suspensions on the market, (2) study the dissolution profiles of these preservatives after reconstituting in water, (3) evaluate the activity of the preservatives by performing the PET on the wet suspension, and (4) describe some simple analytical procedures for these analytes in dry powders. The different HPLC methods used were validated for each analyte.

MATERIALS AND METHODS

Potassium dihydrogenphosphate and sodium hydroxide (both Ph. Eur. grade) were obtained from Merck (Darmstadt, Germany) and HPLC grade methanol and acetonitrile were supplied by Fisher Scientific (Leicestershire, UK). Glacial acetic acid was obtained from JT Baker (Deventer, The Netherlands) while ammonia (pro analysi) was supplied by Merck (Darmstadt, Germany). Methylparaben and propylparaben were obtained from Federa (Brussels, Belgium), while benzoic acid (pro analysi) was supplied by Merck (Darmstadt, Germany). Sorbic acid was bought from Certa (Braine l'Alleud, Belgium). De-ionized milli-Q water was used throughout the experiment.

Thin Layer Chromatography (TLC) for the Identification of Preservatives

Of the seven dry suspensions, only the Artenam® and Artesiane® samples indicated the type of preservative(s) used on the package insert. From the literature, the commonly used preservatives in oral aqueous pharmaceuticals were retrieved and used to identify the preservatives in the other samples. The TLC procedure described in the Ph. Eur. IV for the identification of parabens was initially tested to separate the four preservatives.

The Ca 100 mg of each of the reference preservative powder was weighed in separate 100-ml flasks and dissolved to the mark with methanol. The stationary phase was 10 × 20 cm RP-18 F_{254S} silica gel plates from Merck (Darmstadt, Germany). The initial eluent was composed of 70 volumes of methanol, 30 volumes of water, and 1 volume of glacial acetic acid. Several other compositions were tested to efficiently separate the four components on a single plate (see Table 1). Five μl of each standard solution was manually spotted using a glass capillary pipette at 2 cm spot distance. The plates were then developed in Camag® TLC tanks presaturated with mobile phase. Development time was dependent on eluent composition, but ± 30 min was sufficient for most. The plates were allowed to dry in a well ventilated room. Visualization was on UV at 254 nm with a Camag® Universal UV Lamp (Muttenz, Switzerland).

Table 1. Mobile phase compositions for the separation of preservatives by TLC (detected at 254 nm).

	Retardation Factor (R_F)			
Mobile Phase (v/v/v)	**Methylparaben**	**Propylparaben**	**Sorbic Acid**	**Benzoic Acid**
CH_3OH/H_2O (80/20)	0.70	0.57	0.68	0.69 (Faints spot)
$CH_3OH/H_2O/CH_3COOH$ (70/30/1)	0.47	0.28	0.47	0.50 (Faint spot)
$CH_3OH/H_2O/CH_3COOH$ (80/20/1)	0.75	0.67	0.75	0.75
$CH_3OH/H_2O/CH_3COOH$ (80/20/3)	0.57	0.48	0.64	0.64 (Faints spot)
$CH_3OH/H_2O/NH_3$ (80/20/1)	0.80	0.70	0.87	Highly faint spot
$CH_3CN/H_2O/CH_3COOH$ (95/5/1)	0.88	0.81	0.84	Highly faint spot

UV Spectrophotometry

To identify the preservatives in the other suspensions, methanol was added to each powder bottle, mixed and centrifuged at 3,000 rpm (g = 1,512) for 15 min. The supernatant was collected and appropriate dilutions were made in methanol. Spectra acquisition of the samples was done against a standard solution on Uvikon 860 spectrophotometer (Kontron Instruments, Massachusetts, USA) connected to a Plotter 800 Integrator (Kontron Instruments, Massachussetts, USA). Pure methanol was used as the blank.

HPLC Instrumentation

The chromatographic system for the preservatives (MP, PP, BA, and SA) consisted of a Merck-Hitachi L-6000 pump, a Perkin-Elmer LC 90 UV spectrophotometric detector connected to a Merck-Hitachi D-2500 Chromato-Integrator. The stationary phase in each case was a reversed-phase Nucleosil® 120-4 C_{18} column, 125 mm long by 4 mm (i.d), and 5 µm particle size from Macherey-Nagel (Düren, Germany) except for sorbic acid where a Lichrospher® 250 × 4 mm, 5 µm particle size column from Merck (Darmstadt, Germany) was used. The eluent for the parabens consisted of an acetonitrile: KH_2PO_4 (0.05 M, pH 5.0) buffer (300:700, v/v) mixture. The mobile phase of sorbic acid was composed of a mixture of acetonitrile:water:KH_2PO_4 (0.05 M, pH5.0) buffer, (100:690:240, v/v/v) and benzoic acid was separated using acetonitrile :KH_2PO_4 (0.05 M, pH 5.0) buffer (100:900, v/v) mixture. Detection of MP and PP was achieved on UV at 254 nm, 290 nm for sorbic acid, and 226 nm for benzoic acid. All analyses were done isocratically at a flow rate of 1.0 ml/min and 20 µl of each sample was injected. In all experiments, the buffer was adjusted to their required pH with sodium hydroxide and filtered using a 0.45 µm pore size membrane filter before use.

Standard Solutions Preparation

A bulk powder mixture comprising Ca 0.08% MP and 0.02% PP was prepared and from this mixture about 50 mg was accurately weighed in a 50-ml flask. This was completely dissolved to the mark with pure methanol. The solution was then diluted (100×) with the same solvent for analysis. Sorbic acid standard solution was prepared by weighing ca. 160 mg of it and dissolving in 50 ml methanol. Appropriate dilutions were then made, first 10× in methanol: water (4:1, v/v) mixture and then 2.5× with the mobile phase for injection. Benzoic acid standard was prepared by accurately weighing 60 mg of it in a 50-ml volumetric flask and dissolving to the mark with a methanol:water (900:100, v/v) mixture. From this a 20× dilution was made with a methanol: KH_2PO_4 (0.05 M, pH 5.0) buffer (50:50 v/v).

Preservative Content in Dry Powders

All powders analyzed in this study were anonymously obtained from pharmacies within Nairobi in Kenya (East Africa). An Artenam® semi-industrial batch dry powder suspension containing artemether (180 mg/60 ml) was added to the study. From each product the following were noted: type and dose of active ingredient and type of preservative (if indicated) and registration status. All analyses were performed before the expiry dates of the product.

Powder in each bottle was shaken to free the particles. For the dihydroartemisinin dry powders, exactly 200 ml of methanol:water (80:20, v/v) mixture was added to reduce the influence of the matrix and powder volume on the analysis. This solvent mixture was necessary to dissolve both the active and the preservative in order to use the content of the same bottle for both analyses. For the artemether dry powders, exactly 200 ml of pure methanol was added to the content. All the bottles were then thoroughly mixed and left on the shaking apparatus for at least 1 hr followed by ultrasonication for 15 min. Part of the suspension was transferred to 5-ml Falcon® tubes and centrifuged at 3000 rpm (g = 1,512) for 15 min.

Dissolution of Preservatives in the Reconstituted Suspensions

The instructions described by each manufacturer were followed for reconstitution. The Milli-Q water was added to each powder, well mixed till complete dispersion and part of the suspension was taken to determine its pH. From the rest a suitable volume was transferred to Falcon® tubes and centrifuged at 3,000 rpm (g = 1,512) for 15 min. For the more viscous suspensions, the centrifugation step was repeated on the supernatant. The density of the supernatant was measured and subsequent volumes were determined by sample weighing. Appropriate dilutions of the supernatant were done for HPLC analysis at the following time points: immediately after reconstitution (t_0), 6 hr, 24 hr, 4 days, and 7 days respectively; the maximum period necessary for a complete treatment of severe malaria and during which the suspension is supposed to be stable.

Preservative Efficacy Test

The method described in the Ph. Eur. IV 5.1.3 "Efficacy of Antimicrobial Preservation" was used (European Pharmacopoeia IV, 2003). The test consisted of challenging the reconstituted suspensions in their final containers with a prescribed inoculum of the following microorganisms: *Pseudomonas aeruginosa ATCC 9027*, *Staphylococcus aureus ATCC 6538*, *Escherichia coli ATCC 8739*, *Candida albicans ATCC 10231*, *Zygosaccharomyces rouxii NCYC 381*, and *Aspergillus niger ATCC 16404*. The inoculated preparations were then stored at ambient temperature and samples were withdrawn at specified time intervals and the remaining microorganisms counted.

DISCUSSION

Artemisinin and its semi-synthetic derivatives are currently the most effective anti-malarial compounds on the market. The dry suspension preparations of these drugs are of particular importance since they are specifically made for children (though the dose can also be adapted to an adult patient). This is a very vulnerable age group and more precaution is, therefore, necessary in formulating their medicines. In all such preparations a suitable preservative has to be added. In the tropics, where temperatures tend to be high in addition to high relative humidity, microbial contamination of the reconstituted suspension (and possible patient co-infection) can be common. In fact, in view of the possibility of using contaminated drinking water, most of the drug manufacturers advised that only boiled and cooled water should be used to reconstitute the suspension.

Regulatory law requires that preservatives must be listed by their common or usual names on ingredient labels of all drugs that contain them. Most manufacturers failed to indicate the type of preservative and the composition of other excipients in the formulation. This practice shades vital drug information, which is necessary for the patient, medical practitioners, researchers, and the regulatory authorities.

It was not possible to use TLC alone to identify the preservatives present in the preparations due to the difficulty in separating methylparaben from sorbic acid as their RFvalues were nearly always the same (Table 1). With normal phase plates similar separation problems were encountered. The UV lamp used in spot visualization was set at two standard wavelengths only, 254 nm and 366 nm hence, the faint spots observed with benzoic acid would probably be due to its low absorption at 254 nm (λ_{max} BA = 226 nm).

It is unclear what the recommended concentration of a preservative in a dry suspension is supposed to be. Nothing is mentioned in the United States Pharmacopoeia (USP) or the Ph. Eur. on the actual limits necessary hence, this leaves room for the formulators to employ different amounts of the same preservative; sometimes to detriment of the patient. This disparity in concentration is clearly observed in all the products (Table 2). The total amount of a preservative present in a dry powder is required to be available in the wet suspension. None of the paraben formulations met this criterion. In some drugs, values containing as low as 30% only of preservative were released after reconstitution. This leaves the drug susceptible to contamination. The ICH recommends that content limits of the preservative between 90–110% at release should be acceptable. However, Ofner III et al. (1996) suggested that degradation of the preservative is acceptable as long as sufficient preservative is present to maintain effectiveness. To accomplish this, the use of the right type and quality of the preservative is primordial. For instance, esters of parahydroxybenzoic acids are slightly soluble in water and there is the danger that in the dry powders they may not dissolve fast enough after adding water. For such preparations, their acid salts such as sodium alkylparabens are preferred. Because the parabens took several days to reach their end concentration in the wet suspension, this may suggest that only the acid form of the preservative was used. Secondly, 100% of the dissolved preservative could not be retrieved due to the possibility of preservative adsorption on the solids and/or complex formation on the macromolecules in the suspension such as suspending agents (Martin et al., 1983). Studies have shown that parabens adsorb to the surface of the container-closure system especially plastic containers. The latter are commonly employed in pediatric formulations (Rowe et al., 2005). All products used this packaging except the Artexin® preparation which employed a brown bottle packaging. Due to the possibility of the interactions mentioned above, only the free fraction of the preservative can be active. Thus, the formulator has to be able to strike a balance between a level high enough to pass the PET and low enough to prevent adverse reactions.

The efficacy of a preservative depends not only on its concentration but also on the pH of the suspension. For preservatives that are carboxylic acids, only the unionized species is microbicidal. The pK_a of such preservatives therefore determines the pH range in which the preservative is effective. The antimicrobial activity of the parabens, benzoic acid, sorbic acid, and others certainly decreases as pH increases past their respective pK_a (Anger et al., 1996). It is, therefore, possible that though Artexin® contained high amount of benzoic acid (0.148%), its antimicrobial efficacy was not adequate since the pH of the reconstituted suspension of 5.90 exceeded the pK_a of BA. This high pH dissociates the acid into the salt form leaving only a small undissociated fraction. On the other hand, Santecxin® contained a very low amount of benzoic acid (only 0.031%) which probably was insufficient to impart the preservative's activity. The pH of all paraben formulations (Artesiane®, Gvither®, and Alaxin®) was lower than their pK_a; hence inadequate antimicrobial efficiency could not be due to chemical dissociation. Though the Gvither® sample contained the least dissolved parabens, its PET passed the requirements. This is probably due to the very high amounts of these substances present in the original formulation (0.178% MP and 0.057% PP respectively).

Though there are not many antimalarial dry powders on the market, a more prospective and large scale study involving samples collected in different endemic regions is necessary to ascertain the impact of preservation on the products. This initial study portrays the importance of preservation in aqueous antimalarial compounds.

RESULTS

Preservative Identification

The TLC experiments were done using the standard solutions of methylparaben, propylparaben, benzoic acid, and sorbic acid to rapidly check the possibility of separating and identifying all four preservatives on a single plate. Visualization was done at 254 nm. The spots of MP, PP, and SA were clearly visible on the plates. Only benzoic acid showed faint spots. Methylparaben and propylparaben were well separated from each other but there was more or less a constant retardation factor (RF) value for methylparaben and sorbic acid when different solvent systems were tried (Table 1). Changing eluent compositions did not effectively resolve all four analytes. A system that came close to a good separation was methanol:water:ammonia (80:10:1, v/v/v) with RF values of 0.80, 0.70, and 0.87 for MP, PP, and SA respectively (Figure 1). The manufacturers and origin of the different powders are presented in Table 2. The UV spectra revealed the presence of four different preservative in the dry powders; MP and

PP in Artesiane®, Gvither®, and Alaxin®, benzoic acid in Artexin® and Santecxin®, and sorbic acid in Artenam® respectively. Cotecxin® did not exhibit any clear UV spectrum however, a personal correspondence with the manufacturers stated chlorbutanol as the preservative used. For quantification, spectrophotometry was not a good method since preservatives that exist in combination such as the parabens will absorb at the same wavelength (Koundourellis et al., 2000). In addition, an excipient that can interfere with the analyte cannot be separated on UV thus, HPLC-UV was used in subsequent experiments.

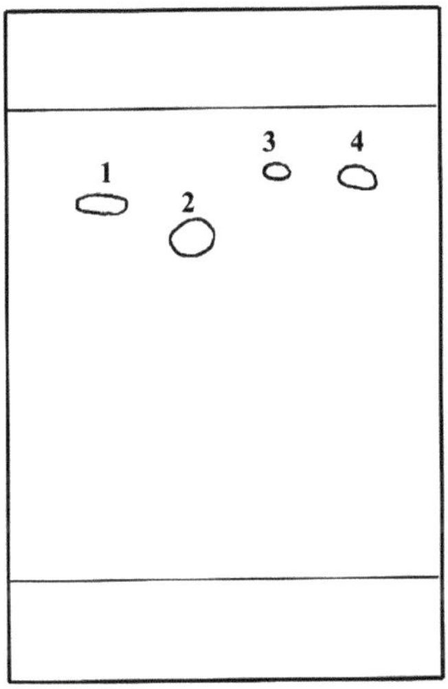

Figure 1. The TLC plate showing the separation of preservatives (1 = methylparaben, 2 = propylparaben, 3 = benzoic acid, 4 = sorbic acid) using a solvent mixture of methanol:water:ammonia (80:20:1, v/v/v).

Table 2. Concentration of preservative(s) in dry suspensions after reconstitution.

Product/Manufacturer	Active Ingredient/Dose	Preservative(s) Identified	% Preservative Found	Normal Value in H_2O^+ (%)
Artenam®* Arenco, Belgium	Artemether 180 mg/60 ml	Sorbic acid	0.27	0.20
Gvither® GVS Labs, India	Artemether 300 mg/100 ml	Methylparaben	0.18	0.08
		Propylparaben	0.06	0.02
Artesiane® Dafra, Belgium	Artemether 300 mg/100 ml	Methylparaben	0.08	0.08
		Propylparaben	0.02	0.02
Alaxin® GVS Labs, India	Dihydroartemisinin 160 mg/80 ml	Methylparaben	0.09	0.08
		Propylparaben	0.01	0.02
Artexin® Sphinx Pharma, Kenya	Dihydroartemisinin 160 mg/80ml	Benzoic acid	0.15	0.10
Santecxin® Shsj, China	Dihydroartemisinin 160 mg/80 ml	Benzoic acid	0.03	0.10
Cotecxin®, Jiaxing Nanhu Pharma, China	Dihydroartemisinin 160 mg/80 ml	Chlorbutanol?	Not tested	0.50

Preservatives Content and Dissolution

In the dry powders, 0.076% MP and 0.020% PP were found in Artesiane®, 0.088% MP and 0.011% PP in Alaxin® while 0.178% MP and 0.057% PP were found in Gvither® respectively. The 0.268% sorbic acid was present in Artenam® while Santecxin® contained 0.031% benzoic acid and Artexin® 0.148% benzoic acid (Table 2). The normal aqua concentrations of parabens used in pharmaceutical products are 0.08% MP and 0.02% PP (when used in combination), 0.10% BA and 0.20% SA respectively (Martindale: The Complete Drug Reference, 1999). However, in a powder mixture with a complex matrix these amounts may vary.

After reconstitution (addition of water) only the benzoic acid (Santecxin® and Artexin®) and the sorbic acid (Artenam®) containing products completely and immediately dissolved their preservatives (Figures 2 and 3) and the levels remained unchanged during the 7 days study period. None of the parabens immediately dissolved and the rate of dissolution differed between MP and PP in the same suspension and within different suspensions (Figures 4 and 5). Artesiane® reached the 90% dissolution rate only after 24 hr in PP and this remained stable for up to day 7. On the other hand, the total level of MP dissolved in the same sample did not exceed 74%. At t_0 the amounts of preservative dissolved were 64.9% MP and 85.3% PP for Artesiane®, 28.8% MP and 30.1% PP for Gvither®, and 78.8% MP and 45.3% PP for Alaxin® respectively. Gvither® possessed the most slowly dissolving parabens and only a maximum of 45.4% MP and 79.2% PP were present after 7 days (Figures 4 and 5). All the drug formulations were registered at the Drug Regulatory Agency of Kenya.

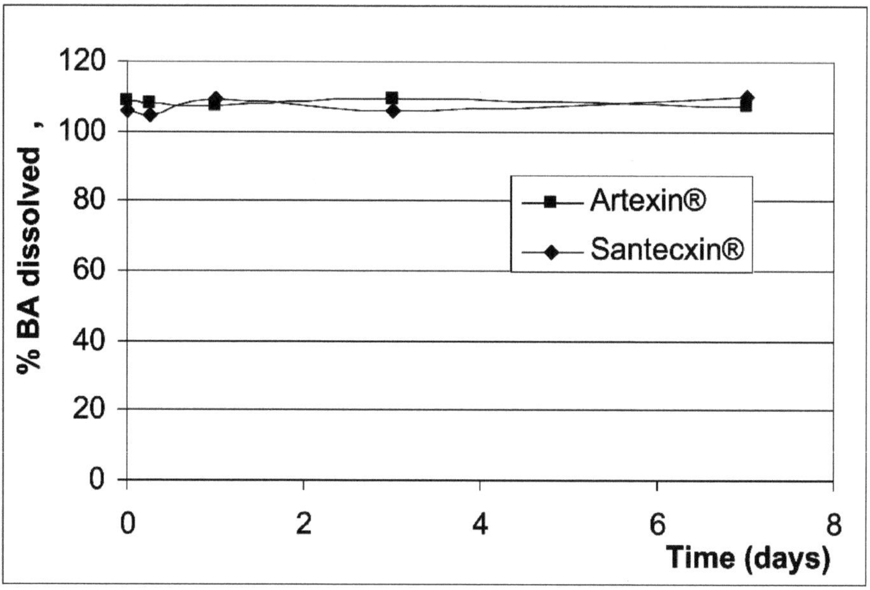

Figure 2. Dissolution profiles of benzoic acid (BA).

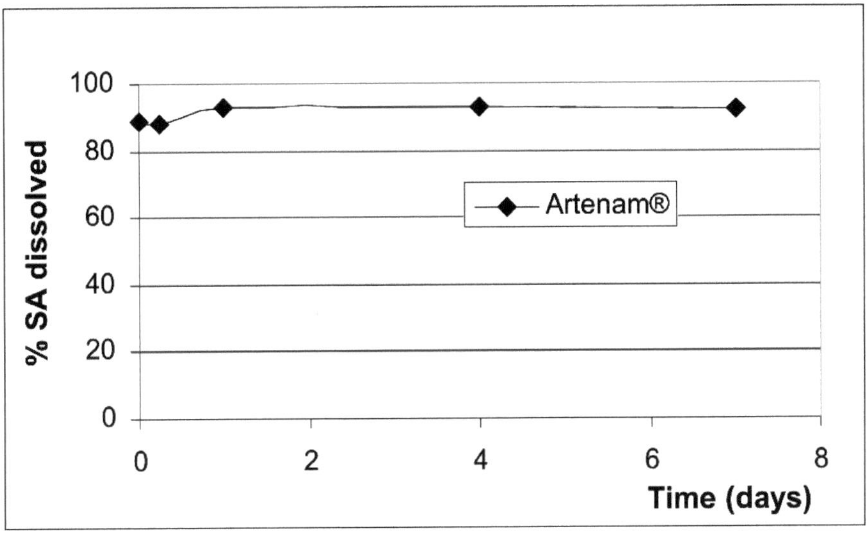

Figure 3. Dissolution profile of sorbic acid (SA).

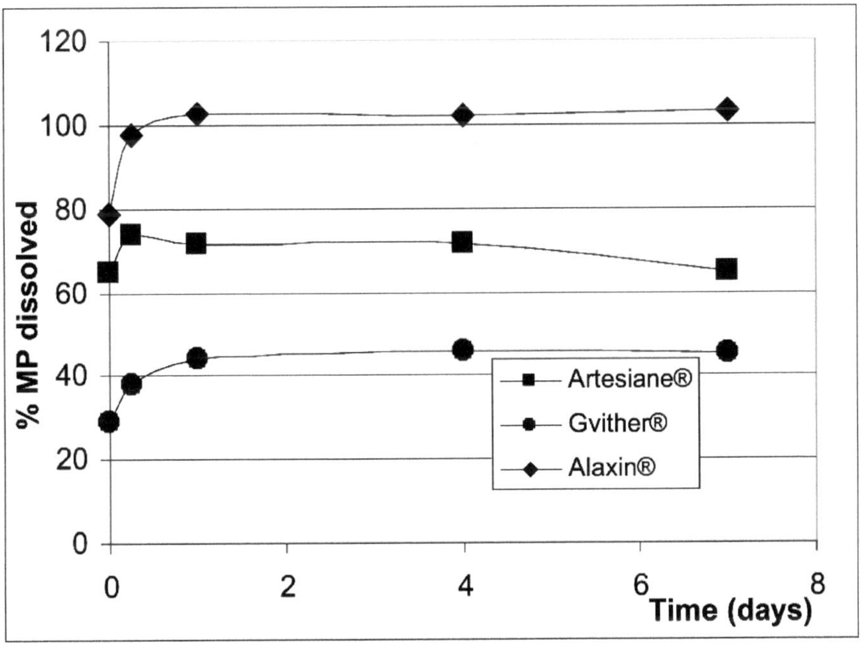

Figure 4. Dissolution profiles of methylparaben (MP).

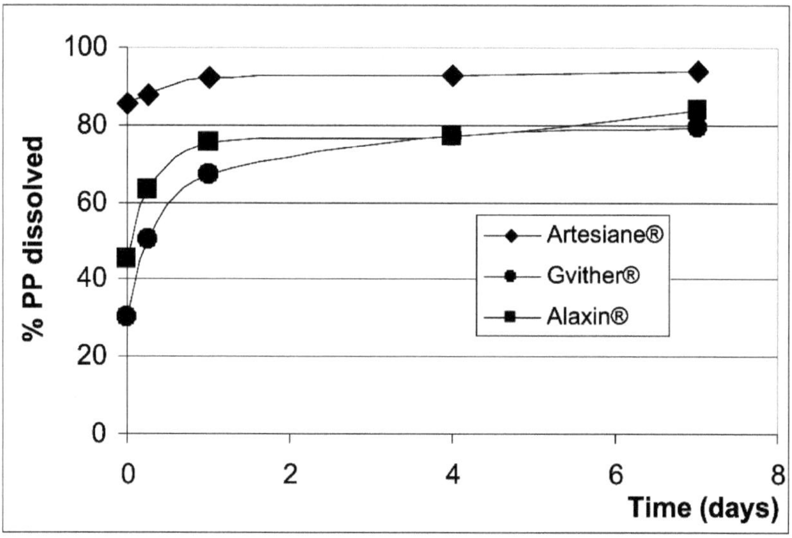

Figure 5. Dissolution profiles of propylparaben (PP).

Efficacy of Antimicrobial Preservation

A PET gives an indication of the antimicrobial activity of a preservative in a preparation. The preservative properties of the preparation were considered adequate if the conditions of the test, there was a significant fall or no increase in the number of microorganisms at the conditions tested. In the tested wet suspensions only two samples, Artenam® and Gvither® met the specific requirements of the European Pharmacopoeia of PET in the killing of the microorganisms. The other five products failed the test (Table 3). In the latter, different pathogen strains were observed with Santecxin® and Cotecxin® retaining the most species of microbes (≥4 out of 6 tested pathogens remained positive). Alaxin® and Artexin® were positive for two microbial species while Artesiane® was positive for one. In all samples, the fungus *Aspergillus niger* was the most positively tested microbe.

Table 3. Efficacy of antimicrobial preservation of the artemisinin-derivative reconstituted suspensions.

	pH Wet Suspension	Preservative	P. aeruginosa	S. aureus	E. coli	C. albicans	Z. rouxii	A. niger	Ph. Eur. Requirements
Artenam®	4.50	Sorbic acid	-	-	-	-	-	-	Conforms
Gvither®	4.30	MP/PP	-	-	-	-	-	-	Conforms
Artesiane®	5.43	MP/PP	-	-	-	-	-	+	Does not conform
Alaxin®	4.40	MP/PP	-	+	-	-	-	+	Does not conform
Artexin®	5.90	Benzoic acid	+	-	+	-	-	-	Does not conform
Santecxin®	5.55	Benzoic acid	+	-	+	+	+	+	Does not conform
Cotecxin®	not tested	Chlorbutanol?	-	-	+	+	+	+	Does not conform

pH of Reconstituted Suspensions

Since a suitable pH is inevitable for the proper functioning of the preservatives, the pH of each reconstituted suspension was measured. The pH ranged from 4.50 to 5.90 in all wet suspensions (Table 3). The pH of two suspensions (Santecxin® pH 5.55 and Artexin® pH 5.90) exceeded by far the pK_a of their preservative, benzoicacid (pK_a4.20). The pH of Artenam® wet suspension was 4.50(pK_a sorbic acid 4.76) while the pH of the Artesiane®, Alaxin®, and Gvither® formulations were respectively 5.43, 4.40, and 4.30(pK_a parabens 8.4).

CONCLUSION

The high number of failures of the artemisinin-derivatives dry suspensions with respect to their antimicrobial preservation suggests that the surveillance of the marketed drugs may be ineffective in Kenya.

Effective preservation of pediatric formulations developed in multi-dose containers is necessary, as it contributes to the microbiological stability of the suspension as well as safeguard patient infection due to the formulation. Especially for children, pediatric medicines requiring a water phase need strict control on the content and efficacy of both the active ingredient as well as the preservative prior to registration. Above all, monitoring should continue after the drugs are on the market.

KEYWORDS

- **Alaxin®**
- **Artemisinin**
- **Artesiane®**
- **Artexin®**
- **European pharmacopoeia**
- **Santecxin®**
- **UV spectrophotometry**

AUTHORS' CONTRIBUTIONS

Magnus A. Atemnkeng participated in the study design, analysis and interpretation of data and wrote the manuscript. Katelijne De Cock participated in the conception, experimental analysis of the study and revision of the manuscript. Jacqueline Plaizier-Vercammen participated in the overall supervision of the study and critically revised the content of the chapter.

ACKNOWLEDGMENTS

The Vlaamse Interuniversitaire Raad (VLIR-UOS), Belgium is acknowledged for financial support.

Chapter 6

Inhibition of Cell Growth and Invasion by Epidermal Growth Factor-targeted Phagemid Particles

Xiu-Mei Cai, Hai-Long Xie, Ming-Zhu Liu, and Xi-Liang Z.

INTRODUCTION

Previous studies demonstrated the EGF-targeted phagemid particles carrying small interfering RNA (siRNA) against Akt could be expressed efficiently in the presence of hydroxycamptothecin (HCPT). However, no significant cell growth inhibition was obtained. This study was to further investigate whether the EGF-targeted phagemid particles carrying siRNA would be a promising tool for anti-cancer siRNA delivery.

We found that pSi4.1-siFAK phagemid particles could significantly inhibit the expression of focal adhesion kinase (FAK) in the HCPT-treated cells. Moreover, we also observed that the particles could potently suppress cell growth and cell invasion.

These results indicated that EGF-targeted phagemid particles might be a promising tool for anti-cancer siRNA delivery in the presence of HCPT.

The siRNA molecules are capable of interrupting the translation of a specific protein by inducing post-transcriptional gene silencing. It is a promising method for silencing therapeutic target genes. A variety of delivery systems are proposed for the delivery of siRNA into cells *in vitro* and *in vivo*. Since phage-based vectors do not exhibit natural tropism towards mammalian cells and can be genetically modified for specific applications, modified phage-based vectors are an attractive alternative strategy for gene delivery. They have been successfully modified to deliver genes to target cells by the effective use of targeting ligands such as growth factors, antibodies, and viral capsid proteins (Burg et al., 2002; Giovine et al., 2001; Kassner et al., 1999; Larocca et al., 1998; Li et al., 2005; Poul and Marks, 1999). To increase the density of ligand display on the phages, an epidermal growth factor (EGF)-modified helper phage genome M13EGFKO7CT was established, which could produce EGF-targeted phagemid particles (Li et al., 2006). The phagemid particles could deliver reporter genes into target cells; however, the efficiency of delivery was limited (Li et al., 2006). A topoisomerase I inhibitor such as camptothecin or HCPT could substantially enhance the transduction of the phagemid gene delivery particles (Burg et al., 2002; Liang et al., 2006). The recent studies showed that the cell-targeted phagemid particles could efficiently deliver siRNA against Akt into cell in the presence of HCPT (Jiang et al., 2008). But, no significant growth inhibition was observed. Thus, to be an effective anti-cancer siRNA delivery vector, more studies should be performed, such as carrying siRNA against other oncogenes.

The FAK, a non-receptor tyrosine kinase, has been implicated in several cellular processes such as proliferation, apoptosis, motility, and invasion. Increased expression of FAK has been found in various malignant tumors, including tumors derived from the lungs, breasts, head and neck, and ovaries (Carelli et al., 2006; Oktay et al., 2003; Kornberg, 1998; Sood, 2005). Therefore, FAK is recognized as an important therapeutic target in the treatment of cancer. Delivery of siFAK by lipofectamine could significantly block the expression of FAK and trigger cell death and block cell migration (Han et al., 2004). But, the siFAK could not be delivered to target cells. To further investigate whether the EGF-targeted phagemid particles in combination with RNA interference (RNAi) would represent an effective therapeutic approach, we used phagemid particles carrying siRNA against FAK to infect H1299 cells and examined the therapeutic potential of this approach.

MATERIALS AND METHODS

Reagents

Dulbecco's Modified Eagle's Medium (DMEM), Dulbecco's phosphate-buffered saline and fetal bovine serum (FBS) were obtained from *Invitrogen* (Grand Island, USA). Restriction endonucleases were obtained from TaKaRa Biotechnology (Dalian, China).

Cell Culture

The H1299 (human lung carcinomas) cells and U87 (human glioblastoma) cells were cultured at 37°C in DMEM containing 10% FBS in a humidified atmosphere containing 5% CO_2.

Plasmid Construction

The modified pSilencer4.1 plasmid was obtained from Dr. Z. Li (Shanghai Jiao Tong University, Shanghai, China). FAK siRNA (target sequence, 5'-GAACCTCGCAGTCATTTAT-3') has been proven to be effective for inhibiting FAK (Mitra et al., 2006). A 59-nt oligo-DNA duplex (5'-AGCTTGAACCTCGCAGTCATTTATTTCAAGAGAATAAATGACTGCGAG GTTCTTTTTTG-3'/5'-GATCCAAAAAAGAACCTCGCAGTCATTTATTCTCTTG AAATAAATGACTGCGAGGTTCA-3') was inserted into the pSilencer4.1 vector digested with BamHI and HindIII. The mock siRNA sequence is 5'-GTCTCCGAACGTGTCACGT-3' (Mitra et al., 2006). Another 59-nt oligo-DNA duplex (5'-AGCTTGTCTCCGAACGTGTCACGTTTCAAGAGAACGTGACACGTTCGGAGACTTTTTTG-3'/5'-GATCCAAAAAAGTCTCCGAACGTGTCACGTTCTCTTGAAACGTGACACGTTCGGAGACA-3') was inserted into the modified pSilencer4.1 vector digested with BamHI and HindIII.

Preparation of Phagemid Particles

Briefly, M13KO7EGFCT was transformed into *Escherichia coli* to create LMP cells (Li et al., 2006). The phagemid carrying siFAK was transformed into the LMP cells. The cells were then plated on Luria-Bertani (LB) agar containing 70 μg/ml kanamycin and 50 μg/ml ampicillin and incubated at 37°C overnight. A cell clone was picked up and transferred into 1 l of LB solution containing 70 µg/ml kanamycin and 50 µg/ml ampicillin. After shaking at 37°C for 15 hr, the supernatant of the culture was collected and the phagemid particles were purified with polyethylene glycol (PEG)/NaCl precipitation. Then, they were quantified by ELISA as previously described (Rondot et al., 2001).

Purification of Single-stranded DNA from Phagemid Particles

Single-stranded DNA (ssDNA) was extracted from the phagemid particles by using the Ph.D.-12 phage display peptide library kit (New England Biolabs, USA) according to the manufacturer's protocol. Briefly, the phagemid particles were precipitated by PEG/NaCl. The pellet was then suspended in iodide buffer. Ethanol (250 ml in total) was added to the buffer, and the pellet was incubated in it for 10 min. The pellet was collected after centrifugation at 12,000 g for 10 min. It was finally dissolved in 30 µl Tris-EDTA (TE) buffer (10 mM Tris-HCl (pH 8.0) and 1 mM EDTA) and analyzed by agarose gel electrophoresis.

Immunocytochemistry

Monolayer cells were grown on glass cover slips and fixed with 4% paraformaldehyde. Endogenous peroxidase activity was quenched with 2% hydrogen peroxide in methanol for 45 min. After the cells were blocked with 5% normal serum for 30 min, they were incubated with primary antibodies to the epidermal growth factor receptor (EGFR) (Cell Signaling Technology, MA) diluted to 1:500 in phosphate-buffered saline (PBS) for 1 hr at room temperature. Then, the cells were rinsed and incubated with horseradish peroxidase (HRP)-conjugated secondary antibodies (Watson Biotech, China) diluted to 1:500 in PBS for 1.5 hr at room temperature. The reaction was developed with diaminobenzidine (Dako, Japan), and then the slides were counterstained with Mayer's hematoxylin. After a final wash, the slides were mounted and the cells were examined using an Olympus photomicroscope (400× magnification).

In Vitro Phagemid Particle Transfection

The cells were plated onto 24-well plates at a density of 10,000 cells per well 24 hr prior to the addition of phage particles. The phages were added at 1,011 pfu/ml and incubated with the cells for 48 hr at 37°C in complete media. Then, the medium was removed and the cells were incubated in fresh medium containing 2.5 µM HCPT for 6 hr at 37°C. Following this, the medium was replaced with fresh medium, and the cells were incubated for 18 hr at 37°C. All the transfections were performed in triplicate at least two times.

Western Blot Analysis

In total, 10_6 H1299 cells transfected with a variety of phagemid particles were lysed after the HCPT treatment. The cells were washed with PBS and lysed in a buffer containing 50 mM Tris (pH 7.5), 5 mM EDTA, 300 mM NaCl, 0.1% Igepal, 0.5 mM NaF, 0.5 mM Na_3VO_4, 0.5 mM phenylmethylsulfonyl fluoride, and an antiprotease mixture. Equal amounts of protein were loaded on a SDS-PAGE and transferred onto a nitrocellulose membrane. They were incubated with specific primary antibodies and then with

HRP-conjugated secondary antibodies. Proteins were visualized by fluorography using an enhanced chemiluminescence system (Pierce Biotechnologies, USA). The anti-FAK antibody (Santa Cruz, CA) was used in 1:1,000 dilutions. The monoclonal antibody to GAPDH was purchased from Kang-Chen Biotech (Shanghai, China). The secondary antibody conjugated with HRP was purchased from Watson Biotech (Shanghai, China).

MTT Assay

After the HCPT treatment, H1299 cells transfected with a variety of phagemid particles were seeded onto a 96-well plate overnight in DMEM containing 10% FBS, and then grown for 0, 24, 48, and 72 hr. Methyl thiazolyl tetrazolium (MTT) (20 μl) solution (5 mg/ml in PBS) was added to each well and incubated for 5 hr at 37°C. The solution was removed and 200 μl of dimethylsulfoxide (DMSO) was added to each well. These plates were vibrated gently for 10 min; they then underwent detection in the universal microplate reader at 490 nm.

Colony-forming Ability Assay

The efficiency of colony formation was assayed in 35-mm dishes prepared with a lower layer of 0.8% agar (GIBCO/BRL) overlaid with 0.3% agar containing 2×10^4 suspended cells. After 5 days, growth was estimated under a Nikon inverted phase-contrast microscope, and individual colonies of more than 50 cells were counted (Zhou et al., 2000).

Transwell Invasion Assay

Polymerized gels were prepared by neutralization of extracellular matrix (ECM) gel (Sigma, USA) with cold DMEM. Cells in DMEM with 0.5% bovine serum albumin (BSA) were plated on the gel, and DMEM with 0.5% BSA and 0.5% FBS was added to the bottom of the chambers. Photographs were taken 36 hr later to capture the cells that had invaded below the gel surface. The number of invading cells in five fields was counted under a 200× magnification. Each value represents the average of three individual experiments, and the error bars represent SD. The p-values were calculated by the ANOVA test in SAS8.2 (Cai et al., 2005).

RESULTS AND DISCUSSION

Studies showed that the cell-targeted phagemid particles were efficient siRNA delivery vectors in the presence of HCPT and they could efficiently deliver siRNA against Akt into targeted cells in the presence of HCPT (Jiang et al., 2008). But, no significant growth inhibition was observed. Thus, to be an effective anti-cancer siRNA delivery vector, more studies should be performed, such as carrying siRNA against other oncogenes. In this study, we made phagemid particles carrying siRNA against FAK to infect H1299 cells and examined the therapeutic potential of this approach. First, the short hairpin RNA (shRNA) against FAK was subcloned into pSi4.1CMV-f1, thus forming pSilencer4.1-siFAK (pSi4.1-siFAK) (Figure 1A). Then, we purified ssDNA from phagemid particles to analyze the ratio of phagemids to helper phage genomes packaged in the phagemid particles. The results indicated that almost all the DNA packaged comprised phagemids (Figure 1B). Previously, the modified helper phage genome (plasmid) M13EGFKO7CT was created to produce EGF-targeted phagemid particles (Jiang et al., 2008; Li et al., 2006). The M13EGFKO7CT plasmid was used to package pSi4.1-siFAK phagemid particles, following which the phagemid particles displayed the EGF ligand. In the immunocytochemical assay, we found that H1299 cells showed a strong positive EGFR immunoreactivity, while very light immunostaining was observed in the U87 cells that were used as negative controls (Figure 2A). Therefore, we infected H1299 cells with pSi4.1-siFAK phagemid particles. Western blotting assay showed that the pSi4.1-siFAK plasmid transfected by lipofectamine could significantly block the expression of FAK. This was not observed in cells transduced with pSi4.1-siFAK phagemid particles without HCPT treatment. Surprisingly, in HCPT treated-cells, the pSi4.1-siFAK phagemid particles could inhibit FAK expression to a great extent. Inhibition of FAK expression was not found in the cells infected with mock phagemid particles (Figure 2B). Taken together, the vectors could deliver siRNA to human carcinoma cells efficiently in the presence of HCPT. The HCPT had been shown to increase the efficiency of transduction of the phagemid vectors (Burg et al., 2002; Chen et al., 1998; Liang et al. 2006). However, the mechanism by which HCPT increased transgene expression was not fully understood (Burg et al., 2002; Liang et al., 2006). It was thought to involve the activation of the host cell repair machinery in response to DNA damage (Burg et al., 2002; Chen et al., 1998; Qing et al., 1997); however, further studies are required to confirm this.

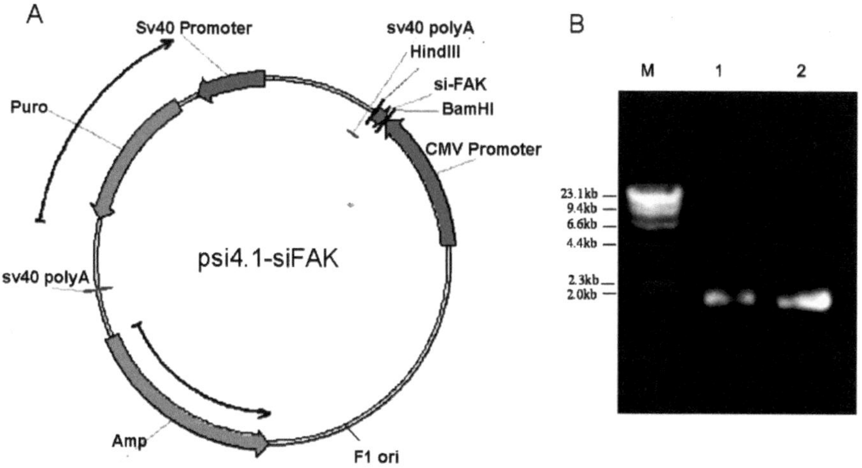

Figure 1. The map of pSi4.1-siFAK phagemid particle and analysis of the ssDNA released from phagemid particles. (A) The pSi4.1-siFAK phagemid particle was constructed as follows: the shRNA against FAK was inserted into the modified pSilencer4.1 vector digested with BamHI and HindIII. (B) The ssDNA was purified from phagemid particles to analyze the ratio of phagemids to helper phage genomes packaged in the phagemid particles. The results indicated that almost all the DNA packaged comprised phagemids. Lane M: λ DNA/HindIII; Lane 1: pSi4.1-siFAK phagemid particles; Lane 2: pSi4.1-simock phagemid particles.

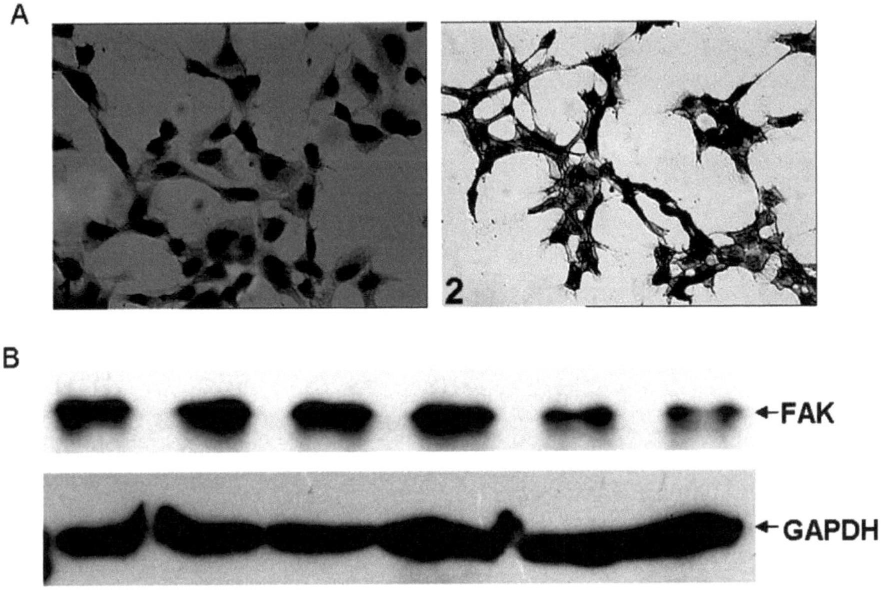

Figure 2. Immunocytochemistry assay of EGFR expression and Western blot analysis of the specific FAK gene silencing by EGF-targeted phagemid particles mediated RNA interference. (A) In the immunocytochemical assay, H1299 cells showed a strong positive EGFR immunoreactivity, while very light immunostaining was observed in the U87 cells that were used as negative controls. 1, H1299; 2, U87. (B) The H1299 cells were infected with pSi4.1-siFAK phagemid particles. In HCPT treated-cells, the pSi4.1-siFAK phagemid particles could inhibit FAK expression to a great extent. 1, H1299; 2, H1299 infected with pSi4.1-simock phagemid particles; 3, H1299 infected with pSi4.1-simock phagemid particles in the presence of 2.5 μM HCPT; 4, H1299 infected with pSi4.1-siFAK phagemid particles; 5, H1299 infected with pSi4.1-siFAK phagemid particles in the presence of 2.5 μM HCPT; 6, H1299 transfected with pSi4.1-siFAK using Lipofectamine 2000.

A series of experiments were performed to determine whether the pSi4.1-siFAK phagemid particles could arrest H1299 cell growth. Cell growth was monitored by the MTT assay, and it was observed that all the cells grew at a similar rate at 0 and 24 hr. However, a great difference began to appear at 48 and 72 hr. In the presence of HCPT, the inhibitory rates were approximately 12–19% in parent and mock cells, compared with parent cells without HCPT. Amazingly, the inhibitory rates reached approximately 52–61% in HCPT-treated cells infected with pSi4.1-siFAK phagemid particles, compared with the control cells. No significant growth inhibition was found in the cells infected with the mock vector or pSi4.1-siFAK phagemid particles in the absence of HCPT (Figure 3A). In addition, we examined the growth arrest of the pSi4.1-siFAK phagemid particles at the 3-dimensional level. In the colony-forming ability assay, the number of colonies of pSi4.1-siFAK phagemid particles decreased by almost 54% in the presence of HCPT, compared with the control cells. In contrast, cells in other groups exhibited little change in the number of colonies (Figure 3B). These data suggested that the treatment of pSi4.1-siFAK phagemid particles could dramatically reduce cell viability in the presence of HCPT.

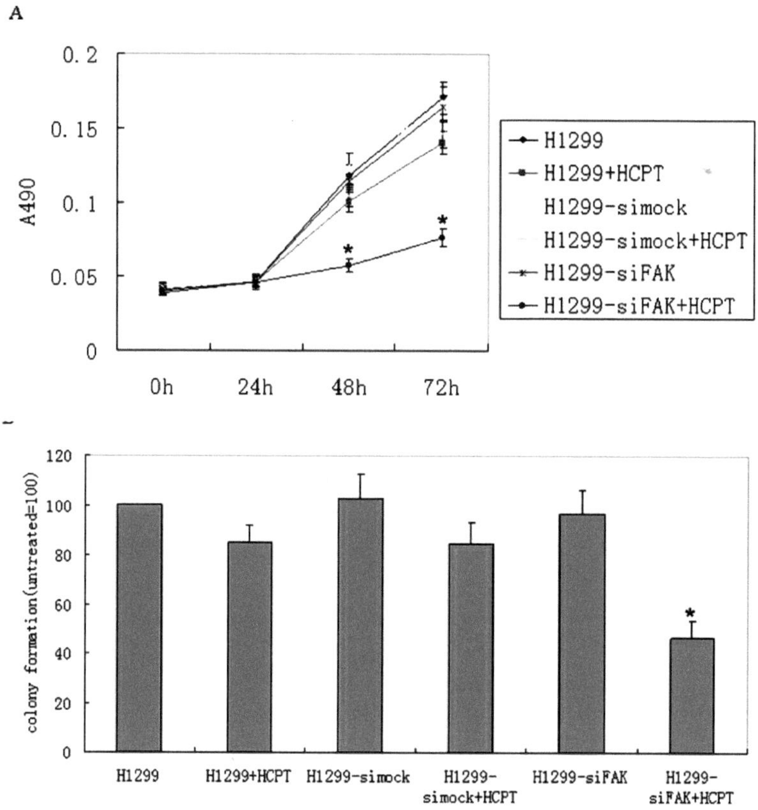

Figure 3. Phagemid particles of pSi4.1-siFAK could inhibit H1299 cell growth. (A) The MTT assay. (B) Colony-forming Ability Assay. The results shown were representative of at least three independent experiments. The HCPT-treated cells that were infected with pSi4.1-siFAK phagemid particles exhibited a significant inhibition of proliferation (*, $p < 0.01$) compared with H1299 cells.

Furthermore, we quantified the effect of pSi4.1-siFAK phagemid particles on cell invasion. In the transwell invasion assay, the number of pSi4.1-siFAK phagemid particles transduced-cells (HCPT treatment) invading through the membrane coated with ECM gel was less than that of the control cells (Figure 4A). The cell invasion was markedly reduced by approximately 50% in pSi4.1-siFAK phagemid particles transduced-cells (HCPT treatment), compared with the control cells; the other groups however showed no obvious change (Figure 4B). Thus, the above data indicated that the transfection of H1299 cells with pSi4.1-siFAK phagemid particles and the HCPT treatment could dramatically inhibit cell invasion.

The RNAi has revolutionized the biological sciences because it can selectively silence messenger RNA (mRNA) expression. However, the delivery of this RNA into target cells represents the main barrier for using siRNA as a novel drug against tumor targets. Since filamentous phages only showed tropism for cells that expressed the appropriate receptors, this tropism could be conferred to phage particles by the expression of a targeting ligand on the phage coat (Kassner et al., 1999; Larocca et al., 1999; Poul and Marks, 1999). Therefore, phages would be an attractive alternative strategy for siRNA delivery. This study demonstrated that EGF-targeted phagemid particles in combination with RNAi and the HCPT treatment represent a new therapeutic approach for silencing oncogenes. However, in order to act as a cancer gene-delivery vector, phage vectors should display other targeting ligands to increase their specificity for different types of tumors.

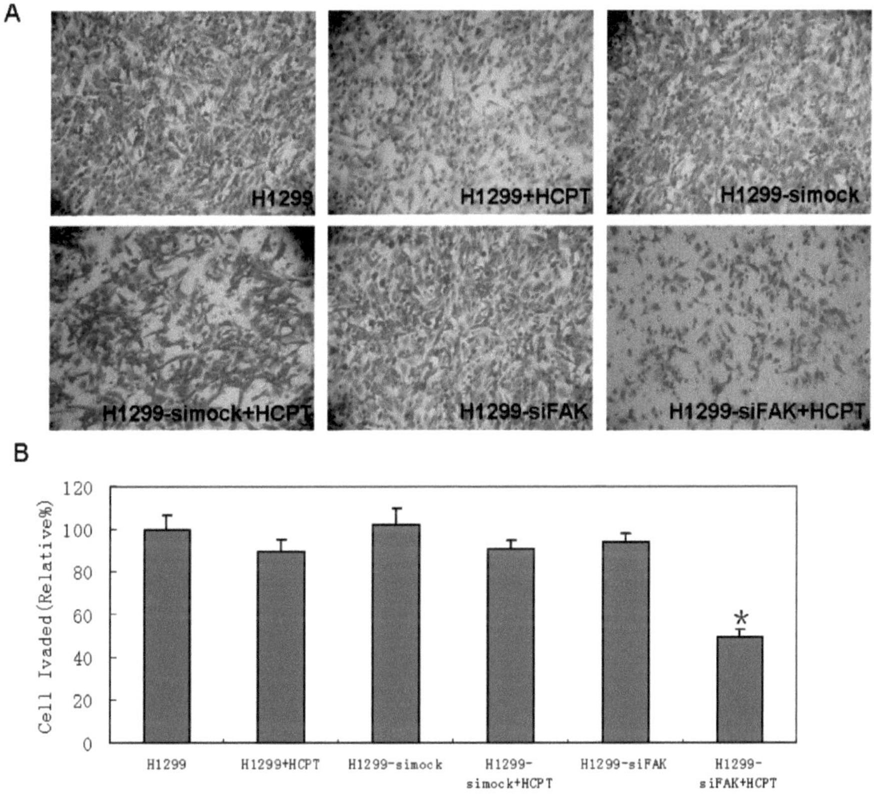

Figure 4. Phagemid particles of pSi4.1-siFAK could inhibit H1299 cell invasion. (A) Cells that invaded after 36 hr through ECM-Gel-coated transwell inserts were stained with crystal violet stain. (B) Cell invasion assay. The HCPT-treated cells that were infected with pSi4.1-siFAK phagemid particles exhibited a significant inhibition of invasion (*, $p < 0.01$) compared with H1299 cells.

CONCLUSION

Therefore, phages would be an attractive alternative strategy for siRNA delivery. This study demonstrated that EGF-targeted phagemid particles in combination with RNAi and the HCPT treatment represent a new therapeutic approach for silencing oncogenes. However, in order to act as a cancer gene-delivery vector, phage vectors should display other targeting ligands to increase their specificity for different types of tumors.

KEYWORDS

- **Epidermal growth factor**
- **Focal adhesion kinase**
- **Hydroxycamptothecin**
- **Phagemid particles**
- **Therapeutic target genes**

AUTHORS' CONTRIBUTIONS

Xiu-Mei Cai carried out the molecular genetic studies, participated in the preparation of phagemid particles and drafted the manuscript. Hai-Long Xie carried out the immunoassays and performed the statistical analysis. Ming-Zhu Liu participated in transwell invasion assay. Xi-Liang Z conceived of the study, and participated in its design and coordination and helped to draft the manuscript. All authors read and approved the final manuscript.

ACKNOWLEDGMENTS

The authors thank Dr. Li ZH for his gifts of plasmids. The project is supported by the National Natural Science Foundation of China (No. 30600336) and Shanghai Leading Academic Discipline Project, Project Number: B110.

Chapter 7

PET-PLA/Drug Nanoparticles Synthesis for Controlled Drug Release

K. Sathish Kumar, V. Selvaraj, and M. Alagar

INTRODUCTION

Polyethylene terephthalate-polylactic acid copolymer (PET-PLA) was synthesized from bis (2-hydroxyethyl terephthalate) and L-lactic acid oligomer in the presence of manganese antimony glycoxide as a catalyst. The synthesized PET-PLA copolymer was used for controlled drug release systems with gold nanoparticles. Fluorouracil containing PET-PLA nanocapsules was prepared in the presence of gold nanoparticles by solvent evaporation method. The morphologies of the nanocapsules were characterized using scanning electron microscopy and transmission electron microscopy. Controlled release of Fu and Fu@Au was carried out in 0.1 M phosphate buffer (pH 7.4) and 0.1 M HCl solution. The results indicated that the drug release for gold nanoparticles/fluorouracil (Au@Fu) incorporated PET-PLA nanocapsules was controlled and slow compared to Fu incorporated PET-PLA nanocapsules. This may be due to the interaction between the gold nanoparticles and fluorouracil in PET-PLA nanocapsules.

Nanotechnology provides a novel route for many biomedical applications especially in the case of incurable diseases such as cancer, diabetes, and so forth. Cancer can affect just every organ in human body. The various treatments of cancer are chemotherapy, radiation therapy, surgery, biological therapy, hormone, and gene therapies. Chemotherapy uses chemical agents (anticancer or cytotoxic drugs) to interact with cancer cells to eradicate or control the growth of cancer. Depending on the type of cancer and kind of drug used, chemotherapy drugs may be administered differently. The 5-Fluorouracil (5-Fu) is one of the oldest chemotherapy drugs and has been used for decades. It is an active medicine against many cancers. Over the past 20 years, increased understanding of the mechanism of action of 5-Fu has led to the development of strategies that increase its anticancer activity. The 5-Fu is given for treatment of cancers like bowel, breast, stomach, and gullet cancer (Bruijn et al., 1989). However, anticancer drugs normally attack both normal cells and cancerous cells when the drug was given as an injection or tablet form for a long time. In order to overcome this side effect, targeting the drug delivery and sustained release of drugs are required. Many research investigations are focused in the preparation of drug encapsulated polymer nanoparticles for the controlled release applications. Biodegradable polymers have become increasingly important in the development of drug delivery systems (Eldrige et al., 1991; O'Hagan et al., 1993; Salhi et al., 2004; Uchida et al., 1994). There are several methods that can be used to make microcapsules (Lai et al., 2006) from biodegradable polymers. Polyethylene terephthalate (PET) is a semicrystalline polymer with high mechanical strength and an excellent thermal stability. Copolyesters such as PET-PLA are biodegradable materials used for tissue engineering, bone reconstruction, and controlled drug delivery systems (van Nostrum et al., 2004; Yuan et al., 2002, 2003). Further gold nanoparticles play an important role in cancer therapy to detect or to deliver the drug to the cancerous cell without affecting the normal cells and have good ability to form complex with many drugs through chemical bonding. Nanoparticles have uniform shape and size and are soluble in an aqueous medium. With this view in mind, the present work is undertaken to synthesize PET-PLA copolyester and the preparation of PET-PLA/Fu and PET-PLA/Fu-Au nanocapsules to study their drug release behavior. A comparative study of sustained release of 5-Fu under different pH conditions was also carried out. The present work is the continuation of our previous work with gold nanoparticles (Selvaraj and Alagar, 2007; Selvaraj et al., 2006).

MATERIAL AND METHODS

Synthesis of PET-PLA Copolyester

The bis (2-hydroxy ethyl terephthalate) and L-lactic acid oligomers (30/70) wt% were reacted in the presence of 10 mg of manganese antimony glycoxide catalyst (Kennay, 1978). The reaction mixture was placed (Olewnik et al., 2007) in a 500 ml flask connected to a vacuum line (0.4 kPa) and immersed in an oil bath at 180°C for 6 hr. As the reactants were stirred, glycol and water were slowly distilled out. The copolyesters were dissolved in chloroform, precipitated in methanol, filtered and dried at 70°C. This was used without further purification.

Preparation of Citrate-capped Gold Nanoparticles

Trisodium citrate (38.8 mM, 50 cm^3) was added to a boiling $HAuCl_4$ solution (1 mM, 500cm^3). As a result, the previously yellow solution of gold chloride turned to wine red color and gave a characteristic absorbance at 518 nm in the UV-vis spectrum.

Preparation of Nanocapsules

Nanocapsules were prepared by the solvent evaporation method similar to that reported previously by Beck et al. (1979). For PET/PLA/5Fu-Au experiment, 5-Fu (50 mg) was added in 0.5 ml nanogold aqueous suspension (with a 30-min shaking under ultrasound to help the adsorption of 5-Fu on gold nanoparticles) and this solution was added to an organic polymer solution (300 mg PET-PLA + 5 ml CH_2Cl_2) under stirring condition. This was continued until the organic solvent was completely evaporated. The suspension became clear after all the nanocapsules precipitated out of the solution. These nanocapsules were collected by filtration and washed with deionized water to remove any undesirable residuals. Finally, the clean nanocapsules were dried in a vacuum oven at 40°C for 24 hr to ensure a complete removal of the organic solvent and deionized water. All the nanocapsules were stored in a desiccator at 25°C. The PET PLA/Fu nanocapsules were also prepared under similar conditions.

Encapsulation efficiency (%) = ((Mass of drug added during Nanoparticle (NP) preparation−Mass of free drug in supernatant)/Mass of Drug added during NP preparation) × 100.

Drug loading (%) = (Mass of 5-Fluouracil in NP/Mass of NP recovered) × 100.

DISCUSSION AND RESULTS

UV-vis Characterization

Figure 1 shows the UV-visible spectrum of citrate stabilized gold nanoparticles. The plasmon band observed for the wine red colloidal gold at 518 nm is characteristic of the gold nanoparticles. The pure drug shows a maximum at 273 nm, but with the addition of 5-Fu to colloidal gold, both the bands at 273 and 518 nm pertaining to pure drug and Au colloids decrease in intensity steadily with time.

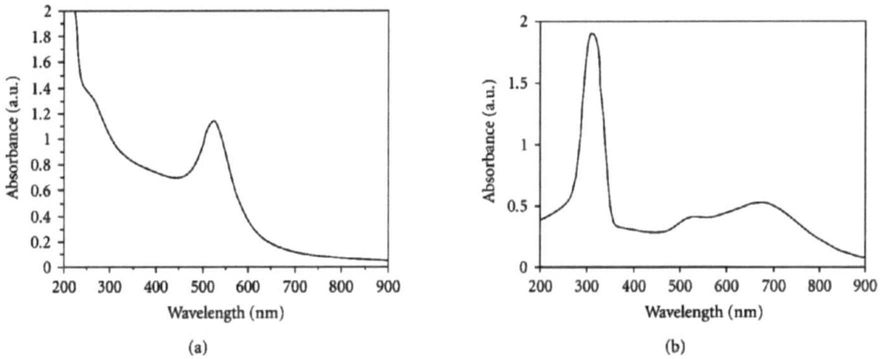

Figure 1. (a) and (b) show the UV-spectrum of Au nanoparticles and Fu@Au nanoparticles.

This decrease is accompanied by the emergence of an additional peak at 650 nm (Figure 1b), that is, a change from wine red to blue with the addition of drug to colloidal gold. The appearance of the new peak is due to the aggregation of gold nanoparticles and the replacement of citrate by 5-Fu, leading to the formation of gold-drug complex. Citrate ions are readily replaced by the –NH ligand on the surface of gold nanoparticles. This ligand exchange reaction provides an important means for the chemical functionalization of the nanoparticles and greatly extends the versatility of these systems.

Morphological Characterization

The PET-PLA/5-Fu-Au and PET-PLA/5-Fu nanocapsules were easily distinguished from PET-PLA/5-Fu nanocapsules by their color. While the color of PET-PLA/5-Fu nanocapsules was white, PET-PLA/5-Fu-Au nanocapsules was purple/blue in color, due to the presence of the gold nanoparticles.

From the TEM (Figures 2a, b) measurements, the average diameters of the gold nanoparticles were found to be in the range of 18–20 nm.

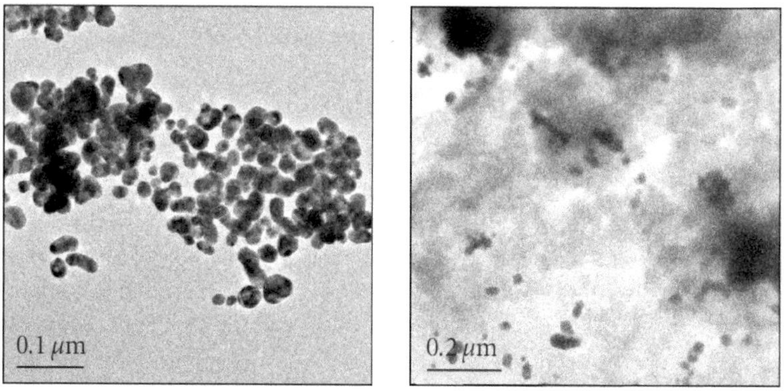

(a) (b)

Figure 2. The TEM images of (a) Au@Fu, and (b) Au-Fu/PET-PLA nanoparticles.

Morphology of nanocapsules (PET-PLA/5-Fu and PET-PLA/5-Fu-Au) prepared was characterized by the SEM analysis (Figures 3a, b).

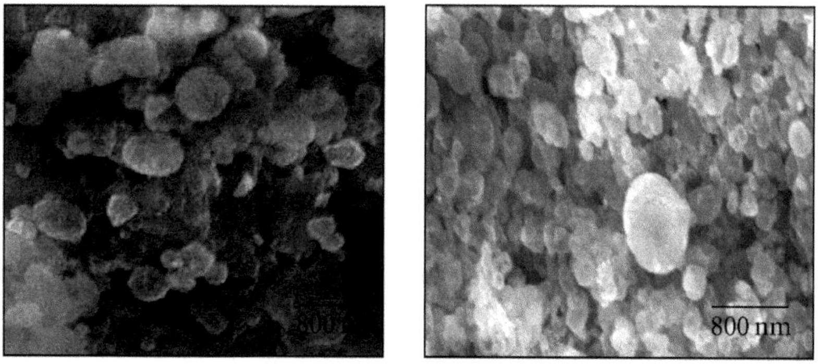

(a) (b)

Figure 3. The SEM images of (a) Fu/PLA-PET nanoparticles, and (b) Fu-Au/PET-PLA nanoparticles.

From the SEM measurements, the size of nanocapsules was found to be in the range of 230–260 nm. The average sizes of the microcapsules to nanocapsules can be prepared by changing the rotational speed from 2,000 to 12,000 rpm.

The average size decreased with an increase in the rotational speed, because of the higher shear stress. However, since the size difference was within the limits of statistical error, this statement remained speculative without further investigations. The surface topography of PET-PLA/5-Fu and PET-PLA/5-Fu-Au nanocapsules was smooth as seen in SEM photographs. The SEM micrographs manifested that nanocapsules prepared in the present study possess a nearly spherical shape.

Encapsulation Efficiency

The encapsulations of PET-PLA/5-Fu-Au and PET-PLA/5-Fu nanocapsules were obtained both in the presence and in the absence of gold nanoparticles. For PET-PLA/5-Fu-Au nanocapsules, the adsorption of 5-Fu on Au led to a larger particle (Fu-Au complex) size and made the diffusion of 5-Fu to the external solution less efficient. Gold nanoparticles also hindered the diffusion of 5-Fu to the external solution because of their insolubility in water and methylene chloride. In addition, each gold nanoparticle was composed of many Au atoms and would absorb more than one 5-Fu molecules. As a result, PET-PLA/5-Fu-Au nanocapsules had a higher encapsulation efficiency (70.21%) and a larger average size than PET-PLA/5-Fu nanocapsules (42.56%). The amount of 5-Fu entrapped within NP was determined by measuring the amount of nonentrapped drug in the supernatant recovered after centrifugation and washing of the nanoparticles, using a UV-visible spectrophotometer (Pignatello et al., 2001).

However, PET-PLA/5-Fu-Au nanocapsules had a higher drug loading (4.63%) than PET-PLA/5-Fu nanocapsules (2.46%).

Drug Release Study

The release profiles of 5-Fu from PET-PLA/5-Fu and PET-PLA/5-Fu-Au nanocapsules in the hydrochloric acid (0.1M) and the phosphate buffered saline (pH 7.4) at 37 ± 0.1°C are shown in Figure 4. Desorption profiles were obtained as follows. The 0.03 g of drug encapsulated polymer nanoparticles was mixed with 10 ml of phosphate buffer solution (pH 7.4) in five fractions. Each fraction was centrifuged as a function of time. The absorbance of each solution was monitored at different times. One sample solution was used only once to ensure that there was no change in the concentration of the solution.

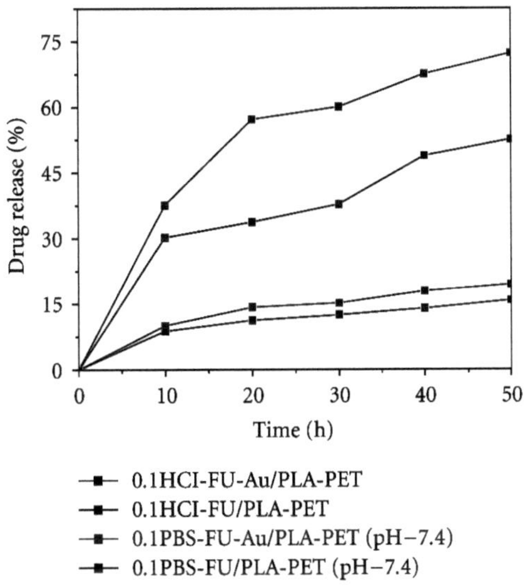

Figure 4. The controlled drug release of Fu@Au in 0.1 M HCl, and 0.1 M PBS.

The intensity of absorption was plotted against time which gave the desorption profile of fluorouracil. In the present study, fluorouracil encapsulated PET-PLA in the presence of gold nanoparticles was used for controlled drug release. In order to find the drug loading, a standard graph was drawn using known concentration of the drug. Figure 4 shows the drug release at different intervals of time using phosphate buffer solution at pH 7.4. The same procedure has been repeated for the drug encapsulated with gold nanoparticles. From Figure 4, it was understood that the drug release was slow and sustained. The release rate of 5-Fu for PET-PLA/5-Fu-Au nanocapsules was slower than that of PET-PLA/5-Fu nanocapsules in the two different dissolution media. The PET-PLA/5-Fu-Au nanocapsules had a slower release behavior mainly because gold nanoparticle in nanocapsules hindered the diffusion of 5-Fu away from the nanocapsules. An initial burst effect (i.e., the rapid release of 5-Fluorouracil) of PET-PLA/5-Fu nanocapsules was observed as shown in Figure 4.

The effect of gold nanoparticles on the release rate was particularly important because the release rates of 5-Fu for PET-PLA/5-Fu nanocapsules were higher than that of PET-PLA/5-Fu-Au nanocapsules in two different dissolution media. Further, the release rates of 5-Fu from PET-PLA/5-Fu and PET-PLA/5-Fu-Au nanocapsules were relatively higher in 7.4 PBS (0.1 M) than in pH 0.1 M HCl. This observation was attributed to the fact that the dissolution medium had a strong influence on the solubility of the drug, and the solubility of 5-Fu in pH 7.4 PBS was higher than that in 0.1 M HCl at the same temperature.

CONCLUSION

The binding of fluorouracil to colloidal gold and encapsulation of Fu to polymer nanoparticles were studied using different analytical techniques. The aggregations of gold nanoparticles were ascertained using UV-visible spectroscopy and TEM analysis. Further, it was observed that the drug release was slow and sustained in the case of PLA-PET/Au-Fu compared to that of PLA-PET/Fu nanoparticles due to the interaction between the drug and gold nanoparticles. The combination of gold and polymer with Fu results in a more potent complex compared to the individual parts, since such a complex can release the drug at controlled rate as well as at the targeted places.

KEYWORDS

- **Nanocapsules**
- **Nanoparticle**
- **Polyethylene terephthalate-polylactic acid copolymer**
- **UV-visible spectroscopy**

Chapter 8

Nanotechnology Approaches to Crossing the Blood-Brain Barrier and Drug Delivery to the CNS

Gabriel A. Silva

INTRODUCTION

Nanotechnologies are materials and devices that have a functional organization in at least one dimension on the nanometer (nm) (one billionth of a meter) scale, ranging from a few to about 100 nm. Nanoengineered materials and devices aimed at biologic applications and medicine in general, and neuroscience in particular, are designed fundamentally to interface and interact with cells and their tissues at the molecular level. One particularly important area of nanotechnology application to the central nervous system (CNS) is the development of technologies and approaches for delivering drugs and other small molecules such as genes, oligonucleotides, and contrast agents across the blood-brain barrier (BBB). The BBB protects and isolates CNS structures (i.e., the brain and spinal cord) from the rest of the body, and creates a unique biochemical and immunological environment. Clinically, there are a number of scenarios where drugs or other small molecules need to gain access to the CNS following systemic administration, which necessitates being able to cross the BBB. Nanotechnologies can potentially be designed to carry out multiple specific functions at once or in a predefined sequence, an important requirement for the clinically successful delivery and use of drugs and other molecules to the CNS, and as such have a unique advantage over other complimentary technologies and methods. This brief review introduces emerging work in this area and summarizes a number of example applications to CNS cancers, gene therapy, and analgesia.

Nanotechnologies are materials and devices that have a functional organization in at least one dimension on the nanometer (one billionth of a meter) scale, ranging from a few to about 100 nm. Nanoengineered materials and devices aimed at biologic applications and medicine in general, and neuroscience in particular, are designed fundamentally to interface and interact with cells and their tissues at the molecular level. The potential of nanotechnological applications to biology and medicine arise from the fact that they exhibit bulk mesoscale and macroscale chemical and/or physical properties that are unique to the engineered material or device and not necessarily possessed by the molecules alone. This supports the development of nanotechnologies that can potentially carry out multiple specific functions at once or in a predefined sequence, which is an important property for the clinically successful delivery of drugs and other molecules to the CNS.

An ability to cross the BBB to deliver drugs or other molecules (e.g., oligonucleotides, genes, or contrast agents) while potentially targeting a specific group of cells (for instance, a tumor) requires a number of things to happen together. Ideally, a nanodelivery-drug complex would be administered systemically (e.g., intravenously) but would find the CNS while producing minimal systemic effects, be able to cross the BBB and correctly target cells in the CNS, and then carry out its primary active function, such as releasing a drug. These technically demanding obstacles and challenges will require multidisciplinary solutions between different fields, including engineering, chemistry, cell biology, physiology, pharmacology, and medicine. Successfully doing so will greatly benefit the patient. Although this ideal scenario has not yet been realized, a considerable body of work has been done to develop nanotechnological delivery strategies for crossing the BBB.

MATERIALS AND METHODS

Applications to Drugs and Other Molecules

A significant amount of work using nanotechnological approaches to crossing the BBB has focused on the delivery of antineoplastic drugs to CNS tumors. For example, radiolabeled polyethylene glycol (PEG)-coated hexadecylcyanoarcylate nanospheres have been tested for their ability to target and accumulate in a rat model of gliosarcoma (Brigger et al., 2002). Another group has encapsulated the antineoplasitc drug paclitaxel in polylactic co-glycolic acid nanoparticles, with impressive results. *In vitro* experiments with 29 different cancer cell lines (including both neural and non-neural cell lines) demonstrated targeted cytotoxicity 13 times greater than with drug alone (Feng et al., 2004). Using a variety of physical and chemical characterization methods, including different forms of spectroscopy and atomic force microscopy, the investigators showed that the drug was taken up by the nanoparticles with very high encapsulation efficiencies and that the release kinetics could be carefully controlled. Research focusing on the delivery of many of the commonly used antineoplastic drugs is important because most of these drugs have poor solubility under physiologic conditions and require less than optimal vehicles, which can produce significant side effects.

In another example, various compounds—including neuropeptides such as enkephalins, the N-methyl-D-aspartate receptor antagonist MRZ 2/576, and the chemotherapeutic drug doxorubicin—have been attached to the surface of poly(butylcyanoacrylate) nanoparticles coated with polysorbate 80 (Alyautdin et al., 1997, 1998; Friese et al., 2000; Gulyaev et al., 1999; Kreuter et al., 1995). The polysorbate on the surface of the nanoparticles adsorb apolipoproteins B and E and are taken up by brain capillary endothelial cells via receptor-mediated endocytosis. Nanoparticle-mediated delivery of doxorubicin is being explored in a rodent model of glioblastoma (Alyautdin et al., 1997, 1998; Friese et al., 2000; Gulyaev et al., 1999; Kreuter et al., 1995; Steiniger et al., 2004). Importantly, recent work in a rat glioblastoma model revealed significant remission with minimal toxicity, setting the stage for potential clinical trials (Steiniger et al., 2004).

The delivery of other drugs is also being investigated. Dalargin is a hexapeptide analog of leucine-enkephalin containing D-alanine, which produces CNS analgesia when it is delivered intracerebroventricularly, but it has no analgesic effects if it is administered systemically, specifically because it cannot cross the BBB on its own

(Alyaudtin et al., 2001; Rousselle et al., 2003). The (3H)-dalargin was conjugated to the same poly(butylcyanoacrylate) nanoparticles described above, injected systemically into mice, and demonstrated by radiolabeling to cross the BBB and accumulate in brain (Alyaudtin et al., 2001). Other, similar studies have also demonstrated delivery of dalargin using polysorbate 80-coated nanoparticles (Schroeder et al., 1998). Other polysorbate 80 nanoparticles have been chemically conjugated to the hydrophilic drug diminazenediaceturate (diminazene) and proposed as a novel treatment approach for second stage African trypanosomiasis (Olbrich et al., 2002). In other work, PEG-treated polyalkylcyanoacrylate nanoparticles were shown to cross the BBB and accumulate at high densities in the brain in experimental autoimmune encephalomyelitis (Calvo et al., 2002), a model of multiple sclerosis (Ercolini et al., 2006; Kanwar, 2005).

For other applications, molecules other than drugs must cross the BBB for therapeutic or diagnostic reasons, including oligonucleotides, genes, and contrast agents. Solid lipid nanoparticles consisting of microemulsions of solidified oil nanodroplets loaded with iron oxide and injected systemically into rats have been shown to cross the BBB and accumulate in the brain with long-lasting kinetics (Peira et al., 2003). Iron oxides are classic superparamagnetic magnetic resonance imaging (MRI) contrast agents. Because iron oxides are insoluble in water, they must be delivered as modified colloids for clinical applications, which is usually achieved by coating them with hydrophilic molecules, such as dextrans (Dupas et al., 1999). Therefore, the delivery vehicle used is critical in determining the functional properties of the contrast agent. By taking advantage of the ability of these solid lipid nanoparticles to cross the BBB, nanoparticles complexed with iron oxides may provide new ways to image the CNS using MRI.

Other work has focused on the delivery of oligonucleotides in an *in vivo* mouse model and an *in vitro* endothelial cell model, with the aim being to develop novel treatments for neurodegenerative disorders (Vinogradov et al., 2004). The investigators synthesized a nanogel consisting of cross-linked PEG and polyethylenimine that spontaneously encapsulated negatively charged oligonucleotides. In their *in vivo* model, they demonstrated that intravenous injections resulted in a 15-fold accumulation of oligonucleotides in the brain after 1 hr, with a concurrent 2-fold decrease in accumulation in liver and spleen when compared with freely administered oligonucleotides (not encapsulated in nanogel particles).

A related area is the delivery of genes to the CNS for gene therapy. A tyrosine hydroxylase (TH) expression plasmid was delivered to the striatum of adult rats using PEG immunoliposome nanoparticles in order to normalize TH expression levels in the 6-hydroxydopamine rat model of Parkinson's disease (Zhanget al., 2003). Using specific antibodies to transferrin receptors conjugated to the nanoparticles, TH plasmids were shown to be expressed throughout the striatum.

CONCLUSION

Nanotechnology-based approaches to targeted delivery of drugs and other compounds across the BBB may potentially be engineered to carry out specific functions as needed.

The drug itself—in other words the biologically active component being delivered, whatever that may be—constitutes one element of a nanoengineered complex. The rest of the complex is designed to carry out other key functions, including shielding the active drug from producing systemic side effects, being prematurely cleared or metabolized, crossing the BBB, and targeting specific cells after it has gained access to the CNS. Implicitly, all of this must be achieved by any drug intended to have CNS effects, regardless of whether it is part of a nanoengineered complex.

An important advantage of a nanotechnological approach, as compared with the administration of free drug or the drug associated with a nonfunctional vehicle, is that these critical requirements do not need to be carried out by the active compound, but by supporting parts of the engineered complex. This allows the design of the active drug to be tailored for maximal efficacy. Currently, most nanoengineered systems for crossing the BBB take advantage of drugs that are already in clinical use and therefore have greater potential for reaching the clinic relatively quickly.

In addition to the delivery of drugs and other compounds across the BBB for therapeutic purposes, the ability to cross the BBB selectively and efficiently in animal models using nanoengineered technologies will have a significant impact on research that focuses on the normal physiology of the CNS and its pathology, by allowing targeted *in vivo* studies of specific cells and processes using methods that take advantage of the intact live organism. Ideally, methods for crossing the BBB will complement other nanotechnological tools being developed to study the CNS, including quantum dot labeling and imaging (Pathak et al., 2006).

KEYWORDS

- **Blood-brain barrier**
- **Central nervous system**
- **Nanoengineered**
- **Polyethylene glycol**

ACKNOWLEDGMENTS

Parts of this chapter were adapted from a more detailed review on nanotechnology approaches for crossing the blood-brain barrier written by the author (Silva et al., 2007). This work was supported by funds from NIH grant NINDS NS054736.

COMPETING INTERESTS

The author declares that they have no competing interests.

Chapter 9

Quantum Dot Imaging for Embryonic Stem Cells

Shuan Lin, Xiaoyan Xie, Manishkumar R. Patel, Yao-Hung Yang, Zongjin Li, Feng Cao, Oliver Gheysens, Yan Zhang, Sanjiv S. Gambhir, Jiang Hong Rao, and Joseph C. Wu

INTRODUCTION

Semiconductor quantum dots (QDs) hold increasing potential for cellular imaging both *in vitro* and *in vivo*. In this report, we aimed to evaluate *in vivo* multiplex imaging of mouse embryonic stem (ES) cells labeled with Qtracker delivered QDs.

Murine ES cells were labeled with six different QDs using Qtracker. The ES cell viability, proliferation, and differentiation were not adversely affected by QDs compared with non-labeled control cells (P = NS). Afterward, labeled ES cells were injected subcutaneously onto the backs of athymic nude mice. These labeled ES cells could be imaged with good contrast with one single excitation wavelength. With the same excitation wavelength, the signal intensity, defined as (total signal-background)/exposure time in millisecond was 11 ± 2 for cells labeled with QD 525, 12 ± 9 for QD 565, 176 ± 81 for QD 605, 176 ± 136 for QD 655, 167 ± 104 for QD 705, and 1,713 ± 482 for QD 800. Finally, we have shown that QD 800 offers greater fluorescent intensity than the other QDs tested.

In summary, this is the first demonstration of *in vivo* multiplex imaging of mouse ES cells labeled QDs. Upon further improvements, QDs will have a greater potential for tracking stem cells within deep tissues. These results provide a promising tool for imaging stem cell therapy non-invasively *in vivo*.

The QDs are emerging as an exciting new class of fluorescent probes for non-invasive *in vivo* imaging (Akerman et al., 2002; Dubertret et al., 2002; Gao et al., 2004; Kim et al., 2004; Larson et al., 2003). Compared to conventional organic dyes, QDs offer a number of fascinating optical and electronic properties. The QDs are semiconductor nanocrystals that can be excited by a wide range of light, ranging from ultraviolet to near-infrared, and can emit different wavelengths of light, depending on their size and composition. The QDs have broad excitation spectra and narrow emission spectra (Figure 1). Because QDs can be excited by one single wavelength and can emit light of different wavelengths, they are ideal probes for multiplex imaging (Han et al., 2011). By contrast, conventional organic dyes cannot be easily synthesized to emit different colors and have narrow excitation spectra and broad emission spectra that often cross into the red wavelengths, making it difficult to use these dyes for multiplexing. In addition, QDs have exceptional photostability (reviewed by Medintz et al. (2005)). Due to their extreme brightness and resistance to photobleaching (Wu et al., 2003), The QDs are ideal for live cell imaging wherein cells must be kept under the excitation light source for long periods of time. Their intense brightness is also helpful for single particle detection (reviewed by Michalet et al. (2005)). By comparison, conventional dyes often photobleach, making longitudinal tracking difficult.

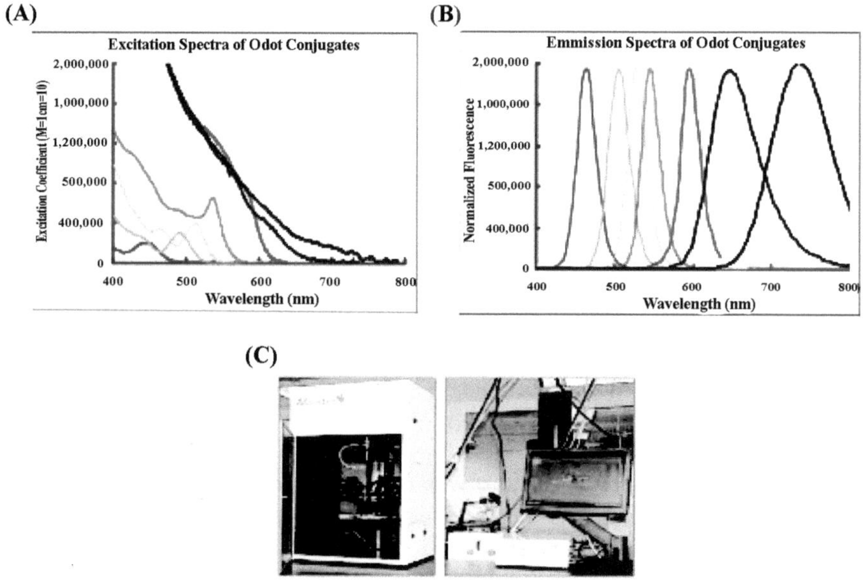

Figure 1. Emission and excitation spectra of QDs (provided by Quamtum Corp.) and Maestro optical system. (A) Excitation and (B) emission spectra of QDs used in the labeling experiments. Dark green = QD 525; green = QD 565; yellow = QD 585; orange = QD 605; red = QD 655; brown = QD 705; blue = QD 800. (C) The Maestro Optical imaging system.

The QDs' photophysical properties have broadened their application and shown great promise as imaging probes in bioimaging, drug discovery, and diagnosis. To keep up with their burgeoning utility, current QD technology has rapidly evolved. The QDs have been used for tumor targeting and imaging (Gao et al., 2004), lymph node (Kim et al., 2004) and vascular mapping (Akerman et al., 2002), and cellular trafficking (Jaiswal et al., 2003; Wu et al., 2003). The QDs can be delivered in a targeted fashion by conjugating them with ligands and antibodies. The QDs can also be introduced into cells non-specifically, which serves as a potential tracking marker for cellular imaging.

Stem cell therapy holds promise for treatment of intractable conditions such as Parkinson's disease, ischemic heart disease, diabetes, and degenerative joint diseases (Bruder et al., 1998; Lindvall et al., 2004; Soria et al., 2011; Strauer and Kornowski, 2003). There are two types of cells used in stem cell therapy, adult stem cells and ES cells. Of the two, ES cells are the ultimate source for use in cell-based therapy because they posses a virtually unlimited capacity for self-renewal and pluripotency, which is defined as the ability to differentiate into all cell types, including neurons, cardiomyocytes, hepatocytes, islet cells, skeletal muscle cells, and endothelial cells (Fuchs and Segre, 2000). In stem cell therapy, monitoring of cell survival and location after transplantation is important for determining their efficacy. Because the absorption and scattering of light in biological tissue can be considerable, any optical signal transmitted from deep tissues to the surface tends to diminish in strength (reviewed by Choy et al. (2003)). With QDs' many advantages over traditional organic dyes, QDs may provide an excellent tool for imaging stem cell therapy.

In this study, we use the peptide-based reagent QTracker to label mouse ES cells with QDs and evaluate the utility of QDs for imaging stem cell therapy. We next show that labeling mouse ES cells with QDs does not adversely affect ES cell viability, proliferation, and differentiation. Finally, we examine QDs' potential for imaging ES cells *in vitro* and *in vivo*.

MATERIALS AND METHODS

Culture of Undifferentiated ES Cells

The murine ES-D3 cell line (CRL-1934) was obtained from the American Type Culture Collection (ATCC; Manassas, VA). The ES cells were kept in an undifferentiated, pluripotent state with 1,000 IU/ml leukemia inhibitory factor (LIF; Chemicon. ESGRO, ESG1107) and grown on top of the murine embryonic fibroblasts feeder layer inactivated by 10 ug/ml mitomycin C (Sigma). The ES cells were cultured on 0.1% gelatin-coated plastic dishes in ES medium containing Dulbecco Modified Eagle Medium supplemented with 15% fetal calf serum, 0.1 mmol/l β-mercaptoethanol, 2 mmol/l glutamine, and 0.1 mmol/l non-essential amino acids as described previously (Boheler et al., 2002; Cao et al., 2006).

Flow Cytometry and Fluorescent Microscopy

Trypsinized mouse ES cells were labeled with QD 655 (10 nM) using Qtracker according to the manufacturer's protocol. Briefly, 10 nM of labeling solution was prepared according to the kit direction. Trypsinized mouse ES cells (1×10^6) were added to the 0.2 ml of labeling solution. After incubating at 37°C for 60 min with intermittent mixing, the ES cells were washed twice with PBS to remove any free QDs and plated on 0.01% gelatin coated plates. Fluorescence microscopy (Carl Zeiss Axiovert 200M) was used to image the cells on day 1. Labeled ES cells were analyzed by flow cytometry (FACSCalibur; BD Biosciences, San Jose, CA) using the FL3 channel to detect QD 655 labeled cells on days 1, 4, and 7 post-labeling. Acquisition data were analyzed by the FlowJo software.

Effect of QDs on ES Cell Viability and Proliferation

The ES cells labeled with six different QDs (10 nM each) and control unlabeled ES cells were plated uniformly in 96-well plates at a density of 5,000 cells per well. Cells were treated according to the manufacturer's protocol and read out on a fluorescence microplate reader (SpectraMax Gemini EM, Molecular Devices Corporation, Sunnyvale, CA) at 24, 48, and 72 hr post-labeling. For Trypan blue exclusion assay (indicative of cell death), aliquots of labeled cells were removed at specific time points and mixed with Trypan blue. The number of dead cells was determined by counting blue cells under a light microscope.

Embryoid Body Formation and Differentiation

The ES cells were differentiated *in vitro* by the "hanging drop" method as described previously (Cao et al., 2006; Keller, 1995; Maltsev et al., 1994). Briefly, the main steps included withdrawal of LIF and cultivation of 400 cells in 18 μl hanging drops to produce embryoid bodies for 3 days, followed by cultivation as suspension in ultra-low-cluster 96-well flat-bottom plates for 2 days. Next, the embryoid bodies were seeded onto 48-well plates.

RT-PCR Analysis of Embryonic and Germ Layer Specific Transcripts

Reverse-transcription polymerase chain reaction (RT-PCR) was used to compare the expression of embryonic marker (Oct4), endoderm (alpha-1-fetoprotein, AFP), mesoderm (fetal liver kinase-1, Flk1), and ectoderm (neural cell adhesion molecule, Ncam) germ layer markers (Abeyta et al., 2004) between control unlabeled ES and QD-labeled ES cells. Total RNA was prepared from cells with Trizol reagent (Invitrogen) according to the manufacturer's protocol. The primer sets used in the amplification reaction were as follow: Oct4 forward primer GGCGTTCTCTTTGCAAAGGTGTTC, reverse primer CTCGAACCACATCCTTCTCT; AFP forward primer TATCAGCCACTGCTGCAACT, reverse primer GTTCAGGCTTTTGCTTCACC; Flk1 forward primer CACCTGGCACTCTCCACCTTC, reverse primer GATTTCATCCCACTACCGAAAG; Ncam forward primer GGAAGGGAACCAAGTGAACA, reverse primer ACGGTGTGTCTGCTTGAACA. The PCR products were separated on 1% agarose gel electrophoresis and quantified with Labworks 4.6 Image Acquisition and analysis software (UVP Bio-Imaging Systems).

In Vivo Fluorescence Imaging of QD-Labeled ES Cells

Right after labeling ES cells with QDs by QTracker, the labeled cells were subcutaneously injected with Matrigel (50 μl, vol. 1:1, BD Biosciences, San Jose, CA) into various locations on the back of athymic nude mice (n = 6). Images were taken with an excitation filter of 465 nm and an emission filter of 510 nm long-pass using the Maestro Optical imaging (CRI Inc, Woburn, MA) as shown in Figure 1B. Detection was set to capture images automatically at 10 nm increments from 500 to 850 nm. The vendor's software (Nuance 2p12_beta) determined the correct exposure time for each QD labeled cells. The resulting TIFF image was loaded into the software and analyzed. Spectral unmixing was done using a user-defined library according to manufacturer's direction for each QD. Briefly, images of six different QD labeled ES cells in 1.5 ml micro-centrifuge tubes were taken separately. Each QD library spectra was decided and set by unmixing autofluorescence spectra and QD spectra manually selected from the image using the computer mouse to select appropriate regions. Images for QD800 sensitivity experiment was taken with an excitation filter of 640 nm and an emission filter of 700 nm long-pass.

Postmortem Immunohistochemical Stainings

After imaging, all animals were euthanized by protocol approved by the Stanford Animal Research Committee. Explanted subcutaneous teratomas were routinely processed for hematoxylin-and-eosin staining. Slides were interpreted by an expert pathologist blinded to the study (AJC).

Statistical Analysis

Data were presented as mean ± SD. For Statistical analysis, the 2-tailed Student t test was used. Differences were considered significant at $P < 0.05$.

DISCUSSION

Stem cells offer an exciting new branch of therapy to treat a variety of conditions and diseases. It is therefore important to develop methods to monitor cell survival and location after transplantation. Due to its many advantages over conventional organic dyes, QDs serve as good candidates to monitor these parameters. In order to evaluate their *in vivo* ability, we delivered them by using commercially available QTracker. Strategies for *ex vivo* cell labeling by QDs include non-specific endocytosis, microinjection, liposome mediated uptake, electroporation, and peptide-based reagents. Previous studies have shown that the liposome-based reagent Lipofectamin 2000 had the highest delivery efficiency, but the QDs were delivered in aggregates (Derfus et al., 2004). Electroporation also delivered QDs in aggregates (Derfus et al., 2004), and may even cause cell death. Peptide-based QTracker (Christoffer et al., 2004) reagents (Invitrogen, CA) deliver QDs into the live cells, and have been shown to be an excellent and easy tool for studying live cell mobility (Davie et al., 2006) and cell fusion (Murasawa et al., 2005).

In this report, we evaluated ES cells labeled with QDs using commercially available Qtracker for non-invasive *in vivo* imaging in living mice. Twenty-four hours after labeling ES cells with QDs, 72% of the cells were positive. However, by day 4 the percentage of positive cells dropped to 4%. This dramatic decrease could be due to the rapid division of ES cells (doubling time of 12–15 hr) or QD diffusion out of dividing cells over time thus causing a dilution of QD signal. The dramatic decrease in signal is consistent with a previous study that used QDs to label human cervical adenocarcinoma cells (Jaiswal et al., 2003).

Another important question is whether QDs affect ES cell properties (i.e., pluripotency and self-renewal) that make them an attractive choice for regenerative therapy. Previous studies have shown that QD toxicity is dose dependent with increasing concentrations affecting cell growth and viability (Hardman, 2006). However, we were interested in any toxicity caused at concentrations used for labeling cells for *in vivo* applications. Therefore, we examined ES cell proliferation and viability at one QD concentration (10 nM) and observed no significant changes between QD labeled ES cells and control unlabeled ES cells. This was true for all QDs tested: QD 525, 565, 605, 655, 705, and 800. These results concur with the study by Jaiswal et al. that also showed no adverse effects by QDs on the viability, morphology, function, and development of various other cells (Jaiswal et al., 2003). Likewise, we confirmed that QDs also had no adverse affect on ES cell differentiation based on RT-PCR analysis of germ layer specific genes. Implanted ES cells are known to form teratoma tumors with a variety of differentiated tissues (Cao et al., 2007). In Figure 6, we found that the teratoma consisted of a variety of tissues including respiratory epithelium, osteochondroid, squamous cell, and immature brain-like neural cell based on histology. This confirmed that QD labeling did not affect *in vivo* differentiation as well. However, although ES cell-derived teratomas were retrieved from the animals, they were not shown to be QD labeled. We believe that the *in vivo* signal could be due to uptake of QD by neighboring host cells. Thus, the poor retention of QDs in targets cells may be a problem for long-term tracking, and more detailed analysis are needed to address this issue in the future.

Another advantage of QDs is their ability to do multiplex imaging of different QDs at the same time. However, in our study, ES cells labeled with different QDs were only capable of being imaged up to day 2 after subcutaneous implantation. A likely cause for this could be the loss of signal due to rapid cell division. Another possible cause could be serum instability of the QDs. Cai et al. reported that QD 705 lost 14% of its original intensity after 24 hr of incubation in mouse serum (Weibo Cai et al., 2006). Any loss of signal could hamper detection of QD labeled cells at later time points, especially those that are not within the near-infrared region since signals from these QDs will also be mostly absorbed by the skin. For those QDs that are in near-infrared region, QD 705 and QD 800, the difference in intensity could be due to transfection efficiency since these two QDs have similar extinction coefficients and quantum yield according to the manufacturer. However, extinction coefficients and quantum yield data were obtained *in vitro* and not in an animal setting. Moreover, the transfection efficiency was similar across all QDs. Therefore, we believe transfection efficiency is unlikely to be the cause of the difference in intensity observed *in vivo*. Due to its higher extinction coefficient and wider emission spectra within near-infrared region, only QD 800 signals were capable to be imaged in the animals for up to 14 days. We observed an increase in signal intensity when using a red shifted excitation laser (640 nm) to image QD 800 labeled ES cells. The normal excitation wavelength is 465 nm. This was somewhat surprising since the excitation coefficient of QD 800 is lower at 640 nm than it is at 465 nm. That is at 640 nm, QD 800 absorbs light with less efficiency than at 465 nm, so less QDs become excited and thus give off lower signal intensities. However, the tissue penetration is much greater at 640 nm. Therefore, labeled cells that would not have been excited at 465 nm could be excited at 640 nm. Thus, these newly excited cells could contribute to the greater signal intensity seen at the detection wavelength of 800 nm.

RESULTS

Qtracker Intracellular QD Delivery

To deliver QDs, we used peptide-based QTracker, which has been shown to be an excellent and easy tool for study live cell mobility (Davie et al., 2006) and cell fusion (Murasawa et al., 2005). In order to determine transfection efficiency in ES cells, labeled ES cells were analyzed by flow cytometry. Figure 2A shows a representative histogram plot based on forward scatter and side scatter gated cells. The red line shows fluorescence intensity of control unlabeled cells and the green line represents the labeled cells. As more QDs were taken up by these cells, the fluorescence intensity increased. Around 72% of the cells were positive 24 hr after labeling and the mean fluorescence intensity (MFI) was 521. However, by day 4 the percentage of positive cells had dropped to ~4% and by day 7 only ~0.7% of the cells were positive by FACS analysis when compared to control unlabeled cells. Fluorescence microscopy (Carl Zeiss Axiovert 200M) was used to image the cells on day 1. Representative brightfield and fluorescent images are shown in Figure 2B. The ES cells can be labeled and monitored by FACS analysis up to 7 days.

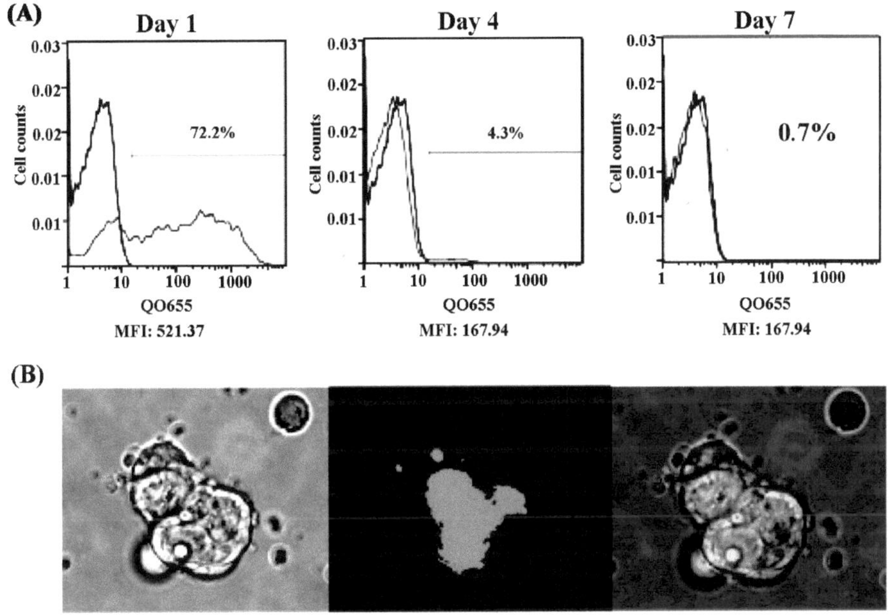

Figure 2. Qtracker intracellular QD delivery quantified by flow cytometry. (A) Flow cytometry detection of QD labeling of mouse ES cells on day 1, day 4, and day 7. Red line = unlabeled cells as control; green line = cells labeled with QD. (B) Fluorescent images of cells labeled with QDs on day 1 post labeling.

QDs Do Not Affect ES Cell Viability and Proliferation

Toxicity of QDs is a key factor in determining whether it will be a feasible probe for both cellular and clinical use. We carefully examined QDs' effect on ES cells by Trypan blue exclusion assay and a CyQuant proliferation assay. Figure 3A shows the percentage of live cells in triplicates at 24, 48, and 72 hr post QD labeling. Overall, there was no significant difference between labeled and unlabeled ES cells (P = NS) for all QDs that were tested: QD 525, 565, 605, 655, 705, and 800. To evaluate cell proliferation, we used the CyQuant assay, which measures the amount of nucleic acids in each well, thereby giving an accurate count of the number of cells in the experimental condition. As shown in Figure 3B, there was also no significant difference between QD labeled ES cells and unlabeled ES cells (P = NS).

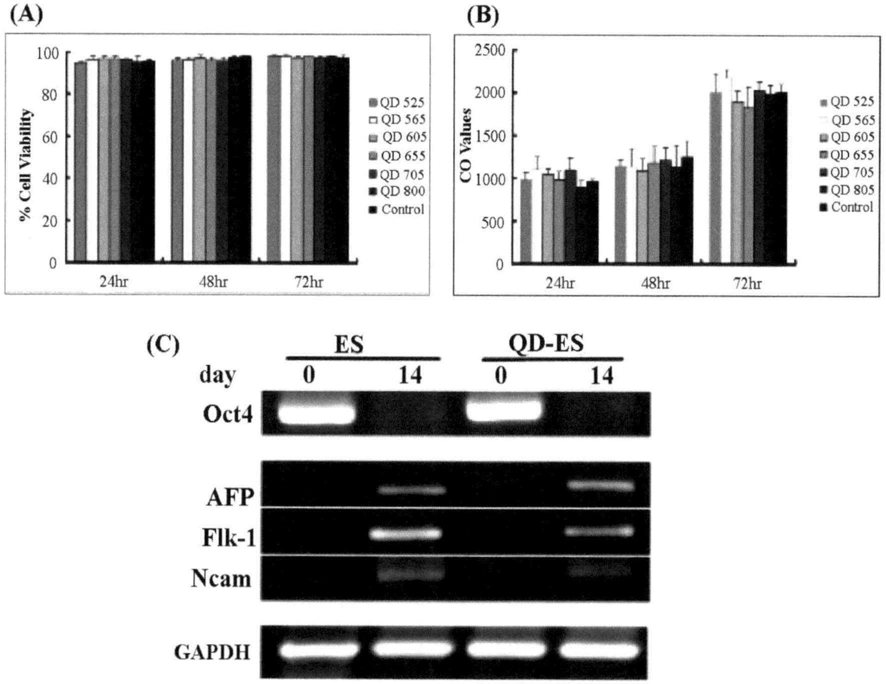

Figure 3. Effects of QDs on ES cell viability, proliferation, and differentiation. (A) Trypan blue exclusion assay and (B) CyQuant cell proliferation assay both showed no significant difference between unlabeled ES cells and labeled ES cell at 24, 48, and 72 hr. (C) The RT-PCR analysis showed the levels of endoderm (AFP), mesoderm (Flk-1), and ectoderm (Ncam) germ layer marker increased from day 0 to day 14 of spontaneous ES cell differentiation using the hanging drop assay. The stem cell marker Oct4 decreased during the same period as expected. The GAPDH is a loading control for all cells. Both QD labeled and unlabeled ES cells showed similar pattern on RT-PCR analysis.

QDs Have No Profound Effects on ES Cell Differentiation *In Vitro*

Having demonstrated that QD labeling had no detectable effect on ES cell growth, we next tested its effect on cellular development and differentiation. Dubertret et al. showed that at high concentrations, QDs injected into an individual blastomere of Xenopus during very early cleavage stages can cause apparent abnormalities in late stage embryos (Dubertret et al., 2002). Therefore, we examined the pluripotency of QD labeled mouse ES cells to ascertain if any developmental interference would occur. In the literature, both human and murine ES cells have well-documented differentiation and replication capacities (Evans and Kaufman, 1981; Thomson et al., 1998). Mouse ES cells were differentiated *in vitro* by hanging drop assay. We then isolated RNA samples from undifferentiated mouse ES cells and embryoid body at day 14 and analyzed them by RT-PCR. Both labeled and unlabeled undifferentiated ES cells (day 0) expressed ES cell specific marker Oct4. Likewise, both labeled and unlabeled differentiated ES cells (day 14) expressed specific markers for endoderm (AFP), mesoderm (Flk1), and ectoderm (Ncam) germ layers (Abeyta et al., 2004) (Figure 3C).

In Vivo Multiplex Imaging Using QDs

One of the most attractive qualities of QDs is their capability for multiplex imaging (i.e., tracking different cell populations with different QDs using different emission wavelengths at the same time). In addition, as QDs are larger than organic dyes, they are not transferred between cells until the cells fuse. Therefore, QDs can provide an excellent tool for studying cell–cell interactions (Murasawa et al., 2005). Here we used QD 525, 565, 605, 655, 705, and 800 to label 1×10^6 ES cells as described. Right after QD labeling, the labeled cells were subcutaneously injected into various locations on the back of athymic nude mice. Images were taken right after injection and the resulting stacked image shown in Figure 4A. The fluorescent intensity was directly proportional to the product of extinction coefficient and the quantum yield. Even though the QDs were excited by the same wavelength, the energy absorbed was different for each QD, causing some QDs to absorb less energy than others. This observation is due to the QDs' ability to produce different light levels at the same excitation wavelength as shown in Figure 1A. Therefore, QDs with longer emission wavelengths will appear brighter. With the same excitation wavelength, the signal intensity (defined as: (total signal-background)/exposure time in millisecond) was 11 ± 2 for cells labeled with QD 525, 12 ± 9 for QD 565, 176 ± 81 for QD 605, 176 ± 136 for QD 655, 167 ± 104 for QD 705, and $1{,}713 \pm 482$ for QD 800. Quantification of these results is shown in Figure 4B. In order to evaluate which QD was better for non-invasive imaging, we imaged the same transplanted mice longitudinally. After day 2, ES cells labeled with QD 525, 565, 605, 655, and 705 could not be detected *in vivo* using the Maestro system. In contrast, QD 800 signal could be detected up to 14 days in animals post injection, which is likely due to its higher extinction coefficient and wider emission spectra within near-infrared region.

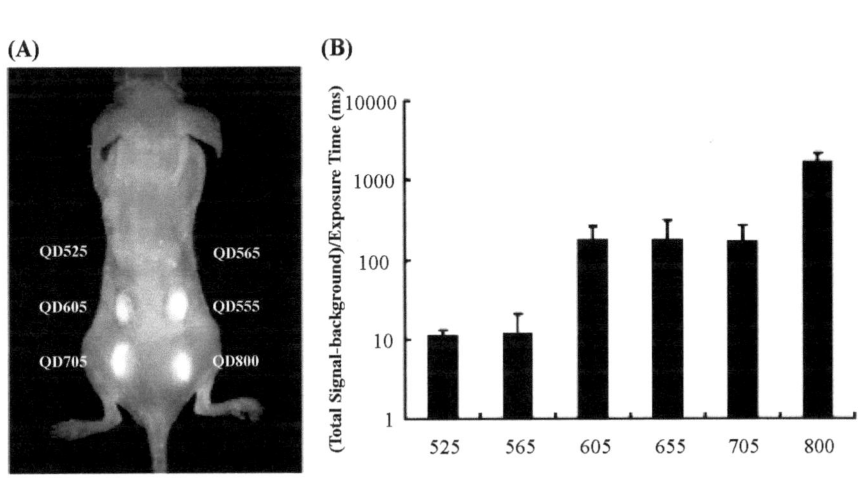

Figure 4. Multiplex imaging capability of QD in live animals. (A) 1 x 10^6 ES cells labeled with QD 525, 565, 605, 655, 705, and 800 were subcutaneously injected on the back of the athymic nude mice right after labeling and the image was taken with a single excitation light source right after injection. The quantification of fluorescent signal intensity defined as total signal-background/exposure time in millisecond was shown in (B).

Detection Sensitivity for *In Vivo* Imaging Using QD800

We have shown that QD 800 offers greater fluorescent intensity than the other QDs tested. However, its detection sensitivity is currently unknown. In particular, what are the fewest number of labeled cells that can be detected by the Maestro system and for what duration? In order to determine the detection sensitivity for *in vivo* imaging, we subcutaneously injected different numbers of QD 800 labeled ES cells (1×10^4, 1×10^5, and 1×10^6) into the back of the mice right after labeling. Images were taken 1 hr post injection and then daily thereafter for 2 weeks using the Maestro Optical imaging system (excitation: 465 nm, emission: 515 long-pass). Figure 5A showed that $\sim 1 \times 10^5$ subcutaneously injected QD labeled cells could be seen through the Maestro system. The signal intensity quantification is shown in Figure 5B. Since QD 800 could also be excited by red light, which offered better tissue penetration, we also imaged the mice using excitation filter 640 nm and emission filter 700 long-pass (Figure 5C). We compared the resulting image to that obtained from earlier settings. Although we still could not visualize the 1×10^4 labeled cells, the signal intensity from 1×10^6 labeled cells did increase with the red light excitation (from 1538 ± 793 to 2378 ± 352) (Figure 5D). Again, signals were still present in the animals up to day 14 using excitation filter 640 nm as shown in Figure 5E.

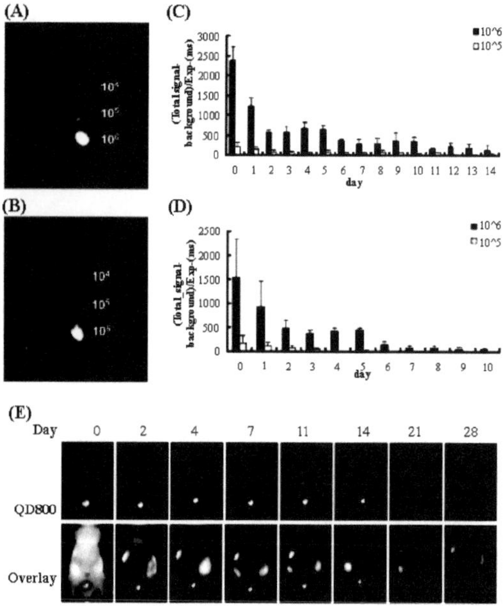

Figure 5. Detection sensitivity of QD 800 imaging in live animals. (A) 1 x 10^4, 1 x 10^5, and 1 x 10^6 QD 800 labeled ES cells were subcutaneously injected on the back of the mice right after labeling. The image was taken 1 hr post injection with excitation filter 465 nm and emission filter 510 nm long-pass, and the quantification of the fluorescent intensity (total signal-background/exposure time (ms) was shown in (B). (C) After images were taken, the mice were imaged again with red excitation light source (640 nm) and the quantification of the fluorescent intensity was shown in (D). Longitudinal imaging of the same representative animal for 1 month shows detection of QD signals up to day 14 (E).

Postmortem Histologic Analysis of QD Labeled ES Cells

After imaging, animals were sacrificed and the subcutaneous tumor developed from 1×10^6 QD800 labeled ES cells was removed for detailed postmortem analysis at day 28 post-injection. Conventional histology using H&E stains confirmed the intact *in vivo* differentiation ability of QD labeled ES cells in living animals (Figure 6). These *in vivo* histologic data are concordant with previous *in vitro* RT-PCR data shown in Figure 4, which further suggest that QDs do not affect the developmental pluripotency of ES cells. However, we could not observe any QDs under microscopic level at day 28, likely due to dilution and diffusion effects.

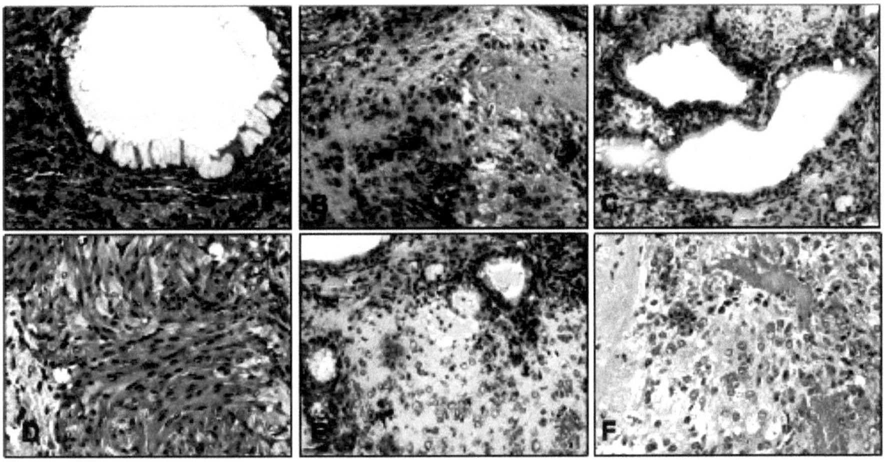

Figure 6. Postmortem histological analysis of transplanted ES cells. (A,D) respiratory epithelium with ciliated columnar and mucin producing goblet cells; (B,E) osteochondroid formation; (C) squamous cell differentiation with keratin pearl; and (F) immature brain-like neural cell formation.

CONCLUSION

In summary, we report the successful demonstration of labeling ES cells with QDs and imaging these labeled cells *in vivo*. We have shown that it is feasible to label ES cells with QDs by Q-Tracker with high efficiency. After labeling, QDs did not affect the viability, and proliferation of ES cells, and have no profound effect on differentiation capacity of ES cells within the sensitivities of the screening assays used. We tested multiplex imaging *in vivo* using the Maestro system and showed that QD 525, QD 565, QD605, QD 655, QD 705, and QD 800 labeled ES cells can be detected *in vivo* using a single excitation wavelength (465 nm). This versatility makes them good candidates for tumor targeting (Gao et al., 2004), lymph node (Kim et al., 2004) and vascular mapping (Akerman et al., 2002), and cell trafficking (Jaiswal et al., 2003; Wu et al., 2003) in small animal imaging. Nevertheless, the use of QD in stem cells is only beginning to be explored. To our knowledge, this is the first demonstration of *in vivo* multiplex imaging of mouse ES cells labeled QDs. Upon further improvements (e.g., near-infrared QDs, better serum stability, and improved cell retention), QDs will have greater potential for tracking of stem cells within deep tissues.

KEYWORDS

- **Embryonic stem**
- **Mean fluorescence intensity**
- **Quantum dots**
- **Reverse-transcription polymerase chain reaction**
- **Trypan blue**

AUTHORS' CONTRIBUTIONS

Shuan Lin carried out the QTracker transfection efficiency studies (FACS and fluorescence imaging), the cell viability assay, the ES cell differentiation assay, the *in vivo* multiplex imaging, and the *in vivo* sensitivity study, participated in the cell proliferation assay, and drafted the manuscript. Xiaoyan Xie carried out the cell proliferation studies, the histology studies, and RT-PCR analysis, and participated in the *in vivo* multiplex imaging and the *in vivo* sensitivity studies. Manishkumar R. Patel participated in the *in vivo* multiplex imaging, and the *in vivo* sensitivity study, and helped to draft the manuscript. Yao-Hung Yang and Zongjin Li participated in the QTracker transfection efficiency studies. Feng Cao and Oliver Gheysens participated in the *in vivo* multiplex imaging and *in vivo* sensitivity study. Yan Zhang participated in the QTracker transfection efficiency studies. Sanjiv S. Gambhir and Jiang Hong Rao participated in the design of the study and helped to draft the manuscript. Joseph C. Wu conceived the study, and participated in its design and coordination and helped to draft the manuscript. All authors have read and approved the final manuscript.

ACKNOWLEDGMENTS

This work was supported in part by grants from the NIH HL089027 (Joseph C Wu), NIH HL074883 (Joseph C Wu), CIRM RS1-00322-1 (Joseph C Wu), ACCF-GE (Joseph C Wu) and SNM Bradley-Alavi Fellowship (Shuan Lin).

Chapter 10

Nanoporous Platforms for Cellular Sensing and Delivery

Lara Leoni, Darlene Attiah, and Tejal A. Desai

INTRODUCTION

In recent years, rapid advancements have been made in the biomedical applications of micro and nanotechnology. While the focus of such technology has primarily been on *in vitro* analytical and diagnostic tools, more recently, *in vivo* therapeutic and sensing applications have gained attention. This chapter describes the creation of monodisperse nanoporous, biocompatible, and silicon membranes as a platform for the delivery of cells. Studies described herein focus on the interaction of silicon-based substrates with cells of interest in terms of viability, proliferation, and functionality. Such microfabricated nanoporous membranes can be used both *in vitro* for cell-based assays and *in vivo* for immunoisolation and drug delivery applications.

The application of micro- and nanotechnology to the biomedical arena has tremendous potential in terms of developing new diagnostic and therapeutic modalities and has increasingly been used to solve complex problems at the molecular and cellular level. While the majority of research has focused on the development of miniaturized diagnostic tools such as electrophoretic, chromatographic, and cell micromanipulation systems (Akin and Najafi, 1994; Anderson, 1989; Baxter et al., 1994; Gourley, 1996; Volkmuth et al., 1995), researchers have more recently concentrated on the development of microdevices and constructs for therapeutic applications. Micro- and nanofabrication techniques are currently being used to develop implants that can record from, sense, stimulate, and deliver to biological systems. Micromachined neural prostheses, drug delivery micropumps/needles, and microfabricated immunoisolation biocapsules (Desai et al., 1998, 1999; Henry et al., 1998; Santini et al., 1999) have all been fabricated using precision-based microtechnologies. Microfabrication methods have also been applied to biotechnology in areas such as DNA sequencing by hybridization, protein patterning, and functional cell sorting.

The interfacing of "chip" technology and cell biology has great potential for use in biomedical research. Moreover, the human body seems appropriate as a target of microtechnology since most structures in the body are in the micron to millimeter size range, the same size range as most micro and nanoscale constructs. Few other engineering technologies can so closely parallel the multidimensional size scale of the living cells and tissues, with both precision and accuracy, in the same fabrication process. The miniaturization and reproducibility of platform features greatly facilitates the use of these systems for cell-based applications.

Microfabricated substrates can provide unique advantages over traditional biomaterials used for biosensing and delivery due to the: (1) Ability to control surface microarchitecture, topography, and feature size in the nanometer and micron size scale, and (2) Control of surface chemistry in a precise manner through biochemical coupling or photopatterning processes. Microfabrication technologies, by their very nature, lend themselves to efficient, economic mass-scale replication, as convincingly demonstrated by the microelectronic industry. They also allow for precise control of feature size, chemistry, and topography. The long-term integration of cells with inorganic materials such as silicon provides the basis for novel delivery and sensing platforms. Our recent work has focused on the ability to maintain cells long term in nanoporous silicon-based microenvironments.

MATERIALS AND METHODS

The nanoporous membranes are achieved by applying fabrication techniques originally developed for micro electro mechanical systems (MEMS). Utilizing bulk and surface micromachining and microfabrication, silicon platforms can be engineered to have uniform and well-controlled pore sizes, channel lengths, and surface properties (Desai et al., 1998, 1999a, 1999b, 2000; Leoni and Desai, 2001). We have developed several variants of microfabricated diffusion barriers, containing pores with uniform dimensions as small as 7 nanometers (Leoni and Desai, 2001). One such variation is described below.

Fabrication

The process flow for fabrication of nanoporous membranes is depicted in Figure 1. The starting substrate is a 400 µm-thick, 100 mm-diameter, and double side polished (100)-oriented silicon wafer. The first step is the etching of the support ridge structure into the substrate. A low stress silicone nitride layer (nitride), which functions as an etch-stop, is then deposited. A polysilicon film, that acts as the base structural layer (base layer) is deposited on top of the etch-stop layer (Figure 1a). The next step is the etching of holes in the base layer, which defines the overall shape of the pores. The holes are etched through the polysilicon by chlorine plasma, with a thermally grown oxide layer used as a mask. After the pore holes are defined and etched through the base layer (Figure 1b), the pore sacrificial oxide is grown on the base layer (Figure 1c). The sacrificial oxide thickness determines the pore size in the final membrane, so control of this step is critical to reproducible pores in the membrane.

To mechanically connect the base polysilicon with the plug polysilicon, which is necessary to maintain the pore spacing between layers, anchor points are defined in the sacrificial oxide layer (Figure 1d). After the anchor points are etched through the sacrificial oxide, the plug polysilicon is deposited to fill in the holes. The plug layer is then planarized down to the base layer (Figure 1e), leaving the final structure with the plug layer only in the base layer openings. A protective nitride layer is then deposited on the wafer, completely covering both sides of the wafer (Figure 1f). This layer is completely impervious to potassium hydroxide (KOH) chemical etch used to release the membranes from the bulk silicon wafer in the desired areas, and the wafer is placed at

80°C KOH bath to etch. After the silicon is completely removed up to the membrane, the protective, sacrificial, and etch stop layers are removed by etching in hydrogen fluoride (HF) (Figure 1g). The pores fabricated on the membranes were characterized by scanning electron microscope (SEM). The nanoporous membranes were seeded with islet cells, insulinoma cells, or PC12 cells and characterized in terms of viability, hormone secretion, and/or proliferation.

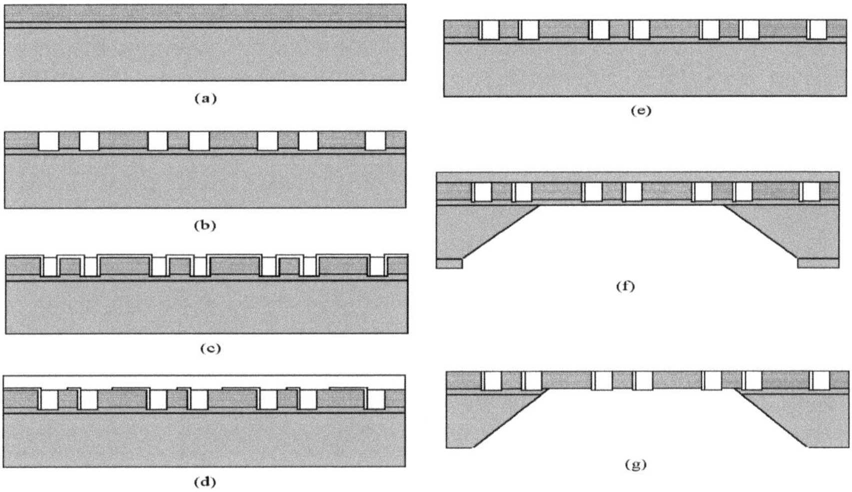

Figure 1. Process flow diagram for nanoporous membrane fabrication.

Insulinoma Cells

Mouse insulinoma βTC3 cells (Efrat et al., 1998) have been obtained from the laboratory of Dr. Shimon Efrat, Department of Molecular Pharmacology, Albert Einstein College of Medicine, Bronx, NY. Cells are cultivated as monolayers in T-flasks in complete medium consisting of DMEM with 25 mM glucose and supplemented with 15% heat-inactivated horse serum (SIGMA) and 2.5% fetal bovine serum (SIGMA). Cultures are maintained at 37°C in a humidified 5% CO_2/95% air atmosphere, and they are passed every 5–10 days. These cells maintain a stable phenotype of glucose responsiveness in the physiological range.

The membrane biocompatibility was characterized by direct contact tests looking at viability of cells in contact with silicon nanoporous membranes. The intracellular fluorescent dye carboxyfluorescein diacetate succinimidyl ester (CFDA, molecular probe) at a concentration of 5 M was used to label cells before *in vitro* culture. First cells were incubated in prewarmed CFDA labeling solution at 37°C in a CO_2 containing incubator for 45 min. The labeling solution was subsequently replaced by prewarmed DMEM medium supplemented with 10% FBS. Then, 10μl of 2×10^7 cells/ml were pipetted onto the membrane well. Cell viability was checked after 24 hr by counting with a hemacytometer under a light microscope. The viability was compared with cells grown on latex (negative control) and standard culture dishes. Cell attachment and proliferation to the various surfaces was also observed and measured.

Neurosecretory Cells (PC12)

The PC12 cells (ATCC, Manassass, VA) of passages three to five were plated and at a density of 1–2 × 10^6 cells per 100 mm dish, maintained at 37°C in 5% CO_2 and re-fed every 2–3 days. To determine the interaction between PC12 cells and silicon nanoporous membranes, the growth patterns of PC12 cells seeded at approximately 3–4 × 10^3 cells into micromachined membrane-based biocapsules and polyurethane (control) capsules (n = 3) contained in 12 well culture dishes were monitored at days 1, 2, and 4. After the designated incubation times, the silicon and control capsules were transferred to empty culture wells and rinsed with PBS to remove loosely adherent cells. Samples were then incubated with 1 × trypsin-EDTA solution to detach the adherent cells. Cell suspensions were then centrifuged at 850 rpm for 5 min. PC12 cell pellets were resuspended in fresh Eagle's minimal essential medium (EMEM) media and counted twice with a hemocytometer. The PC12 viability was monitored by labeling with intracellular fluorescent dye as described above.

In Vivo Biocompatibility

Implantation of nanoporous membranes were done according to the National Institute of Health (NIH) guidelines for the care and use of laboratory animals. Male Lewis rats were anesthetized with inhalation of ether. A laparatomic incision was made and the biocapsules were either sutured on the adbominal wall or wrapped into the momentum and sutured to the same. Incision was closed by suture (polypropylene). Capsules were retrieved after two weeks. Tissue samples were fixed in 10% buffered formalin, paraffin embedded, sectioned, and stained with Hematoxylin-Eosin (H-E).

DISCUSSION AND RESULTS

Silicon nanoporous membranes were fabricated with pore sizes ranging from 7 to 49 nm as described in Leoni and Desai (2001). The pore size was controlled through a sacrificial oxide etching which allows one to create nanoscale features using conventional lithography. Figure 1 shows the overall process flow of the membrane fabrication

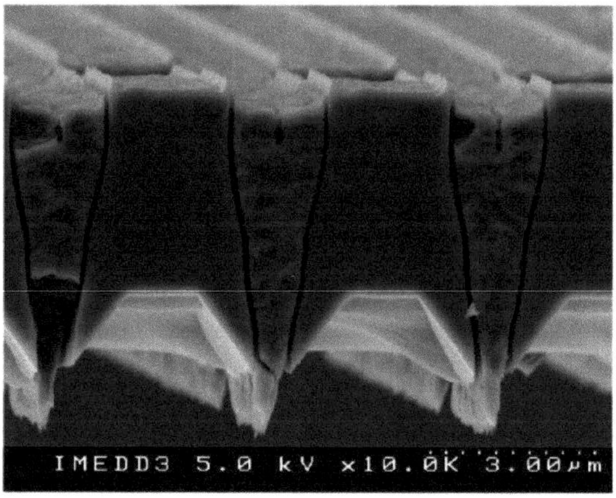

Figure 2. SEM micrograph of microfabricated nanoporous membrane: side view detail.

and is discussed in details in the experimental methods section. Figure 2 shows a cross sectional SEM image of the membrane with the nanoscale channels visible. The membranes can be fabricated in arrays on a single wafer, allowing one to produce multiple nanoporous membranes for *in vitro* or *in vivo* applications.

Insulinoma Cells

Silicon nanoporous membranes, control petri dishes, and latex membranes were seeded with insulinoma cells as described. We found that the insulinoma cells grew without any marked changes on the silicon surfaces. In fact, viability of the cells in the silicon nanoporous environments was equivalent to conventional cell culture surfaces, ranging from 100 to 90% over 8-day period (Figure 3). All cell types had normal morphology. In terms of proliferation, cells seeded in nanoporous microenvironments had similar levels of proliferation compared to control surfaces up to day 4 and then a decreased rate of proliferation at day 8 (Figure 4). This behavior was presumably due to contact inhibition resulting from the limited nanoporous surface area that cells were seeded in as compared to the control surface area. Cells exhibited limited viability and proliferation on the negative control surface of latex. Figure 5 shows an image of insulinoma cells growing on a partially etched nanoporous membrane. It is interesting to note that the cells limit their attachment to the porous regions of the membrane. Such behavior could be due to the nanopores providing a greater surface area for cells to attach. In addition, the etched porous surface is more hydrophilic as its final etch step is in HF solution and therefore may promote greater cell attachment. Figure 6 shows that cells insulinoma cells seeded in silicon nanoporous microenvironments are indeed functional and can secrete insulin over time. Glucose-supplemented medium was allowed to diffuse to the cells, through the membrane, to stimulate insulin production and monitor cell functionality. Results indicate that the insulin secretion by cells and subsequent diffusion of the insulin through the nanoporous membrane channels is similar to that of cell grown in culture.

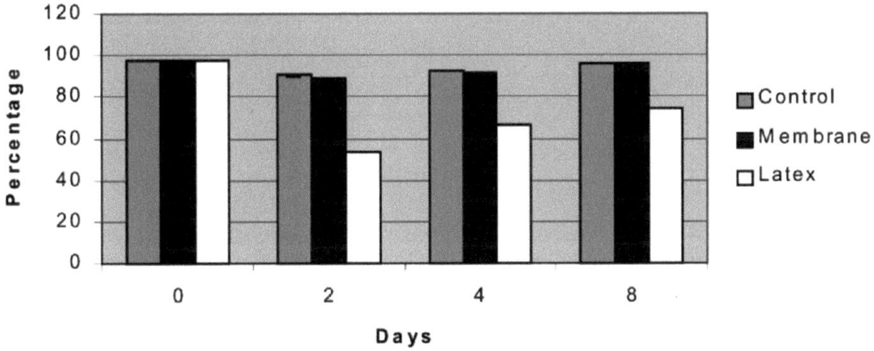

Figure 3. Viability of insulinoma cells over an 8-day period compared to control surface (petri dish) and negative control (latex).

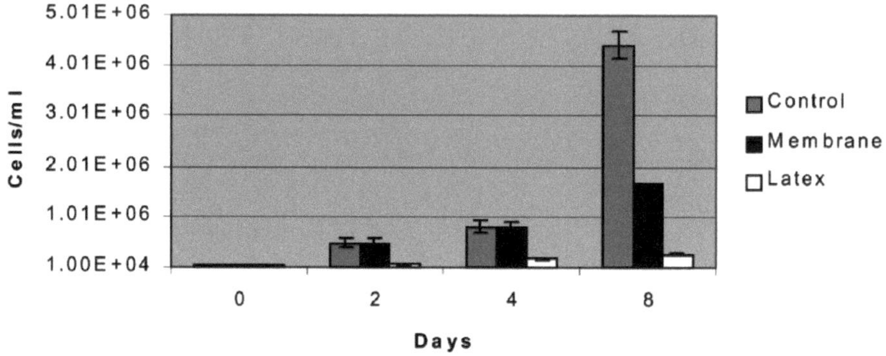

Figure 4. Proliferation of insulinoma cells over an 8-day period compared to control surface (petri dish) and negative control (latex).

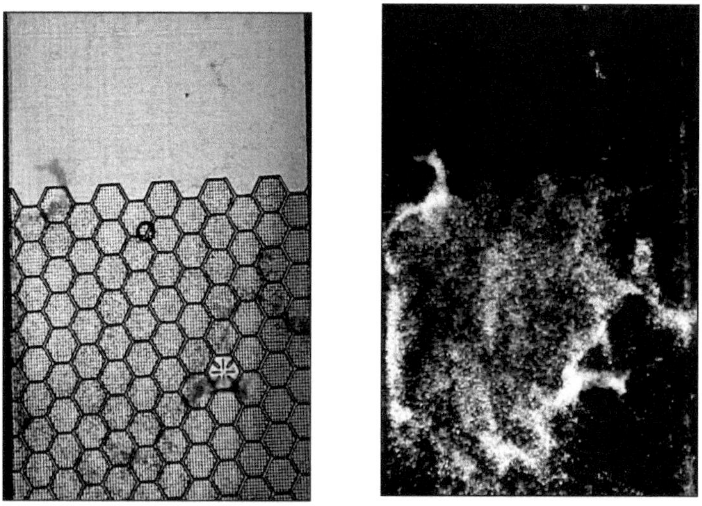

Figure 5. Micrograph of (a) top surface of partially etched nanoporous membrane and (b) nanoporous membrane seeded with fluorescently labeled insulinoma cells. Note the preferential adhesion of the cells to the etched membrane architecture.

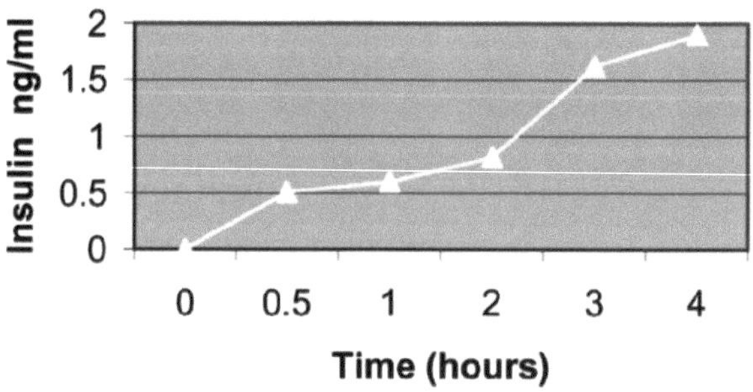

Figure 6. Insulin secretion profile from cells seeded on nanoporous membranes.

Diffusion Properties

When nutrients and time sensitive compounds are diffusing across a membrane, it is highly desirable to be able to precisely control the diffusion characteristics in order to retain the dynamic response of cells seeded on the membrane to external stimuli. The ability of the nanoporous microfabricated membranes to perform size-base exclusion and controlled diffusion of biomolecules has been studied. Membranes exhibited controlled diffusion of glucose and albumin based on membrane pore size. Such control over molecular diffusion was precise and reproducible (Figure 7).

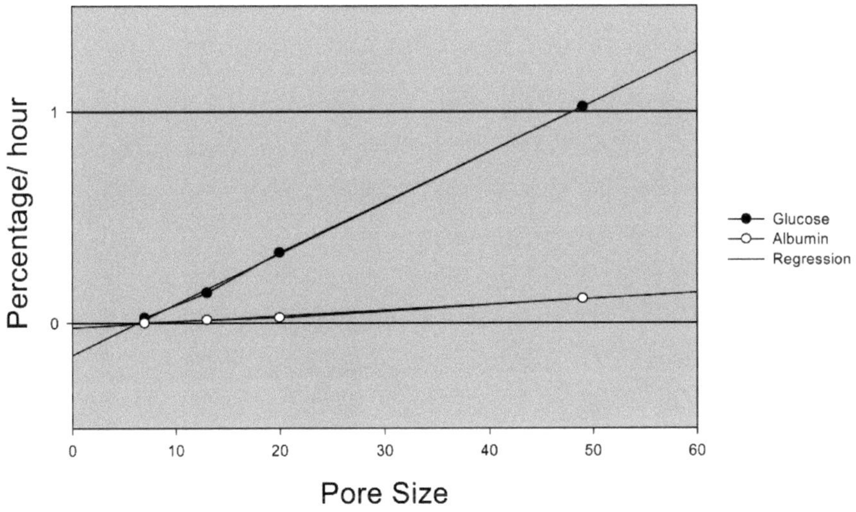

Figure 7. Glucose and albumin diffusion rates.

PC12 Cells

We found that PC12 cells also maintained approximately 100% viability as compared to control surfaces and actually proliferated to a greater extent in silicon nanoporous environments. Figure 8 shows empty nanoporous wells and wells seeded with PC12 cells at day 1 and day 7. The cells are able to become confluent and differentiated within the nanoporous wells. Cells seeded to the silicon nanoporous membranes experienced an approximate 245.31% ± 62.5% growth increase from day 1 to day 4 while those seeded to the polyurethane (control) capsules encountered only a 75.9% ± 21% growth increase (Figure 9). Moreover, cells attached to the silicon nanoporous membranes underwent high proliferation, increasing in number by approximately two-fold every other day of the culture period. At day 1 of cell culture, the number of cells attached to the silicon-based biocapsules and control capsules were observed approximately equal. By day 4, however, the silicon biocapsules exhibited a 110% ± 35.36% greater number of adherent cells. In contrast to the polyurethane capsules, cells that were attached to the silicon biocapsules were noticed to attach firmly to the membrane as they strongly resisted detachment upon trypsinizing.

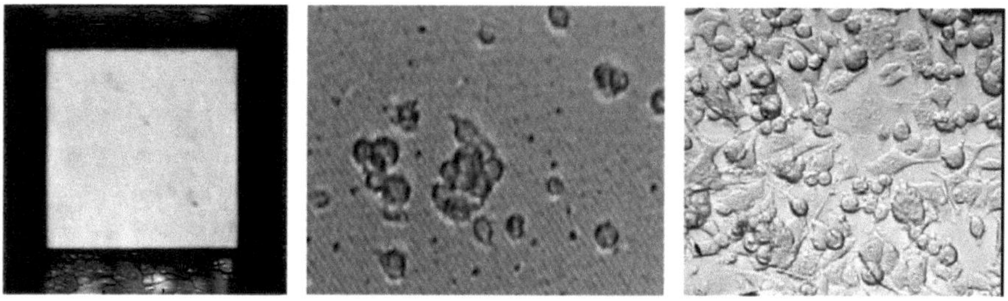

Figure 8. (a) Empty nanoporous membrane and membrane seeded with PC12 cells seeded at (b) day 1 and (c) day 7. Cells show proliferation and differentiation within the nanoporous wells.

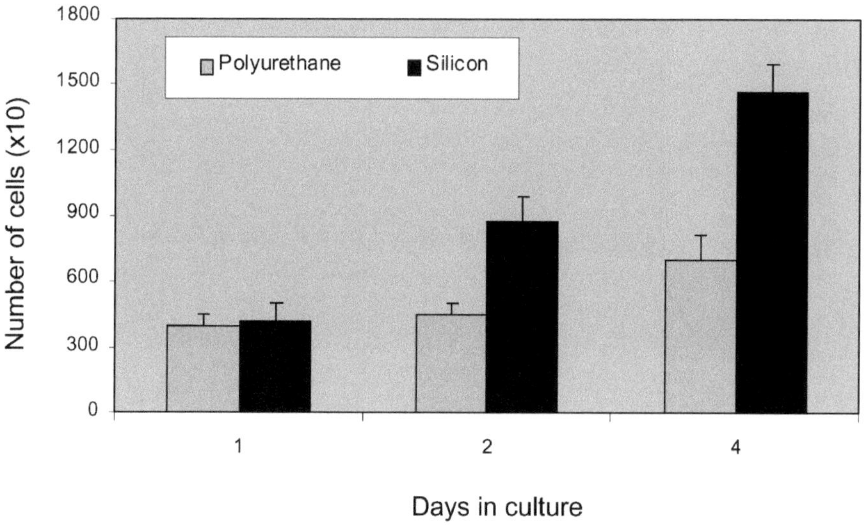

Figure 9. The PC12 proliferation data in polyurethane (control) and silicon-based capsules. Reported are average values of experiments performed with 3x standard deviations.

In Vivo Biocompatibility

At a gross examination, silicon nanoporous membranes seemed free of fibrotic tissue and clean. A rich network of blood vessels surrounded the microfabricated membrane in proximity of the diffusion area, minimizing possible limitations of glucose-insulin exchange due to the lack of a well developed vascular system surrounding the membrane (Figure 10a). Microscopic analysis of tissue sampled from the membrane located in the omentum revealed a non-uniform structure, with prevalence of large round cells typical of adipose tissue (Figure 10b). There was no evidence of macrophages or lymphocytes infiltration. Round structures of different diameters resembling ducts could be seen. Their lumen presented secretion of probable proteinaceous origin. Adenomers were also dispersed in the tissue, as well as small vessels characterized by a thin layer of elongated cells, typical of the lining endothelium in capillaries.

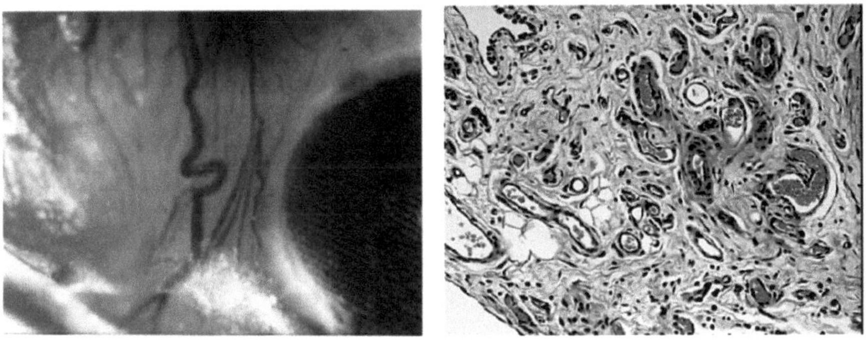

Figure 10. (a) Nanoporous membrane retrieved from the peritoneal cavity: detail; (b) H-E stained tissue (x20). Several blood vessels are visible (arrow).

CONCLUSION

A method to create precise nanoporous membranes via microfabrication technology has been described. Membranes can be fabricated to present uniform and well-controlled pore sizes as small as 7 nm, tailored surface chemistries, and precise microarchitecture. These platforms can be interfaced with living cells to allow for biomolecular separation and immunoisolation. Ideally a membrane in contact with cells should be biocompatible and allow for the free exchange of nutrients, waste products, and secreted therapeutic proteins. Furthermore, where nutrients and time sensitive compounds are diffusing across a membrane it is highly desirable to be able to control the diffusion characteristic precisely in order to retain the dynamic response of seeded cells to external stimuli. Membranes were shown to be sufficiently permeable to support the viability of insulinoma and PC12 cells. Applications of these nanoporous membranes range from cellular delivery to cell-based biosensing to *in vitro* cell-based assays (Figure 11).

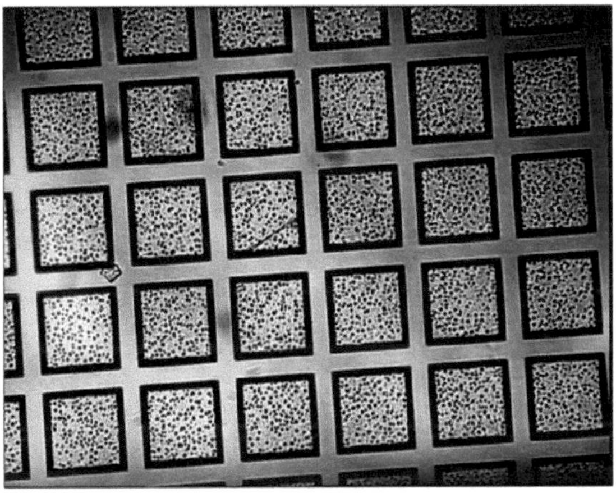

Figure 11. Arrays of nanoporous wells seeded with cell clusters that can potentially be used for high throughput cell-based assays.

In order to retain the same performance *in vivo*, the biohybrid device must be fully biocompatible, which implies that the membrane should elicit little or no foreign body response. The host response is a potentially serious problem to clinical implementation of the technology. The direct consequence of a nonbiocompatible membrane is a fibrotic overgrowth on the surface that interferes with diffusive transport of molecules and oxygenated blood supply. The microfabricated nanoporous membrane proved to be highly biocompatible. After 2 weeks implantation into rat peritoneal cavity, there was no or minimal fibrotic tissue, no significant host response was elicited, and a rich microvascular system was surrounding the device.

KEYWORDS

- **Microfabricated substrates**
- **Miniaturized diagnostic tools**
- **Nanoporous membranes**
- **Polysilicon film**

ACKNOWLEDGMENTS

Portions of this project were funded by NSF and The Whitaker Foundation. Special thanks to iMEDD, Inc. for technical support and fabrication of the membranes.

Chapter 11

Skin Permeation Mechanism and Bioavailability Enhancement of Celecoxib

Faiyaz Shakeel, Sanjula Baboota, Alka Ahuja, Javed Ali,
and Sheikh Shafiq

INTRODUCTION

Celecoxib, a selective cyclo-oxygenase-2 inhibitor has been recommended orally for the treatment of arthritis and osteoarthritis. Long term oral administration of celecoxib produces serious gastrointestinal side effects. It is a highly lipophilic, poorly soluble drug with oral bioavailability of around 40% (Capsule). Therefore the aim of the present investigation was to assess the skin permeation mechanism and bioavailability of celecoxib by transdermally applied nanoemulsion formulation. Optimized oil-in-water nanoemulsion of celecoxib was prepared by the aqueous phase titration method. Skin permeation mechanism of celecoxib from nanoemulsion was evaluated by Fourier transform infra-red (FTIR) spectral analysis, differential scanning calorimeter (DSC) thermogram, activation energy measurement, and histopathological examination. The optimized nanoemulsion was subjected to pharmacokinetic (bioavailability) studies on Wistar male rats.

The FTIR spectra and DSC thermogram of skin treated with nanoemulsion indicated that permeation occurred due to the disruption of lipid bilayers by nanoemulsion. The significant decrease in activation energy (2.373 kcal/mol) for celecoxib permeation across rat skin indicated that the stratum corneum (SC) lipid bilayers were significantly disrupted ($p < 0.05$). Photomicrograph of skin sample showed the disruption of lipid bilayers as distinct voids and empty spaces were visible in the epidermal region. The absorption of celecoxib through transdermally applied nanoemulsion and nanoemulsion gel resulted in 3.30 and 2.97-fold increase in bioavailability as compared to oral capsule formulation.

Results of skin permeation mechanism and pharmacokinetic studies indicated that the nanoemulsions can be successfully used as potential vehicles for enhancement of skin permeation and bioavailability of poorly soluble drugs.

By many estimates up to 90% of new chemical entities (NCEs) discovered by the pharmaceutical industry today and many existing drugs are poorly soluble or lipophilic compounds (Kommuru et al., 2001). The solubility issues obscuring the delivery of these new drugs also affect the delivery of many existing drugs (about 40%). Relative to compounds with high solubility, poor drug solubility often manifests itself in a host of *in vivo* consequences like decreased bioavailability, increased chance of food effect, more frequent incomplete release from the dosage form, and higher intersubject variability. Poorly soluble compounds also present many *in vitro* formulation development hindrances, such as severely limited choices of delivery technologies and increasingly complex dissolution testing with limited or poor correlation to the *in vivo* absorption. However, important advances have been made in improving the bioavailability of poorly soluble compounds, so that promising drug candidates need no longer be neglected or have their development hindered by sub optimal formulation. In addition to more conventional techniques, such as micronization, salt formation, complexation, and so forth, novel solubility/bioavailability enhancement techniques have been developed. The recent trend for the enhancement of solubility/bioavailability is lipid-based system such as microemulsions, nanoemulsions, solid dispersions, solid lipid nanoparticles, liposomes, and so forth. This is also the most advanced approach commercially, as formulation scientists increasingly turn to a range of nanotechnology-based solutions to improve drug solubility and bioavailability.

Nanoemulsions have been reported to make the plasma concentration profiles and bioavailability of poorly soluble drugs more reproducible (Constantinides, 1995; Kawakami et al., 2002a, 2002b; Kommuru et al., 2001; Lawrence and Rees, 2000). Nanoemulsions have also been reported as one of the most promising techniques for enhancement of transdermal permeation and bioavailability of poorly soluble drugs (Baboota et al., 2007a, 2007b; Karande et al., 2004; Shafiq et al., 2007a, 2007b; Shakeel et al., 2007a, 2007b). Nanoemulsions are thermodynamically stable transparent (translucent) dispersions of oil and water stabilized by an interfacial film of surfactant and cosurfactant molecules having a droplet size of less than 100 nm (Shafiq et al., 2007a, 2007b, 2007c). Many formulation scientists have investigated skin permeation mechanism of many drugs using chemical enhancers (Cole and Heard, 2007; Cotte et al., 2004; Goodman and Barry, 1989; Narishetty and Panchagnula, 2004; Stott et al., 2001; Vaddi et al., 2002; Yamane et al., 1995; Zhao and Singh, 1998) and microemulsion technique (Changez et al., 2006; Dreher et al., 1997). Best of our knowledge, skin permeation mechanism of celecoxib has not been reported using microemulsion or nanoemulsion technique although these techniques have been known to enhance skin permeation of drugs effectively (Baboota et al., 2007a, 2007b; Shakeel et al., 2007a, 2007b). Celecoxib (CXB), a selective cyclo-oxygenase-2 (COX-2) inhibitor has been recommended orally for the treatment of arthritis and osteoarthritis (Gaurel et al., 1997). Long term oral administration of CXB produces serious gastrointestinal side effects (Gaurel et al., 1997). It is a highly lipophilic, poorly soluble drug with oral bioavailability of around 40% (Capsule). Therefore the aim of the present investigation was to evaluate the mechanism of skin permeation and bioavailability of CXB using nanoemulsion technique.

MATERIALS AND METHODS

Celecoxib was a kind gift sample from Ranbaxy Research Labs (India). Propylene glycol mono caprylic ester (Sefsol 218) was a kind gift from Nikko Chemicals (Japan). Diethylene glycol monoethyl ether (Transcutol-P) was gift sample from Gattefosse (France). Glycerol triacetate (Triacetin) and acetonitrile (HPLC grade) were purchased from E-Merck (India). Cremophor-EL was purchased from Sigma Aldrich (USA). Deionized water for HPLC analysis was prepared by a Milli-Q-purification system. All other chemicals used in the study were of analytical reagent grade.

Preparation of Nanoemulsion

Various nanoemulsions were prepared by aqueous phase titration method (spontaneous emulsification method). Optimized nanoemulsion formulation (C2) of CXB was prepared by dissolving 2% w/w of CXB in 15% w/w combination of Sefsol-218 and Triacetin (1:1). Then 35% w/w mixture of Cremophor-EL and Transcutol-P (1:1) were added slowly in oil phase. Then 50% w/w of distilled water was added to get the final preparation.

Preparation of Nanoemulsion Gel

Nanoemulsions gel (NGC2) was prepared by dispersing 1% w/w of Carbopol-940 in sufficient quantity of distilled water. This dispersion was kept in dark for 24 hr for complete swelling of Carbopol-940. 2% w/w of CXB was dissolved in 15% w/w mixture of Sefsol-218 and Triacetin (1:1). CXB solution was added slowly to Carbopol-940 dispersion. 0.5% w/w of triethanolamine (TEA) was added in this mixture to neutralize Carbopol-940. Then 35% w/w mixture of Cremophor-EL and Transcutol-P (1:1) were added slowly. Then remaining quantity of distilled water was added to get the final preparation 100% w/w.

The composition of nanoemulsion and nanoemulsion gel are given in Table 1.

Table 1. Compositions of nanoemulsion (C2) and nanoemulsion gel (NGC2).

Ingredients	C2	NGC2
CXB (% w/w)	2.0	2.0
Carbopol-940 (% w/w)	-	1.0
Sefsol 218 (% w/w)	7.5	7.5
Triacetin (% w/w)	7.5	7.5
Cremophor-EL	17.5	17.5
Transcutol-P (% w/w)	17.5	17.5
Triethanolamine (% w/w)	-	0.5
Distilled water to (% w/w)	100.0	100.0

Droplet Size Analysis

Droplet size distribution of optimized nanoemulsion was determined by photon correlation spectroscopy, using a Zetasizer 1000 HS (Malvern Instruments, UK). Light scattering was monitored at 25°C at a scattering angle of 90°. A solid state laser diode was used as light source. The sample of optimized nanoemulsion was suitably diluted with distilled water and filtered through 0.22 μm membrane filter to eliminate mutiscattering phenomena. The diluted sample was then placed in quartz couvette and subjected to droplet size analysis.

Preparation of Full Thickness Rat Skin

Approval to carry out these studies was obtained from the Animal Ethics Committee of Jamia Hamdard, New Delhi, India. Male Wistar rats were sacrificed with prolonged ether anaesthesia and the abdominal skin of each rat was excised. Hairs on the skin of animal were removed with electrical clipper, subcutaneous tissues were surgically removed and dermis side was wiped with isopropyl alcohol to remove residual adhering fat. The skin was washed with distilled water, wrapped in aluminum foil and stored in a deep freezer at –20°C till further use.

Preparation of Epidermis and Stratum Corneum

The skin was treated with 1 M sodium bromide solution in distilled water for 4 hr (Panchagnula et al., 2001). The epidermis from full thickness skin was separated using cotton swab moistened with water. Epidermal sheet was cleaned by washing with distilled water and dried under vacuum and examined for cuts or holes if any. The SC samples were prepared by floating freshly prepared epidermis membrane on 0.1% trypsin solution for 12 hr. Then SC sheets were cleaned by washing with distilled water.

FTIR Spectral Analysis of Nanoemulsion Treated and Untreated Rat Skin

The SC was cut into small circular discs. 0.9% w/v solution of sodium chloride was prepared and 0.01% w/v sodium azide was added as antibacterial and antimycotic agent. 35 ml of 0.9% w/v of sodium chloride solution was placed in different conical flasks and SC of approximate 1.5 cm diameter was floated over it for 3 days. After 3 days of hydration, these discs were thoroughly blotted over filter paper and FTIR spectra of each SC disc was recorded before nanoemulsion treatment (control) in frequency range of 400 to 4,000 cm^{-1} (Perkin Elmer, Germany). After taking FTIR spectra, the same discs were dipped into CXB nanoemulsion formulation present in 35 ml of methanolic phosphate buffer saline (PBS) pH 7.4 (30:70). This was kept for a period of 24 hr (equivalent to the permeation studies) at 37 ± 2°C. Each SC disc after treatment was washed, blotted dry, and then air dried for 2 hr. Samples were kept under vacuum in desiccators for 15 min to remove any traces of formulation completely. The FTIR spectra of treated SC discs were recorded again. Each sample served as its own control.

DSC Studies of Nanoemulsion Treated and Untreated Rat Skin

Approximately 15 mg of freshly prepared SC was taken and hydrated over saturated potassium sulphate solution for 3 days. Then the SC was blotted to get hydration between 20 and 25%. Hydrated SC sample was dipped into nanoemulsion formulation present in 35 ml of methanolic PBS pH 7.4 (30:70). This was kept for 24 hr (equivalent to the permeation studies) at 37 ± 2°C. After treatment, SC was removed and blotted to attain hydration of 20–25%, cut (5 mg), sealed in aluminum hermatic pans and equilibrated for 1 hr before the DSC run. Then, the SC samples were scanned on a DSC6 DSC (Perkin Elmer, Germany). Scanning was done at the rate of 5°C/min over the temperature range of 30–200°C (Cumming and Winfield, 1994; Panchagnula et al., 2001).

Determination of Activation Energy

In vitro skin permeation study of CXB across rat skin was carried out at 27, 37, and 47°C in the methanolic PBS pH 7.4 (30:70). These studies were performed on a modified

Keshary-Chien diffusion cell with an effective diffusional area of 4.76 cm^2 and 35 ml of receiver chamber capacity. In the donor compartment, 1 ml of nanoemulsion formulation was taken (containing 20 mg of CXB). Receiver compartment was composed of the vehicle only (methanolic PBS pH 7.4). Permeability coefficients were calculated at each temperature and activation energy of CXB was then calculated from Arrhenius relationship given as follows (Golden et al., 1986; Narishetty and Panchagnula, 2004):

$$P = P_o e^{-Ea/RT} \; or$$
$$\log P = Ea / 2.303RT + \log P_o$$

where, Ea is the activation energy, R is gas constant (1.987 kcal/mol), T is absolute temperature in K, P is the permeability coefficient, and P_0 is the Arrhenius factor.

Histopathological Examination of Skin Specimens

Abdominal skins of Wistar rats were treated with optimized CXB nanoemulsion (C2) in methanolic PBS pH 7.4. After 24 hr, rats were sacrificed and the skin samples were taken from treated and untreated (control) area. Each specimen was stored in 10% formalin solution in methanolic PBS pH 7.4. The specimens were cut into section vertically. Each section was dehydrated using ethanol, embedded in paraffin for fixing and stained with hematoxylin and eosin. These samples were then observed under light microscope (Motic, Japan) and compared with control sample. In each skin sample, three different sites (epidermis, dermis, and subcutaneous fat layer) were scanned and evaluated for mechanism of skin permeation enhancement. These slides were interpreted by Dr. Ashok Mukherjee, Professor, Department of Pathology, All India Institute of Medical Sciences (AIIMS), New Delhi, India.

Pharmacokinetic Studies

Approval to carry out pharmacokinetic studies was obtained from the Animal Ethics Committee of Jamia Hamdard, New Delhi, India. Guidelines of ethics committee were followed for the studies. Pharmacokinetic studies were performed on optimized nanoemulsion (C2), nanoemulsion gel (NGC2) and marketed capsule. The male Wistar rats were kept under standard laboratory conditions (temperature 25 ± 2°C and relative humidity of 55 ± 5%). The rats were kept in polypropylene cages (six per cage) with free access to standard laboratory diet (Lipton feed, Mumbai, India) and water ad libitum. About 10 cm^2 of skin was shaved on the abdominal side of rats in each group except group treated with marketed capsule. They were fasted for the period of 24 hr for observations on any unwanted effects of shaving. The dose for the rats was calculated based on the weight of the rats according to the surface area ratio (Ghosh et al., 2005). The rats were divided into three groups (n = 6). Group I received C2 transdermally, group II received NGC2 transdermally and group III received marketed capsule orally. The dose of CXB in all groups was 1.78 mg/kg of body weight. The rats were anaesthetized using ether and blood samples (0.5 ml) were withdrawn from the tail vein of rat at 0 (pre-dose), 1, 2, 3, 6, 12, 24, 36, and 48 hr in microcentrifuge tubes in which 8 mg of EDTA was added as an anticoagulant. The blood collected was mixed with the

EDTA properly and centrifuged at 5,000 rpm for 20 min. The plasma was separated and stored at –21°C until drug analysis was carried out using HPLC.

Plasma samples were prepared by adding 500 µl of plasma, 50 µl standard solution of CXB, 50 µl of internal standard solution (ibuprofen), 50 µl of phosphate buffer (pH 5; 0.5 M), and 4 ml of chloroform in small glass tubes. The tubes were vortex for 1 min and centrifuged for 20 min at 5,000 rpm. Upper layer was discarded and the chloroform layer was transferred to a clean test tube and evaporated to dryness at 50°C under the stream of nitrogen. The residue was reconstituted in 100 µl of mobile phase, mixed well and 20 µl of the final clear solution was injected into the HPLC system.

The CXB in plasma was quantified by the reported HPLC method with slight modifications (Jalalizadeh et al., 2004). The method was validated in our laboratory. A Shimadzu model HPLC equipped with quaternary LC-10A VP pumps, variable wavelength programmable UV/VIS detector SPD-10AVP column oven (Shimadzu), SCL 10AVP system controller (Shimadzu), Rheodyne injector fitted with a 20 µl loop and Class-VP 5.032 software was used. Analysis was performed on a C_{18} column (25 cm × 4.6 mm ID SUPELCO 516 C_{18} DB 5 µm RP-HPLC). The mobile phase consisted of acetonitrile:water (40:60). The mobile phase was delivered at the flow rate of 0.9 ml/min. Detection was performed at 260 nm. Injection volume was 20 µl. The concentration of unknown plasma samples was calculated from the calibration curve plotted between peak area ratios of CXB to IS against corresponding CXB concentrations.

Pharmacokinetic and Statistical Analysis

The plasma concentration of CXB at different time intervals was subjected to pharmacokinetic (PK) analysis to calculate various parameters like maximum plasma concentration (C_{max}), time to reach maximum concentration (T_{max}), and area under the plasma concentration-time curve ($AUC_{0\to t}$ and $AUC_{0\to\omega}$). The values of C_{max} and T_{max} were read directly from the arithmetic plot of time and plasma concentration of CXB. The AUC was calculated by using the trapezoidal method. The relative bioavailability of the CXB after the transdermal administration versus the oral administration was calculated as follows:

$$F\% = \frac{AUC\ sample}{AUC\ oral} \cdot \frac{Dose\ oral}{Dose\ sample} \times 100$$

The PK data between different formulations was compared for statistical significance by one-way analysis of variance (ANOVA) followed by Tukey-Kramer multiple comparisons test using GraphPad Instat software (GraphPad Software Inc., CA, USA).

DISCUSSION AND RESULTS

Droplet Size Analysis

The mean droplet size of optimized nanoemulsion (C2) was found to be 16.41 ± 1.72 nm. All the droplets were found in the nanometer range which indicated the suitability of formulation for transdermal drug delivery. Polydispersity signifies the uniformity of droplet size within the formulation. The polydispersity value of the formulation C2 was very low (0.105) which indicated uniformity of droplet size within the formulation.

FTIR Spectral Analysis of Formulation Treated and Untreated Rat Skin

The FTIR spectrum of untreated SC (control) showed various peaks due to molecular vibration of proteins and lipids present in the SC (Figure 1a). The absorption bands in the wave number of 3,000–2,700 cm^{-1} were seen in untreated SC. These absorption bonds were due to the C-H stretching of the alkyl groups present in both proteins and lipids (Figure 1a). The bands at 2,920 cm^{-1} and 2,850 cm^{-1} were due to the asymmetric $-CH_2$ and symmetric $-CH_2$ vibrations of long chain hydrocarbons of lipids respectively. The bands at 2,955 cm^{-1} and 2,870 cm^{-1} were due to the asymmetric and symmetric CH_3 vibrations respectively (Babua and Pandit, 2005). These narrow bands were attributed to the long alkyl chains of fatty acids, ceramides and cholesterol which are the major components of the SC lipids.

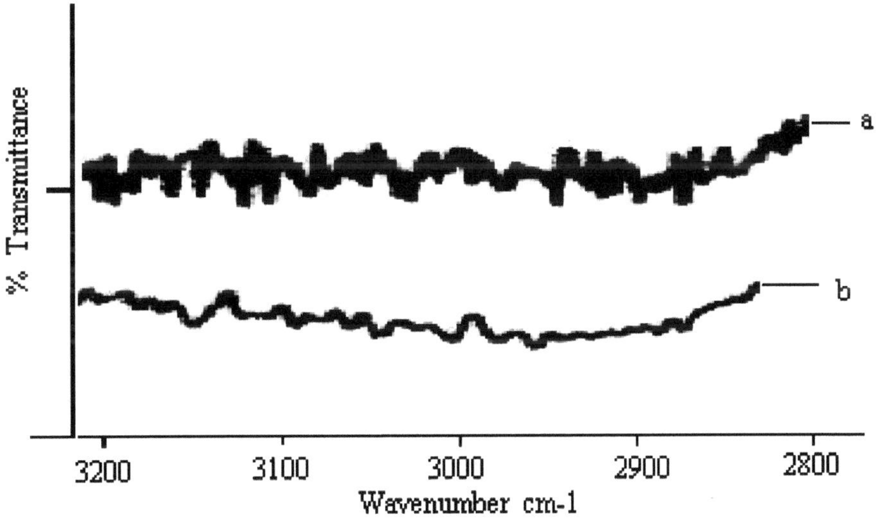

Figure 1. FTIR spectra of rat SC.
Change in lipid C-H stretching (2,920 cm^{-1}) vibrations after 24 hr treatment with (a) control (b) C2.

The two strong bands (1,650 cm^{-1} and 1,550 cm^{-1}) were due to the amide I and amide II stretching vibrations of SC proteins (Figure 2a). The amide I and amide II bands arisen from C = O stretching vibration and C-N bending vibration respectively. The amide I band consisting of components bands, represented various secondary structure of keratin.

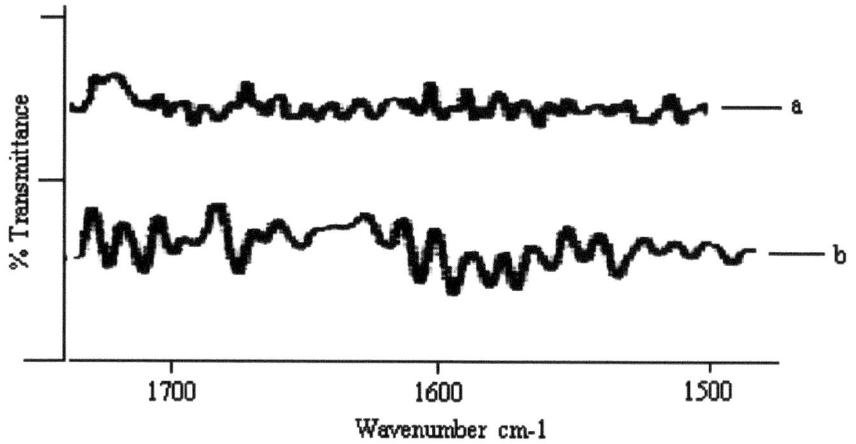

Figure 2. FTIR spectra of rat SC.
Change in amide I (1,640 cm^{-1}) and amide II (1,550 cm^{-1}) stretching vibrations after 24 hr treatment with (a) control (b) C2.

There was clear difference in the FTIR spectra of untreated and nanoemulsion treated SC with prominent decrease in asymmetric and symmetric CH- stretching of peak height and area (Figure 1b).

The rate limiting step for transdermal drug delivery is lipophilic part of SC in which lipids (ceramides) are tightly packed as bilayers due to the high degree of hydrogen bonding. The amide I group of ceramide is hydrogen bonded to amide II group of another ceramide and forming a tight network of hydrogen bonding at the head of ceramides. This hydrogen bonding makes stability and strength to lipid bilayers and thus imparts barrier property to SC (Panchagnula et al., 2005). When skin was treated with nanoemulsion formulation (C2), ceramides got loosened because of competitive hydrogen bonding leading to breaking of hydrogen bond networks at the head of ceramides due to penetration of nanoemulsion into the lipid bilayers of SC. The tight hydrogen bonding between ceramides caused split in the peak at 1,650 cm^{-1}(amide I) as shown in the control skin spectrum (Figure 2a). Treatment with nanoemulsion resulted in either double or single peak at 1,650 cm^{-1}(Figure 2b) which suggested breaking of hydrogen bonds by nanoemulsion.

DSC Studies

The DSC thermogram of untreated rat epidermis revealed four endotherms (Figure 3a). The first three endotherms were recorded at 34°C (T_1), 82°C (C2), and 105°C (T_3) respectively, whereas fourth endotherm (T_4) produced a very sharp and prominent peak at 114°C which is attributed to SC proteins. The first endotherm (having the lowest enthalpy) was attributed to sebaceous section (Lee et al., 2005) and to minor structural rearrangement of lipid bilayer (Xiong et al., 1996). The second and third endotherm (T_2 and T_3) appeared due to the melting of SC lipids and the fourth endotherm (T_4)

has been assigned to intracellular keratin denaturation (Goodman and Barry, 1989). It was observed that both T_2 and T_3 endotherms were completely disappeared or shifted to lower melting points in thermograms of SC treated with nanoemulsion formulation (C2). This indicated that the components (oil, surfactant or cosurfactant) of nanoemulsion enhanced skin permeation of CXB through disruption of lipid bilayers. Nanoemulsion formulation (C2) also decreased the protein endotherm T_4 to lower melting point, suggesting keratin denaturation and possible intracellular permeation mechanism in addition to the disruption of lipid bilayers (Figure 3b). Thus it was concluded that the intracellular transport is a possible mechanism of permeation enhancement of CXB. Another observation was that T_4 increased up to 122°C in case of nanoemulsion formulation with broadening of the peak. Shift to higher transition temperature (T_m) and peak broadening has been attributed to dehydration of SC as another mechanism of permeation enhancement in addition to disruption of lipid resulting in higher permeation of CXB (Vaddi et al., 2002).

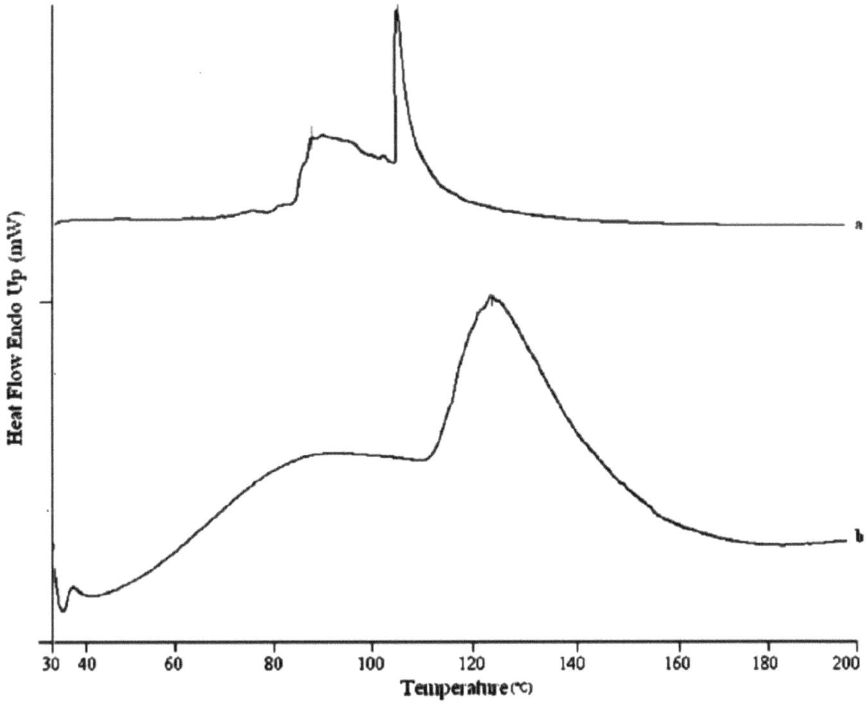

Figure 3. DSC thermogram of control SC and nanoemulsion treated SC for 24 hr. (a) control (b) C2.

Determination of Activation Energy

The activation energy (E_a) for diffusion of a drug molecule across skin (rat or human) depends on its route of diffusion and physicochemical properties. Nanoemulsions can change this value of E_a to greater extent by their action on SC lipids. The activation energy for ion transport has been reported as 4.1 and 10.7 kcal/mol across human epidermis (Pagano et al., 1968) and phosphatidylcholine bilayers respectively (Monti et al., 1995). The Arrhenius plot between logarithms of permeability coefficient (log P_b) and reciprocal of absolute temperature (1/T) was found to be linear in the selected temperature range between 27 and 47°C, indicating no significant structural or phase transition changes within the skin membrane (Figure 4). The value of E_a for permeation of CXB across rat skin was calculated from the slope of Arrhenius plot. The E_a of CXB from nanoemulsion formulation C2 was found to be 2.373 kcal/mol. The significant decrease in E_a for CXB permeation across rat skin indicated that the SC lipid bilayers were significantly disrupted ($p < 0.05$).

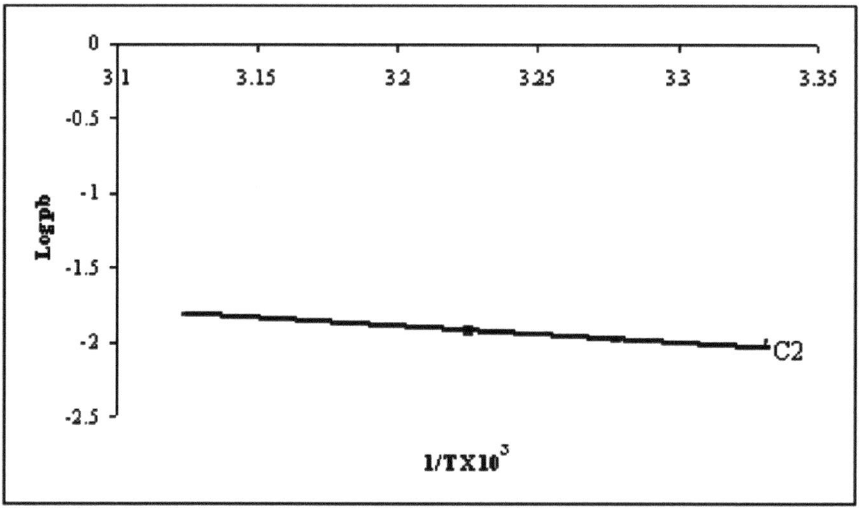

Figure 4. Arrhenius plots of C2 permeation across rat skin.

It is also well established that ion transport across skin occurs mainly via aqueous shunt pathways (Cullander and Guy, 1991). In the light of these reports it can be anticipated that if a molecule moves via polar pathways across human cadaver epidermis then E_a value would be akin to that of ion transport across skin. In our study, E_a of CXB from formulation C2 was 2.373 kcal/mol. Therefore it was concluded that nanoemulsions create pathways in the lipid bilayers of SC resulting in enhanced transdermal permeation of CXB (Clarys et al., 1998).

Histopathological Studies

The photomicrographs of control (untreated skin) showed normal skin with well defined epidermal and dermal layers. Keratin layer was well formed and lied just adjacent to the topmost layer of the epidermis. Dermis was devoid of any inflammatory cells. Skin appendages were within normal limits (Figures 5a, b). When the skin was treated with nanoemulsion formulation (C2) for 24 hr, significant changes were observed in the skin morphology. Low power photomicrograph of skin sample showed epidermis with a prominent keratin layer, a normal dermis and subcutaneous tissues. High power photomicrograph of skin sample showed a thickened and reduplicated stratum corneum with up to eight distinct layers. The epidermis showed increase in its cellular layers to four to six cells. Dermis does not show any edema or inflammatory cell infiltration. The disruption of lipid bilayers was clearly evident as distinct voids and empty spaces were visible in the epidermal region (Figures 6a, b). These observations support the *in vitro* skin permeation data of CXB (unpublished data).

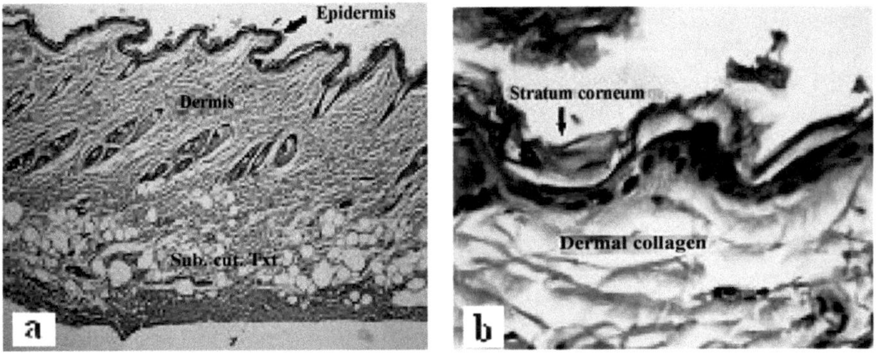

Figure 5. Photomicrographs of skin sample from control group animal showing normal epidermis, dermis and subcutaneous tissues at (a) low power view (HE Ч 100) (b) high power view (HE x 400).

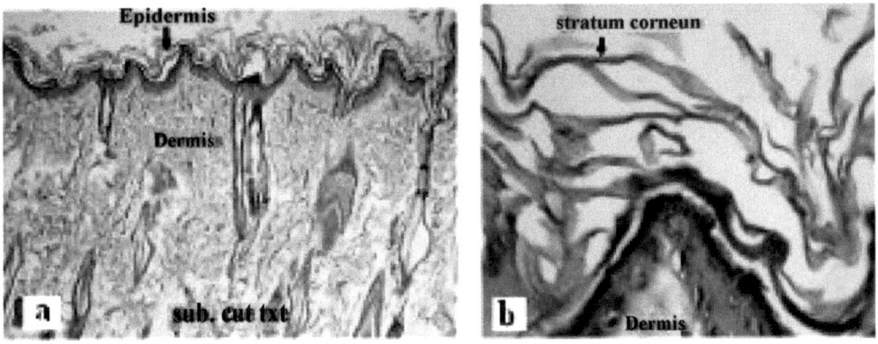

Figure 6. Photomicrographs of skin sample from nanoemulsion treated animal at (a) low power view (HE x 100) (b) high power view (HE x 400).

There were no apparent signs of skin irritation (erythma and edema etc.) observed on visual examination of skin specimens treated with nanoemulsion formulation.

Pharmacokinetic Studies

Plasma concentration of CXB from formulations C2, NGC2, and capsule at different time intervals was determined by reported HPLC method. The graph between plasma concentration and time was plotted for each formulation (Figure 7). It was seen from

Figure 7 that the plasma concentration profile of CXB for C2 and NGC2 showed greater improvement of drug absorption than the oral capsule formulation. Peak (maximum) plasma concentration (C_{max}) of CXB in C2, NGC2 and capsule was 680 ± 100, 610 ± 148, and 690 ± 180 ng/ml respectively whereas time (t_{max}) to reach C_{max} was 12 ± 2.1, 12 ± 2.4, and 3 ± 0.8 hr respectively (Table 2 and Figure 7). $AUC_{0\rightarrow t}$ and $AUC_{0\rightarrow\omega}$ in formulations C2, NGC2 and capsule were 14,435 ± 1,741, 13,005 ± 1,502, and 4,366 ± 1,015 ng/ml.h respectively and 19,711.3 ± 2,012, 17,507.3 ± 1,654, and 4,688.5 ± 1,293 ng/ml.h respectively (Table 2). These pharmacokinetic parameters obtained with formulations C2 and NGC2 were significantly different from those obtained with oral capsule formulation ($p < 0.05$). The significant AUC values observed with C2 and NGC2 also indicated increased bioavailability of the CXB from C2 and NGC2 in comparison with oral capsule formulation ($p < 0.05$). The formulations C2 and NGC2 were found to enhance the bioavailability of CXB by 3.30 and 2.97 folds (percent relative bioavailability 330 and 297) with reference to the oral capsule (Table 2). This increased bioavailability from transdermal formulations (C2 and NGC2) may be due to the enhanced skin permeation and avoidance of hepatic first pass metabolism.

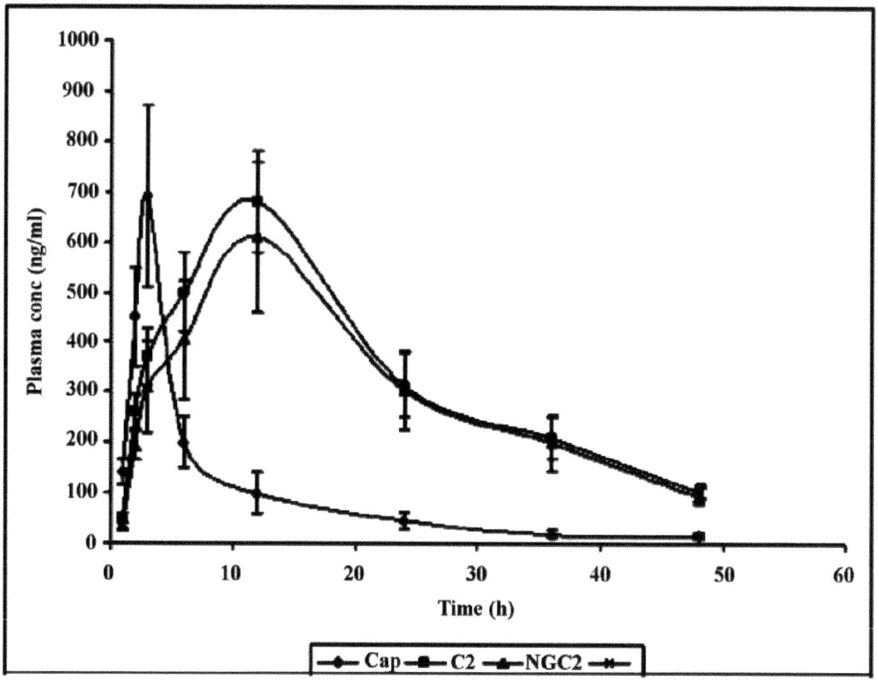

Figure 7. Plasma concentration (Mean ± SD) time profile curve of CXB from C2, NGC2, and capsule (n = 6).

Table 2. Pharmacokinetic parameters (Mean ± SD, n = 6) of CXB from C2, NGC2, and capsule.

Formulation	t_{max}^{a} **± SD (h)**	C_{max}^{b} **± SD (ng/ml)**	$AUC_{0\to t}^{c}$ **± SD (ng/ml.h)**	$AUC_{0\to \alpha}^{d}$ **± SD (ng/ml.h)**
C2	12 ± 1.8	680 ± 100	14435 ± 1741	19711.3 ± 2012
NGC2	12 ± 2.0	610 ± 148	13005 ± 1502	17507.3 ± 1654
Capsule	3 ± 0.8	690 ± 180	4366 ± 1015	4688.5 ± 1293

CONCLUSION

The FTIR spectra and DSC thermogram of skin treated with nanoemulsion indicated that permeation occurred due to the extraction of SC lipids by nanoemulsion. The significant decrease in activation energy for CXB permeation across rat skin indicates that the SC lipid bilayers were significantly disrupted ($p < 0.05$). Photomicrograph of skin sample showed the disruption and extraction of lipid bilayers as distinct voids and empty spaces were visible in the epidermal region. There were no apparent signs of skin irritation observed on visual examination of skin specimens treated with nanoemulsion formulation. The pharmacokinetic studies revealed significantly greater extent of absorption than the oral capsule formulation ($p < 0.05$). The absorption of CXB from C2 and NGC2 resulted in 3.30 and 2.97-fold increases in bioavailability as compared to the oral capsule formulation. Results of these studies indicate that nanoemulsions can be successfully used for enhancement of skin permeation as well as bioavailability of poorly soluble drugs.

KEYWORDS

- **Celecoxib**
- **Differential scanning calorimeter**
- **Fourier transform infra-red**
- **Nanoemulsions gel**
- **Pharmacokinetic**
- **Stratum corneum**

AUTHORS' CONTRIBUTIONS

Faiyaz Shakeel performed pharmacokinetic studies. Sanjula Baboota and Alka Ahuja prepared skin for histopathological examination and activation energy measurement. Javed Ali took FTIR spectra and DSC thermogram. Sheikh Shafiq validated HPLC method for analysis of drug in plasma samples. Sanjula Baboota, Alka Ahuja, and Javed Ali guided the studies. Finally manuscript has been checked and approved by all the authors.

ACKNOWLEDGMENTS

The authors are thankful to Dr. Ashok Mukherjee, for observation and interpretation of photomicrographs of skin samples. The authors are also thankful to Nikko Chemicals (Japan) and Gattefosse (France) for gift samples of Sefsol 218 and Transcutol-P respectively.

COMPETING INTERESTS

The authors declare that they have no competing interests.

Chapter 12

Raft-dependent Endocytosis of Autocrine Motility Factor/Phosphoglucose Isomerase

Liliana D. Kojic, Sam M. Wiseman, Fariba Ghaidi, Bharat Joshi, Hinyu Nedev, H. Uri Saragovi, and Ivan R. Nabi

INTRODUCTION

Autocrine motility factor/phosphoglucose isomerase (AMF/PGI) is the extracellular ligand for the gp78/AMFR receptor over-expressed in a variety of human cancers. We showed previously that raft-dependent internalization of AMF/PGI is elevated in metastatic MDA-435 cells, but not metastatic, caveolin-1-expressing MDA-231 cells, relative to non-metastatic MCF7, and dysplastic MCF10A cells suggesting that it might represent a tumor cell-specific endocytic pathway.

Similarly, using flow cytometry, we demonstrate that raft-dependent endocytosis of AMF/PGI is increased in metastatic human colon adenocarcinoma grade II cell line (HT29) cancer cells expressing low levels of caveolin-1 relative to metastatic, caveolin-1-expressing, human **colon** tumor (HCT116) colon cells and non-metastatic Caco-2 cells. Therefore, we exploited the raft-dependent internalization of AMF/PGI as a potential tumor-cell specific targeting mechanism. We synthesized an AMF/PGI-paclitaxel conjugate and found it to be as efficient as free paclitaxel in inducing cytotoxicity and apoptosis in tumor cells that readily internalize AMF/PGI compared to tumor cells that poorly internalize AMF/PGI. Murine K1735-M1 and B16-F1 melanoma cells internalize FITC-conjugated AMF/PGI and are acutely sensitive to AMF/PGI-paclitaxel mediated cytotoxicity *in vitro*. Moreover, following *in vivo* intratumoral (i.t.) injection, FITC-conjugated AMF/PGI is internalized in K1735-M1 tumors. The i.t. injection of AMF/PGI-paclitaxel induced significantly higher tumor regression compared to free paclitaxel, even in B16-F1 cells, known to be resistant to taxol treatment. Treatment with AMF/PGI-paclitaxel significantly prolonged the median survival time (MST) of tumor bearing mice. Free AMF/PGI exhibited a pro-survival role, reducing the cytotoxic effect of both AMF/PGI-paclitaxel and free paclitaxel suggesting that AMF/PGI-paclitaxel targets a pathway associated with resistance to chemotherapeutic agents. The AMF/PGI-FITC uptake by normal murine spleen and thymus cells was negligible both *in vitro* and following intravenous (i.v.) injection *in vivo* where AMF/PGI-FITC was selectively internalized by subcutaneous B16-F1 tumor cells. The raft-dependent endocytosis of AMF/PGI may therefore represent a tumor cell specific endocytic pathway of potential value for drug delivery to tumor cells.

Endocytosis is the general mechanism by which cells regulate entry of external substances into the cell and represents an important route for delivery of targeted therapeutics for a variety of pathologies including cancer (Bareford and Swaan, 2007).

Clathrin-mediated endocytosis represents the best characterized endocytic pathway, however a number of clathrin-independent endocytic routes, in particular raft-dependent pathways, have recently come under intense scrutiny. Various raft pathways showing differential caveolin, dynamin, and small G protein dependence have been characterized and shown to be coopted by various viruses, toxins, and extracellular pathogens (Kirkham and Parton, 2005; Lajoie and Nabi, 2007; Marsh and Helenius, 2006). Caveolae-mediated uptake is a well-characterized endocytic mechanism in endothelial cells (Predescu et al., 2007), but whether other raft-dependent pathways represent selective portals into specific cell types, such as tumor cells, remains to be demonstrated.

A novel promising target for anti-cancer agents is the receptor for AMF/PGI, known as gp78/AMFR, that was recently identified as one of 189 genes mutated at significant frequency in breast and colorectal cancer (Sjoblom et al., 2006). Increased expression of gp78/AMFR in human cancers is significantly correlated with more advanced tumor stage and decreased patient survival (Chiu et al., 2008). The gp78/AMFR is the cell surface receptor for AMF/PGI and also an E3 ubiquitin ligase localized to a distinct mitochondria-associated smooth subdomain of the endoplasmic reticulum (Benlimame et al., 1995; Goetz and Nabi, 2006; Goetz et al., 2007; Wang et al., 2000). The recent identification of the KAI1 metastasis suppressor as a gp78/AMFR endoplasmic reticulum-associated degradation (ERAD) substrate strongly supports a role for gp78/AMFR up-regulation in metastasis promotion (Tsai et al., 2007).

The AMF/PGI is a glycolytic enzyme that has been shown to exhibit extracellular cytokine function, under the aliases neuroleukin, maturation factor and AMF, targeting neurons, lymphocytes, and cancer cells, respectively (Chaput et al., 1988; Faik et al., 1988; Gurney et al, 1986a, 1986b; Watanabe et al., 1996; Xu et al., 1996). The AMF/PGI is selectively secreted by transformed cell lines and has been extensively implicated in the autocrine stimulation of tumor cell motility and proliferation through activation of PKC, Rho, Rho-GDI, and p27Kip1 inducing reorganization of focal contacts and loss of E-cadherin via upregulation of the E-cadherin transcription repressor Snail (Kanbe et al., 1994; Liotta et al., 1986; Niinaka et al., 1998; Silletti et al., 1996; Tsutsumi et al, 2002, 2004; Yanagawa et al., 2004). The AMF/PGI exhibits anti-apoptotic activity by downregulating, apoptotic protease activating factor (1Apaf-1) and caspase-9 expression (Haga et al., 2003). The AMF/PGI is also an angiogenic factor, whose expression is induced under hypoxic conditions in response to expression of HIF-1, and crosstalk between AMF/PGI and vascular endothelial growth factor (VEGF) regulates both induction of AMF/PGI and AMF/PGI promotion of angiogenesis (Funasaka et al., 2001, 2002, 2005). The AMF/PGI overexpression induces cellular transformation and promotes tumorigenicity as well as the formation of larger tumors and metastases upon orthotopic implantation of PaCa-2 pancreatic tumor cells, while partial AMF/PGI knockdown induces cellular senescence (Funasaka et al., 2007; Tsutsumi et al., 2003, 2004). Increased AMF/PGI levels in the urine and serum of cancer patients is associated with the presence of colorectal, breast, lung, kidney, and gastrointestinal carcinomas (Baumann et al., 1990; Bodansky, 1954; Filella et al., 1991; Guirguis et al., 1990; Patel et al., 1995; Schwartz, 1973). Expression of both AMF/PGI and gp78/AMFR are therefore strongly associated with tumor progression and metastasis.

Upon binding of AMF/PGI to cell surface gp78/AMFR, it is endocytosed via a dynamin-dependent raft pathway to the smooth endoplasmic reticulum that is negatively regulated by expression of Cav1 (Benlimame et al., 1998; Le et al, 2002). This pathway is distinct from that followed by GM1 ganglioside bound cholera toxin b-subunit (Ct-b) and appears to represent a unique pathway in that it targets directly the smooth endoplasmic reticulum (Lajoie and Nabi, 2003, 2007) The raft-dependent endocytosis of AMF/PGI is upregulated in Ras- and Abl-transformed NIH-3T3 cells that express reduced levels of the raft-associated protein caveolin-1 (Cav1) (Le et al., 2002). Metastatic breast tumor cell lines show increased cell surface gp78/AMFR expression, however AMF/PGI uptake was increased only in metastatic MDA-435 cells that express gp78/AMFR and reduced Cav1 levels and not in MDA-231 cells expressing both gp78/AMFR and high levels of Cav1 (Kojic et al., 2007). The raft-dependent endocytosis of AMF/PGI to the smooth endoplasmic reticulum may therefore represent a specific endocytic pathway for the selective targeting of gp78/AMFR-positive, Cav1-deficient tumors.

In this study, we show that raft-dependent uptake of AMF/PGI is specific for gp78/AMFR-positive/Cav1-negative metastatic colon cancer cells, do not target normal immune cells and occur *in vivo* in subcutaneous K1735-M1 and B16-F1 melanoma tumor models. In addition, we have synthesized and characterized a novel AMF/PGI-paclitaxel conjugate that shows increased tumor selectivity and cytotoxicity compared to free paclitaxel and targets and kills AMF/PGI-internalizing cells, both *in vitro* and *in vivo*. The i.t. injection of AMF/PGI-paclitaxel induced tumor regression and increased survival of tumor bearing mice, identifying AMF/PGI-paclitaxel as a potential targeted therapeutic agent for gp78/AMFR-positive cancers.

MATERIALS AND METHODS

Antibodies and Reagents

Monoclonal rat IgM antibody against gp78/AMFR (3F3A) was used in the form of ascites fluid (Nabi et al., 1990). Rabbit anti-Cav1/2 antibody was purchased from Transduction Laboratories (Greenland, NH) and rabbit anti-pAkt and Akt from Cell Signaling (Danvers, MA). Alexa-488 and Alexa-647 conjugated anti-rat secondary antibodies and Alexa-568-conjugated phalloidin were purchased from Molecular Probes (Eugene, OR). Rhodamine-red-X anti-rat IgM was from Jackson Immunoresearch Laboratories (West Grove, PA) and ACK buffer from Cambrex Bio Science (Walkersville, MD). Methyl-β-cyclodextrin (mβCD), genistein, FITC-conjugated transferrin (Tf-FITC), rabbit PGI (Type XI), propidium iodide (PI), paclitaxel, staurosporin, goat serum, and pronase (from *Streptomyces griseus*, Type XIV) were purchased from Sigma (St. Louis, MO). Annexin V-FITC apoptosis detection kit was purchased from BD Pharmingen. AMF/PGI was conjugated to fluorescein with the Fluorescein-EX protein labeling kit (Molecular Probes).

Synthesis of 2′-Glutaryl-Paclitaxel and Conjugation to AMF/PGI

The 2′-Glutaryl-paclitaxel was synthesized by mixing 39 μM paclitaxel with 3 μM glutaric anhydride each dissolved in pyridine for 3 hr at room temperature (Guillemard and Saragovi, 2001). This reaction forms an ester bond at the C2′ position of paclitaxel. The solvent was then removed *in vacuo*, and the residue was dissolved in $CHCl_3$ and washed with double-distilled H_2O. Purification was achieved by high-performance liquid chromatography on a semipreparative column (Phenomenex); the mobile phase consisted of acetonitrile:water gradient from 35:65 to 75:25 over 50 min.

The 2′-Glutaryl-paclitaxel (1.334 nM) was then derivatized with N,N′-carbonyldiimidazole (13.34 nM; Sigma) for 25 min at 45°C. The carbodiimide reaction activates a carboxylic group on 2′-glutaryl-paclitaxel by removing a hydroxyl. Then, AMF/PGI was added slowly over a 20 min period at room temperature at a 2:1 molar ratio of paclitaxel:AMF/PGI, and the reaction proceeded for 16 hr at 4°C. The reaction forms an AMF/PGI-paclitaxel conjugate via formation of a peptide bond with amino groups in the protein. The solution was then dialyzed for 2 hr against water and overnight against phosphate buffered saline (PBS).

To quantify conjugated paclitaxel, a known mass of AMF/PGI-paclitaxel conjugate was incubated for 48 hr at room temperature in 0.1 M acetate buffer (pH 4) to hydrolyze ester bonds. Paclitaxel was then extracted with chloroform and evaporated to dryness. Quantification of this purified paclitaxel was done by analytical high-performance liquid chromatography (Phenomenex) on a mobile phase of acetonitrile:water from 35:65 to 75:25 over 40 min. Known concentrations of paclitaxel were used as standard control. The measured molar ratio of protein:coupled paclitaxel to AMF/PGI dimer was 4.3:1 (Guillemard and Saragovi, 2001).

Cell Lines and Primary Cells

The Caco-2, HCT116, HT29, MCF7, and MDA-435 were obtained from American Type Culture Collection (ATCC, Manassas, VA) and maintained in complete RPMI 1640 supplemented with 10% fetal bovine serum. The highly metastatic murine melanoma K1735 clone M1 (K1735-M1) was kindly provided by Dr. I. Fidler, M.D. Anderson Cancer Center, Houston, TX). The K1735-M1 and B16-F1 (Nabi and Raz, 1987) cells were maintained in DMEM supplemented with 10% fetal bovine serum. To minimize phenotypic drift, all cell lines were passaged two to three times after recovery from frozen stocks before initiating the experiments and maintained in culture for a maximum of eight to 10 passages.

Primary cells were obtained from mice euthanized by CO_2 asphyxiation and perfused with 0.6 mM EDTA in PBS prior to organ collection. Spleen, thymus and brain tissue was collected and placed in ice-cold PBS/2%FBS. Single cell suspensions were treated with ACK buffer to lyse the red blood cells. An enriched population of spleen macrophages was obtained by incubating spleen suspensions at 37°C and removing non-adherent cells after 3 hr.

Experimental Animals

Six to 10-week-old C3H/HeN (MTV-) and C57/BL6 specific pathogen-free female mice were purchased from Charles River Laboratories (Wilmington, MA) and used for *in vivo* studies. Mice were housed four per cage and maintained under pathogen-free conditions according to international and institutional guidelines. Ambient light was regulated on a 12 hr light–dark cycle. Animals were cared for and used in accordance with protocols (#A04-0360) approved by the Animal Care Committee of the University of British Columbia.

Immunofluorescence Labeling, Flow Cytometry and Western Blotting

Western blotting and flow cytometry of cell surface gp78/AMFR expression and AMF/PGI-FITC internalization, were performed as previously described (Kojic et al., 2007). For uptake studies, cells were incubated with 25 μg/ml AMF/PGI-FITC, or 15 μg/ml Tf-FITC for 30 min at 37°C. Cell surface-bound conjugate was removed with pronase (400 μg/ml) for 10 min. Where indicated, cells were pretreated for 30 min at 37°C with 5 mM mßCD, 100 μg/ml genistein, or 1 mg/ml AMF/PGI and treatments were maintained during incubation with AMF/PGI-FITC. For flow cytometry, at least 50,000 cells were acquired and analyzed using FACSCalibur and Cellquest software (BD Biosciences). Confocal microscopy was performed with the 100× Plan Apochromat objective of an Olympus FV1000 confocal microscope.

In Vitro Growth Inhibition

The growth-inhibitory effects of AMF/PGI-paclitaxel conjugate and free paclitaxel was quantified by measuring cell viability using a crystal violet colorimetric assay (Nabi et al., 1990). Cells were seeded at 5×10^3 cells/well in 96-well microtiter plates and allowed to attach overnight. Paclitaxel was dissolved in dimethyl sulfoxide (DMSO) as a stock concentration of 5 mg/ml. Serial dilutions of either free paclitaxel, or an equimolar paclitaxel concentration of AMF/PGI-paclitaxel conjugate were made with growth medium and added to the wells to achieve concentrations of 0–1,000 nM. Control cells received the same amount of the diluent. Competition of AMF/PGI-paclitaxel growth-inhibition potency was done by adding a 20-fold excess of AMF/PGI to the treated cells. Cell growth inhibition was quantified after 48 hr. Quadruplicate cultures were analyzed in three separate experiments and the results are presented as a percentage of treated versus untreated control cells, considering untreated cells as 100% control values.

In Vitro Apoptosis Assay

To detect apoptosis, cells were treated with the indicated concentration of AMF/PGI-paclitaxel, free paclitaxel, or staurosporine for 48 and 24 hr, respectively. After that, cells were trypsinized, double-stained with Annexin V-FITC and 7-aminoactinomycin (7-ADD) according to the manufacturer's instructions (Annexin V-FITC apoptosis detection kit, BD Parmingen) and analyzed by dual-color flow cytometry. Cells staining positive for Annexin V-FITC but not 7-ADD were considered apoptotic. The loss of cell viability in the analyzed cells was confirmed by propidium iodine (PI) staining.

In Vivo Uptake of AMF/PGI-FITC Conjugate

For *in vivo* uptake studies, syngeneic C3H/HeN mice were injected subcutaneous (s.c.) with K1735-M1 tumor cells (1×10^6 in 50 μl sterile PBS) into the lower flanks near the rib cage. Tumor growth was recorded every other day and when established tumors reached a diameter of 8–10 mm, mice were anesthetized by intraperitoneal (i.p.) injection of ketamine and received i.t. 50 μl injections of either PBS or FITC-conjugated AMF/PGI in PBS. After 6 hr, the animals were sacrificed and tumors excised, weighed, embedded in OCT, quickly frozen and stored at −80°C. The 10 μm thick sections were stained with Hoechst and Alexa568-phalloidin fluorescence and analyzed with an Olympus FV1000 confocal microscopy. To obtain single cell suspensions, the tumors were cut into small pieces in ice cold PBS, resuspended vigorously, pelleted and incubated for 10 min at 37°C in PBS containing pronase (0.4 mg/ml). Tumor cell suspensions were analyzed by flow cytometry for presence of AMF/PGI-FITC positive cells.

In Vivo Efficacy Studies

The C3H/HeN mice were injected s.c. with K1735-M1 mouse melanoma cells and tumor growth was recorded every other day. Tumor nodules were allowed to grow for approximately 11–13 days and the length and width of the tumors were measured by digital calipers, calculating tumor volume by the following formula: length × width2 × Π/6. At this time mice were randomized such that each group had a mean starting tumor volume of 40–50 mm^3 prior to treatment. Mice were divided into four experimental groups with eight mice in each of them: mice in control group received 50 μl diluent (PBS-DMSO); mice in second group received 50 μl free paclitaxel (300 ng/injection); mice in the third group received free paclitaxel (300 ng) and AMF/PGI (18 μg); and mice in group four received AMF/PGI-paclitaxel conjugate (300 ng of paclitaxel-equivalent and 18 μg of AMF/PGI).

The C57/BL6 mice were injected s.c. with B16-F1 (0.5×10^6 in 50 μl sterile PBS) mouse melanoma cells. Well-defined s.c. tumors were formed after 11–12 days, at which time mice were randomized such that each group had a mean starting tumor volume of approximately 60 mm^3. Mice were divided into five experimental groups with 10 mice in each of them: mice in the control group received 50 μl diluent (PBS-DMSO); mice in the second group received 50 μl free paclitaxel (300 ng/injection); mice in the third group received free paclitaxel (300 ng) and AMF/PGI (18 μg); mice in the fourth group received AMF/PGI-paclitaxel conjugate (300 ng of paclitaxel-equivalent and 18 μg of AMF/PGI); and mice in the fifth group received free AMF/PGI (18 μg) concomitantly with AMF/PGI-paclitaxel conjugate.

Animals received a total of five consecutive daily i.t. injections with a 21-gauge needle placed in the center of the tumors. The i.t. injections were infused over 10–15 sec, and the needle was allowed to remain in place for an additional 15–20 sec before removal. After the treatments, all mice were tagged, and tumors were measured three times per week. Animals were weighed at the time of tumor measurement. Mice were monitored for a maximum of 40 days, until the tumor was completely regressed, or until the tumor volume exceeded 10 × 12 mm in diameter, for which the mice were euthanized for excessive tumor load. Then, the excised tumors were resected, weighed, embedded in OCT, quickly frozen and stored at −80°C.

The gp78/AMFR Immunolabeling of Mouse Tissues

Mouse organs, K1735-M1 and B16-F1 tumors were quickly frozen in ornithine carbamyl transferase (OCT; Tissue-Tek, Miles, Elkhart, IN) and stored at −80°C. Human

HCT116 colon carcinoma xenografts and 5-day-old mouse brain sections were kindly provided by Dr. Cal Roskelley and Dr. Tim O'Connor, respectively (Dept. of Cellular and Physiological Sciences, University of British Columbia). Serial frozen sections were cut at 7 μm, fixed in ice-cold methanol for 10 min followed by a short rinse in phosphate-buffered saline. Endogenous peroxidase activity was blocked with 3% H_2O_2 in methanol and non-specific adsorption minimized by pre-incubating the sections in 10% normal rabbit serum/0.3% Triton X-100 in PBS for 20 min. The sections were then incubated for 60 min with anti-gp78/AMFR (1:25), followed by 30 min incubation with rabbit anti-rat IgM-biotinylated secondary antibody (1:1,000). Bound antibody was detected using the avidin biotin complex (ABC Elite kit; Vector Laboratories, Burlingame, CA) with diaminobenzidine (DAB) as a substrate. All sections were stained simultaneously at room temperature. Control sections were treated in the same way with omission of primary antibody. Tissues were counterstained with hematoxylin/eosin solution.

In Vivo Targeting of Fluorescently Labeled AMF/PGI

The C57/BL6 mice were injected s.c. with B16-F1 (0.5×10^6 in 50 μl sterile PBS) mouse melanoma cells. At day 12 after implantation, tumors reached ~60 mm^3 in size, at which point mice were administered AMF/PGI-FITC (250 ug/ml), free FITC or PBS alone i.v. through the tail vein. Two hours later the mice were terminated, tumors, spleens, and thymuses collected, processed as single cell suspensions, treated with pronase, and analyzed by flow cytometry for intracellular uptake of the FITC label.

Statistical Analysis

Unless otherwise stated, all values are presented as mean ± SEM (standard error of the mean) and are representative of at least three independent experiments each performed in duplicate. Statistical significance was calculated using the Student t-test for paired comparison; $p < 0.05$ was considered statistically significant.

DISCUSSION

Tumor heterogeneity is a hallmark of neoplastic disease. Tumor-specific therapies, targeting specific molecular characteristics of human malignancies through a prescreening process, have increasingly become adopted into clinical practice. The AMF/PGI represents an ideal carrier for drug delivery in that it is a native protein circulating at high levels in serum (Baumann et al., 1990; Bodansky, 1954; Filella et al., 1991; Guirguis et al., 1990; Patelet al., 1995; Schwartz 1973), is the ligand for a receptor, gp78/AMFR, significantly associated with malignancy in a broad range of human cancer types (Chiu et al., 2008) and is internalized via a distinct, tumor-associated raft-dependent endocytic pathway (Guillemard and Saragovi, 2001; Kojic et al., 2007). The demonstration here of upregulated gp78/AMFR expression and increased AMF/PGI uptake by tumor cells relative to normal immune cells further supports the tumor specificity of the raft-dependent endocytosis of AMF/PGI. The lack of gp78/AMFR expression in adult thymus and spleen is consistent with previous reports of the reduced expression of gp78/AMFR in adult brain relative to developing brain (Leclerc et al.,

2000). This suggests that gp78/AMFR expression may be enhanced during development and that the role of AMF/PGI in lymphocyte maturation (Gurney et al., 1986) may be absent or limited in normal adult immune tissue. Therefore, while AMF/PGI is a ubiquitous cytokine with multiple cellular targets, increased gp78/AMFR expression in cancer and low expression in normal adult tissue, suggests that circulating AMF/PGI may preferentially interact with gp78/AMFR expressing tumor cells relative to normal cells.

Selectivity of the AMF/PGI raft-dependent pathway for tumor cells is certainly related to expression of its receptor by target cells. However, the sorting mechanism that segregates AMF/PGI-internalizing rafts from other endocytic raft domains and delivers internalized AMF/PGI to the smooth endoplasmic reticulum remains unclear. The selective uptake of AMF/PGI, amongst other studied raft endocytic ligands, via this pathway to the smooth endoplasmic reticulum is consistent with a role for AMF/PGI binding in raft domain segregation and endocytosis. The role of Cav1 as a negative regulator of raft-dependent uptake of AMF/PGI in tumor cells (Kojic et al., 2007; Le et al., 2002) is supported here by the demonstration that metastatic Cav1-expressing HCT116 colon tumor cells show reduced uptake of AMF/PGI relative to HT29 cells. Compilation of data obtained on the same breast cancer tissue microarray probed with antibodies to gp78/AMFR and Cav1 (Joshi et al., 2008; Kojic et al., 2007) shows that gp78/AMFR and Cav1 tumor cohorts do not correlate with one another ($p = 0.421$). Together with the lack of gp78/AMFR correlation with HER2 (Kojic et al., 2007), this suggests that gp78/AMFR labeling defines a substantial cohort of tumors that cannot be treated with HER2-targeted therapy and that should, in the absence of Cav1, internalize AMF/PGI.

Cav1 may function to sequester critical effectors that regulate the raft-dependent endocytosis of AMF/PGI (Lajoie and Nabi, 2007). The positive correlation of gp78/AMFR and pAkt expression in an invasive breast cancer tumor cohort, the PI3K sensitivity of AMF/PGI uptake and the ability of AMF/PGI to stimulate PI3K-dependent cell survival suggests that PI3K is such an effector (Kojic et al., 2007; Tsutsumi et al., 2003). However, the relationship between raft-dependent AMF/PGI uptake and its role as a pro-survival factor remains to be determined. The ability of free AMF/PGI to protect cells from cell death induced not only by AMF/PGI-paclitaxel but also by free paclitaxel suggests that AMF/PGI may be generally exerting a pro-survival effect on tumor cells. Paclitaxel is a common clinically utilized chemotherapeutic drug and elevated levels of circulating AMF/PGI in cancer patients may therefore function to suppress its pro-apoptotic effects, and potentially have similar effects on other chemotherapeutic drugs. The AMF/PGI-paclitaxel may therefore be targeting a PI3K/Akt-dependent pathway that is critical for tumor cell survival and promotes resistance to commonly employed chemotherapeutic drugs. Indeed, the ability of AMF/PGI-paclitaxel to suppress the proliferation of paclitaxel-resistant B16-F1 melanoma cells *in vitro* and to significantly delay B16-F1 tumor growth *in vivo*, suggests that it may bypass or override the drug resistance of these cells.

Paclitaxel is an established chemotherapeutic drug and has been shown to be efficacious when conjugated to various anti-cancer agents (Guillemard and Saragovi, 2004). The data presented here demonstrate that AMF/PGI can mediate drug delivery to gp78/AMFR expressing tumor cells *in vitro* and *in vivo*. Use of AMF/PGI as a carrier of a chemotherapeutic drug represents a novel therapeutic approach unique in that, firstly, it utilizes a native circulating protein that should not elicit an immune response and, secondly, it targets a receptor that is over-expressed and actively internalized via a distinct endocytic pathway by specific cancers. Use of AMF/PGI thereby addresses a major challenge for targeted therapeutics, designing a carrier system for effective intracellular drug delivery. The ability of AMF/PGI-paclitaxel to induce tumor regression and promote survival upon i.t. of K1735-M1 and B16-F1 tumors identifies the raft-dependent endocytosis of AMF/PGI as a novel drug delivery route for tumor cells. AMF/PGI-paclitaxel is therefore a potential therapeutic agent for targeted treatment of select cohorts of tumors resistant to currently utilized chemotherapeutic drugs.

RESULTS

gp78/AMFR Expression and AMF/PGI Internalization in Human Colon Carcinoma Cell Lines

We previously showed that gp78/AMFR expression was elevated in metastatic MDA-435 and MDA-231 cells relative to non-metastatic MCF-7 and dysplastic MCF10A mammary tumor cells and that AMF/PGI-FITC uptake was selectively increased in MDA-435 cells that express reduced levels of Cav1 (Kojic et al., 2007). We have now expanded these studies to three human epithelial colon cancer cell lines, non-metastatic Caco-2 and metastatic HCT116 and HT29 cells. By western blot, significant gp78/AMFR protein expression was detected in invasive HCT116 and HT29 colon cancer cell lines and was very low in Caco-2 cells. Expression of caveolin (Cav1/2) was elevated in HCT116 cells and was minimal in HT29 and Caco-2 cells (Figure 1A). Flow cytometry analysis confirmed abundant cell surface gp78/AMFR expression in metastatic HCT116 and HT29 cells with reduced expression in Caco-2 cells (Figure 1B). Following incubation of the cells with 25 μg/ml AMF/PGI-FITC for 30 min at 37°C, AMF/PGI-FITC was abundantly internalized in gp78/AMFR-positive/Cav1-negative HT29 cells relative to the other colon cell lines (Figure 1B), as determined by flow cytometry. HT29 cells showed significant uptake of AMF/PGI-FITC both in terms of percentage of AMF/PGI-FITC positive cells and mean fluorescence intensity. The AMF/PGI-FITC uptake was slightly increased in HCT116 relative to Caco-2 cells but was significantly lower compared with HT29 cells. Immunofluorescence analysis shows that AMF/PGI-FITC was internalized selectively by HT29 cells to the anti-gp78/AMFR labeled smooth endoplasmic reticulum (Figure 1C). Increased uptake of AMF/PGI-FITC in metastatic colon carcinoma cells is therefore inversely correlated with caveolin expression.

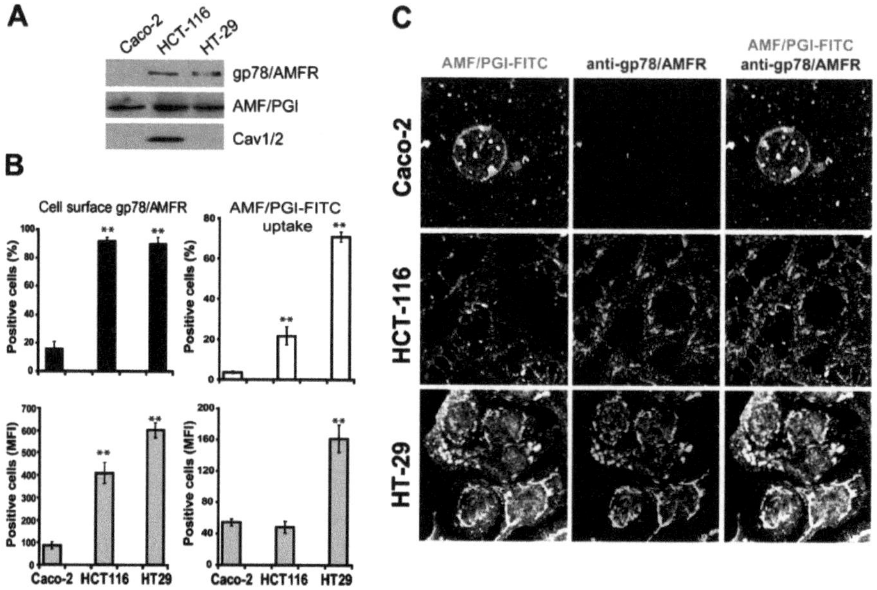

Figure 1. The Gp78/AMFR surface expression and AMF/PGI-FITC endocytosis in human colon tumor cells. (A). TX-100 soluble fractions from Caco-2, HCT116, and HT29 colon cell lines were analyzed by western blot for gp78/AMFR, AMF/PGI, Cav1/2, and β-actin, as indicated. (B). Caco-2, HCT116, and HT29 human colon tumor cells were profiled for surface expression of gp78/AMFR and for AMF/PGI-FITC uptake and analyzed by flow cytometry. Cells were labeled with 3F3A primary antibody followed by Alexa-647 conjugated secondary antibody. Alternatively, the cells were incubated for 30 min at 37°C in the presence of AMF/PGI-FITC and flow cytometry of AMF/PGI-FITC uptake performed after 10 min incubation in DMEM containing pronase (400 μg/ml). Relative quantitative analysis of the percentage of positive cells (top graph) and changes in the Mean Fluorescence Intensity (MFI) (bottom graph) are shown. The data represent the average of at least three separate experiments (mean ± SEM; **, $P \leq 0.001$, relative to Caco-2 cells). (C) Caco-2, HCT116, and HT29 human colon tumor cells were incubated with 25 μg/ml AMF/PGI-FITC for 30 min prior to fixation and labeling with the 3F3A anti-gp78/AMFR monoclonal antibody followed by appropriate secondary antibodies and analyzed by confocal microscopy. The AMF/PGI-FITC labeling is presented in green and the anti-gp78/AMFR labeled smooth endoplasmic reticulum in red.

Cholesterol extraction with mβCD and inhibition of tyrosine kinases with genistein (Le and Nabi, 2003) inhibited the raft-dependent endocytosis of AMF/PGI-FITC in HT29 cells (Figure 2A). Furthermore, unlabeled AMF/PGI competed for AMF/PGI-FITC uptake confirming that uptake in these cell lines is receptor-mediated (Figure 2A). Neither mβCD nor genistein had any impact on the clathrin-dependent uptake of transferrin or cell surface gp78/AMFR expression (Figure 2A). Pretreatment of HT29 cells with these agents also disrupted delivery of AMF/PGI-FITC to the smooth endoplasmic reticulum (Figure 2B). Adenoviral overexpression of Cav1 and the dynamin-K44A mutant but not the clathrin hub, or wild-type dynamin, inhibited AMF/PGI-FITC uptake in HT29 cells (Figure 2C). The receptor-mediated, dynamin-dependent uptake of AMF/PGI-FITC via a raft-dependent endocytic pathway to the smooth endoplasmic reticulum is therefore elevated in metastatic colon carcinoma cells expressing low levels of caveolin.

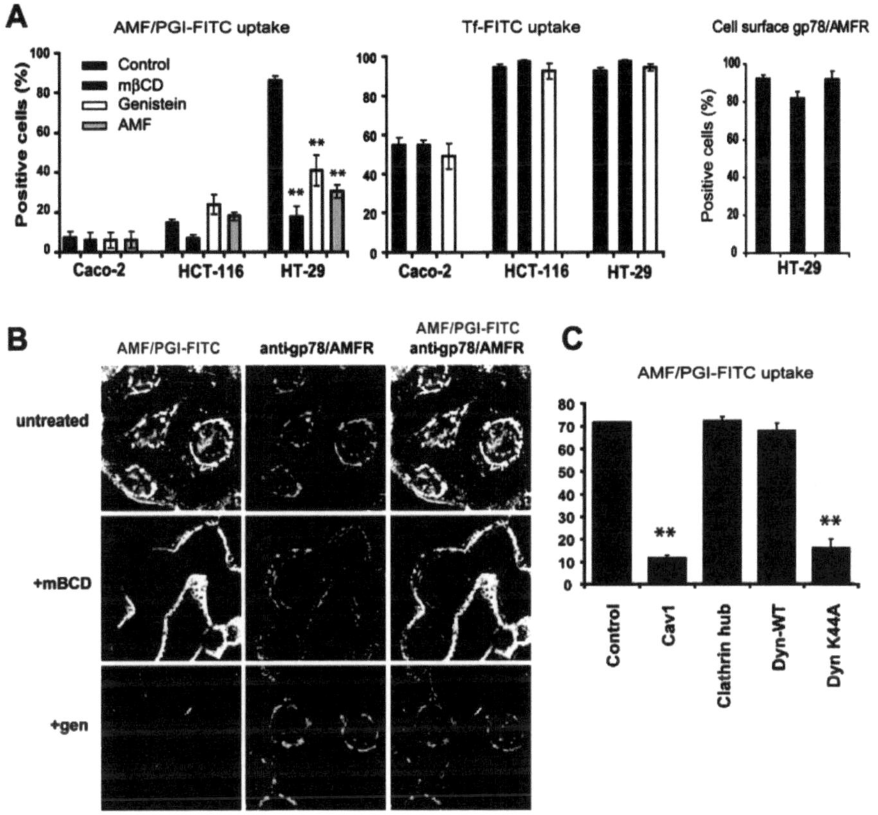

Figure 2. The AMF/PGI-FITC uptake in colon carcinoma cells is raft-dependent, dynamin-dependent, and negatively regulated by Cav1. (A) Caco-2, HCT116, and HT29 colon cells were pretreated for 30 min with 5 mM mЯCD, 100 μg/ml genistein, or an excess of unconjugated AMF/PGI (1 mg/ml) and then incubated with AMF/PGI-FITC (left graph) or Tf-FITC (center graph), followed by incubation with pronase and flow cytometry. Surface gp78/AMFR expression of HT29 cells treated for 30 min with 5 mM mЯCD, or 100 μg/ml genistein, was determined by staining cells at 4°C with 3F3A anti-gp78/AMFR mAb followed by Alexa647-conjugated secondary antibody and analysis by flow cytometry (n = 4; mean ± S.E.; **, P ≤ 0.001 relative to control). (B) The HT29 colon cells were left untreated or pretreated for 30 min with 5 mM mЯCD or 100 μg/ml genistein, incubated with 25 μg/ml AMF/PGI-FITC for 30 min prior to fixation and labeling with the 3F3A anti-gp78/AMFR monoclonal antibody followed by appropriate secondary antibodies. The AMF/PGI-FITC labeling is presented in green and the anti-gp78/AMFR labeled smooth endoplasmic reticulum in red. (C) HT29 cells were infected with adenoviruses expressing the tTA alone (control) or coinfected with the tTA adenovirus and adenoviruses coding for Cav1, clathrin hub, wild-type dynamin-1 (DynWT), or mutant dynamin-1 K44A (DynK44A). After 48 hr, AMF/PGI-FITC uptake was assessed by flow cytometry (percent positive cells; n = 3; ** P ≤ 0.001 relative to control).

AMF/PGI-Paclitaxel is Pro-apoptotic and Growth Inhibitory

The AMF/PGI-paclitaxel conjugate at a 4.3:1 molar ratio of paclitaxel to AMF/PGI dimers was prepared as previously described (Guillemard and Saragovi, 2001) and its specificity assessed by its ability to inhibit uptake of AMF/PGI-FITC in MDA-435 cells. The MDA-435 cells were incubated with 25 μg/ml AMF/PGI-FITC in the presence of excess concentrations of either free AMF/PGI or AMF/PGI-paclitaxel conjugate and the uptake of AMF/PGI-FITC was measured by flow cytometry (Figure 3A, left panel). The ability of both AMF/PGI and AMF/PGI-paclitaxel to compete with AMF/PGI-FITC uptake confirms that paclitaxel conjugation to AMF/PGI preserves the receptor binding properties of paclitaxel conjugated AMF/PGI.

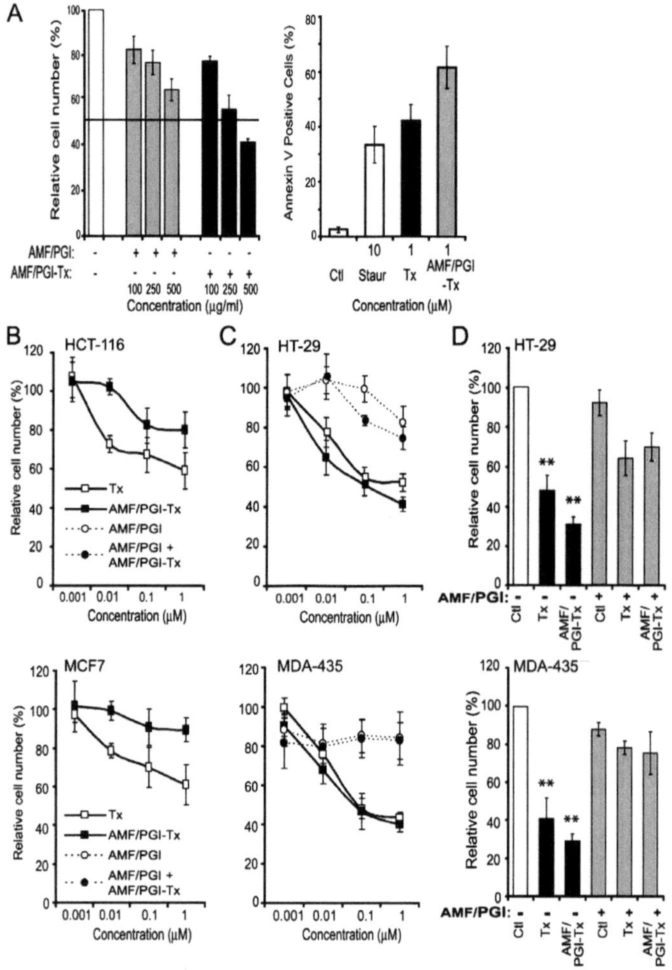

Figure 3. The growth inhibition and pro-apoptotic effects of AMF/PGI-paclitaxel.

(A) The specificity of AMF/PGI-paclitaxel was determined by competitive binding assay. The MDA-435 cells were incubated for 60 min at 4°C in the presence of various concentrations (100–500 μg/ml) of either free AMF/PGI or AMF/PGI-paclitaxel conjugate. Afterwards, cells were stained with anti-gp78/AMFR mAb (3F3A) and Alexa647-conjugated secondary antibody and surface expression of gp78/AMFR determined by flow cytometry (left panel). Results were normalized and expressed as means ± SE (n = 4) compared to the control (untreated cells). Induction of apoptosis by 10 μM staurosporine, 1 μM paclitaxel (Tx), or 1 μM AMF/PGI-paclitaxel conjugate was determined as described in the Materials and Methods by flow cytometry using the Annexin V–FITC assay (right panel). The growth inhibitory ability (B, C) and selectivity (D) of AMF/PGI-Paclitaxel conjugate were

Figure 3. *(Caption Continued)*

assessed on HCT116 and MCF7 cells that poorly internalize AMF/PGI (B) and HT29 and MDA-435 cells that efficiently internalize AMF/PGI (C, D). Cells were treated with increasing log concentrations of paclitaxel equivalent concentrations (0–1 μM) of free paclitaxel, AMF/PGI-paclitaxel conjugate, or controls, as indicated, for 48 hr (B, C). Alternatively, HT29 and MDA-435 cells were treated with 1 μM free paclitaxel or AMF/PGI-paclitaxel in the presence or absence of a 20x fold excess of unconjugated AMF/PGI for 48 hr (D). Cell viability was then measured using crystal violet staining. Each measurement was done in quadruplicate and the results are presented relative to untreated control cells. Results were normalized and expressed as mean ± SE (n = 4) compared to the control (untreated cells), **, $P \leq 0.001$ versus control.

Paclitaxel is well known for its ability to arrest tumor cells in mitosis and promote apoptosis (Kumar, 1981). The pro-apoptotic activity of the AMF/PGI-paclitaxel conjugate was evaluated using an Annexin V-FITC flow cytometry assay (Figure 3A, right panel). AMF/PGI-paclitaxel induced a significant increase in cell surface Annexin V expression, when used at the same molar concentration as free paclitaxel.

The ability of AMF/PGI-paclitaxel to prevent tumor cell proliferation was evaluated *in vitro* on HT29 colon and MDA-435 breast cells that efficiently internalize AMF/PGI-FITC, as well as HCT116 colon and MCF-7 breast tumor cells that show significantly lower uptake of AMF/PGI-FITC (Figure 1) (Kojic et al., 2007). Cells were incubated in the presence of increasing log concentrations (0.001–1 μM) of paclitaxel, or equimolar paclitaxel equivalents of AMF/PGI-paclitaxel conjugate, and cell number determined after 48 hr relative to control cells. AMF/PGI-paclitaxel was less efficient at inhibiting HCT116 and MCF-7 cell proliferation than free paclitaxel (Figure 3B), consistent with the reduced uptake of AMF/PGI-FITC by these cells. However, treatment of HT29 and MDA-435 cells with AMF/PGI-paclitaxel resulted in a significant dose-dependent inhibition of cell proliferation, at least equivalent to that of free paclitaxel (Figure 3C). These results, firstly, confirm that the conjugation of AMF/PGI to paclitaxel did not alter the biochemical properties of free paclitaxel and, secondly, demonstrate the selectivity of the AMF/PGI-paclitaxel conjugate towards tumor cells that efficiently internalize AMF/PGI.

We then tested whether excess free AMF/PGI could prevent the inhibition of cell proliferation by the AMF/PGI-paclitaxel conjugate. Concomitant treatment of HT29 and MDA-435 cells with free AMF/PGI significantly abrogated growth inhibition by AMF/PGI-paclitaxel (Figure 3D). These results suggest that free AMF/PGI may compete with AMF/PGI-paclitaxel for cell surface receptor binding. However, excess free AMF/PGI also reduced the cytotoxic effect of free paclitaxel suggesting that it may generally exhibit a pro-survival role (Tsutsumi et al., 2003). The AMF/PGI-paclitaxel may therefore inhibit cell proliferation by abrogating a prosurvival pathway associated with resistance to chemotherapeutic agents.

AMF/PGI Internalization in Murine Melanoma Cells and Tumors

The B16-F1, the original cell line in which gp78/AMFR was identified, and K1735-M1 are highly metastatic melanoma cells that express gp78/AMFR and respond to AMF/PGI treatment (Nabi and Raz, 1987, 1988; Silletti et al., 1998a, 1998b). By flow cytometry, both K1735-M1 and B16-F1 cells show high levels of gp78/AMFR expression and robust uptake of AMF/PGI-FITC that could be inhibited by mβCD, genistein, or 10-fold excess free AMF/PGI (Figure 4A). Confocal analysis confirmed that internalization of AMF/PGI-FITC to the anti-gp78/AMFR labeled smooth endoplasmic reticulum in both cell lines was effectively disrupted by mβCD and genistein (Figure 4B). Taken together, these results confirm that in metastatic K1735-M1 and B16-F1 murine melanoma cells, AMF/PGI is internalized to the smooth endoplasmic reticulum via a raft-dependent pathway.

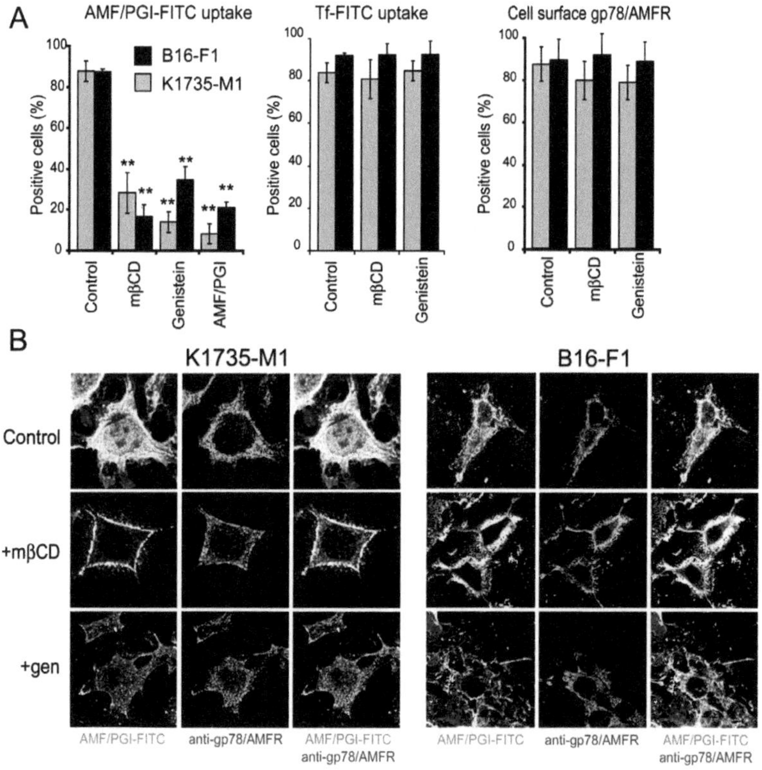

Figure 4. Internalization of AMF/PGI to the smooth endoplasmic reticulum of murine melanoma cells is raft-dependent. (A)The K1735-M1 (grey) and B16-F1 (black) melanoma cells were left untreated (Control) or pretreated for 30 min with 5 mM mβCD, 100 μg/ml genistein, or an excess of unconjugated AMF/PGI (1 mg/ml), then incubated with AMF/PGI-FITC or Tf-FITC, followed by incubation with pronase. Flow cytometry analysis of AMF/PGI-FITC (left panel, mean±SEM; **, $P \leq 0.001$; $n = 4$) and Tf-FITC (middle) containing cells was performed as described in Materials and Methods. Surface gp78/AMFR expression on untreated cells (Control) or cells treated for 30 min with 5 mM mβCD or 100 μg/ml genistein, was determined by labeling with 3F3A anti-gp78/AMFR mAb followed by Alexa647-conjugated secondary antibody at 4°C and analyzed by flow cytometry (right panel). (B) The K1735-M1 (left) and B16-F1 (right) melanoma cells were incubated with 25 μg/ml AMF/PGI-FITC for 30 min prior to fixation. The AMF/PGI-FITC was revealed with rabbit anti-FITC and the smooth endoplasmic reticulum labeled with 3F3A anti-gp78/AMFR antibody followed by appropriate secondary antibodies and confocal imaging. The AMF/PGI-FITC labeling is presented in green and the anti-gp78/AMFR labeled smooth endoplasmic reticulum in red. Where indicated, cells were pretreated for 30 min with 5 mM mβCD (+mβCD; middle row) or 100 μg/ml genistein (+gen; bottom row).

Furthermore, to determine whether tumor cells *in situ* internalize AMF/PGI, we established s.c. K1735-M1 tumors in the flanks of syngeneic C3H mice. Immunohistological examination of 6 μ tumor sections confirmed the high degree and uniform expression of gp78/AMFR by cells within the K1735-M1 tumor (Figure 5A). The AMF/PGI-FITC was then administered directly into well-established K1735-M1 tumors. After 6 hr mice were sacrified and the tumors resected. One-half of each tumor was used for histological analysis. The second-half was processed for flow cytometry of AMF/PGI-FITC uptake in single cell suspensions generated from tumor tissue by mechanical/enzymatic digestion followed by protease treatment. As seen in Figure 5B, AMF/PGI-FITC labeling in tumor sections is localized to both the cell surface and cytoplasmic region of the tumor cells, as defined by phalloidin labeling of F-actin. Furthermore, by flow cytometry, dose-dependent uptake of AMF/PGI-FITC in tumor cells was observed (Figure 5C), demonstrating that K1735-M1 tumor cells *in situ* are able to efficiently internalize fluorescently labeled AMF/PGI.

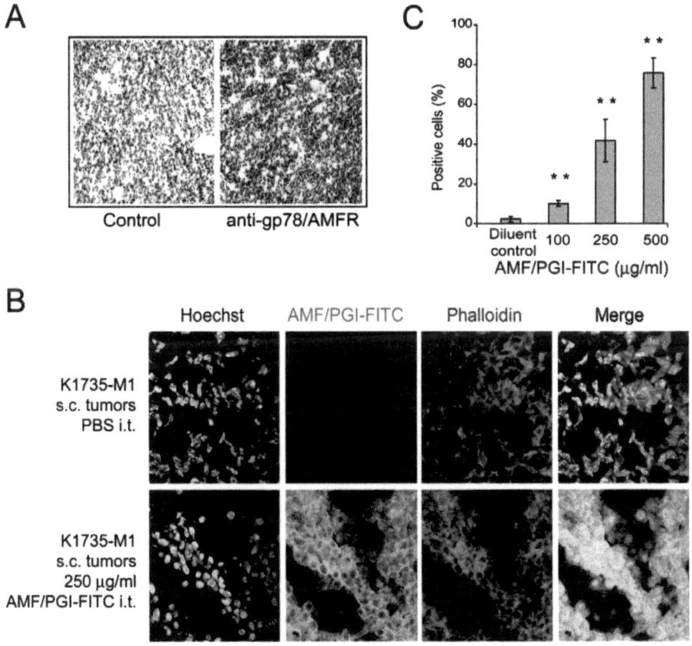

Figure 5. The Gp78/AMFR expression and AMF/PGI-FITC uptake in primary tumors. (A). The K1735-M1 tumor sections were immunohistochemically labeled with anti-gp78/AMFR antibody followed by biotinylated secondary antibody, HRP-conjugated avidin-biotin complex and staining with DAB. Control sections were labeled in parallel in the absence of primary antibody. (B) The K1735-M1 tumor sections from tumors injected with PBS (Control) or 250 μg/ml AMF/PGI-FITC were labeled with Hoechst nuclear stain (blue) and Alexa568-phalloidin (red) and images acquired by confocal microscopy using equivalent acquisition settings. FITC labeling (green) in AMF/PGI-FITC injected tumors overlapped extensively with phalloidin-labeled actin (red). (C) The PBS and AMF/PGI-FITC injected K1735-M1 tumors were mechanically dissociated, treated with pronase and analyzed for AMF/PGI-FITC positivity by flow cytometry. The data represent the average of seven different tumors (mean ± SEM; **, $P \leq 0.001$, relative to PBS injected tumors).

In Vivo Efficacy of AMF/PGI-Paclitaxel

To test our approach in mice, we used two melanoma tumor models, K1735-M1 and B16-F1. *In vitro* treatment of K1735-M1 and B16-F1 cells with increasing log concentrations (0.001–1 μM) of free paclitaxel, or with equimolar concentrations of AMF/PGI-paclitaxel conjugate, resulted in a dose-dependent inhibition of cell proliferation (Figures 6A, B). However, far lower concentrations of AMF/PGI-paclitaxel conjugate, compared to free paclitaxel, were needed to evoke an antiproliferative effect in both cell lines. The concentration at which proliferation of K1735-M1 cells was inhibited by 50% (IC50) was 0.1 μM with AMF/PGI-paclitaxel compared to 1 μM for free paclitaxel ($p < 0.001$; Figure 6A, left panel). The B16-F1 melanoma cells were not sensitive to paclitaxel alone however their proliferation was efficiently inhibited by equimolar concentrations of AMF/PGI-paclitaxel (Figure 6B, left panel). As observed for HT29 and MDA-435 cells (Figure 3), the ability of AMF/PGI-paclitaxel to inhibit cell proliferation of both K1735-M1 and B16-F1 cells was inhibited by the concomitant addition of excess AMF/PGI. The AMF/PGI alone did not affect proliferation of either K1735-M1 or B16-F1 cells but did inhibit paclitaxel-mediated inhibition of cell proliferation of K1735-M1 and B16-F1 cells (Figures 6A, B; right panels).

We next examined the effect of the AMF/PGI-paclitaxel conjugate on tumor growth and survival in the K1735-M1 and B16-F1 syngeneic mouse melanoma tumor models. Well-defined tumors 50–60 mm^3 in volume were formed approximately 11–13 days after s.c. injection of C3H mice with K1735-M1 and of C57/BL6 mice with B16-F1 melanoma cells, at which time the treatment was initiated. The i.t. injections of AMF/PGI-paclitaxel conjugate (300 ng paclitaxel) on five consecutive days resulted in a consistent measurable difference in tumor size between the control and AMF/PGI-paclitaxel treated animals in both K1735-M1 and B16-F1 models (Figures 6C, D).

In the K1735-M1 model, there was significant tumor regression on day 25, with most of the animals treated with AMF/PGI-paclitaxel exhibiting tumors that were much smaller compared to untreated mice (Figure 6C, left panel). Twenty-five days after subcutaneous implantation of K1735-M1 cells, the mean tumor volume was 637 ± 112 mm^3 for the mice that received i.t. injections of diluent compared to 58 ± 27 mm^3 for the mice that received i.t. injections of AMF/PGI-paclitaxel conjugate. Statistical analysis with the Student-T two-sample test confirmed that mean tumor volume was significantly smaller in the group treated with AMF/PGI-paclitaxel, compared with the group treated with diluent alone ($p < 0.001$). The i.t. injections of free paclitaxel also resulted in tumor regression. The mean tumor volume for the eight animals that received i.t. free paclitaxel injections was 229 ± 65 mm^3, however free paclitaxel was significantly less effective compared to AMF/PGI-paclitaxel treatment ($p < 0.05$).

The MST of untreated mice was 21 (17–25) days, and because of tumor burden all mice from this group were terminated by day 25 (Figure 6C, right panel). Mice treated with five consecutive i.t. injections of free paclitaxel (300 ng) showed improved, although not statistically significant, survival compared to untreated mice. The MST for this treatment group was 25 (19–39) days and one of eight mice was still alive after 39 days. The treatment of tumor bearing mice with i.t. injections of AMF/PGI-paclitaxel conjugate significantly prolonged their survival compared with untreated controls (p <

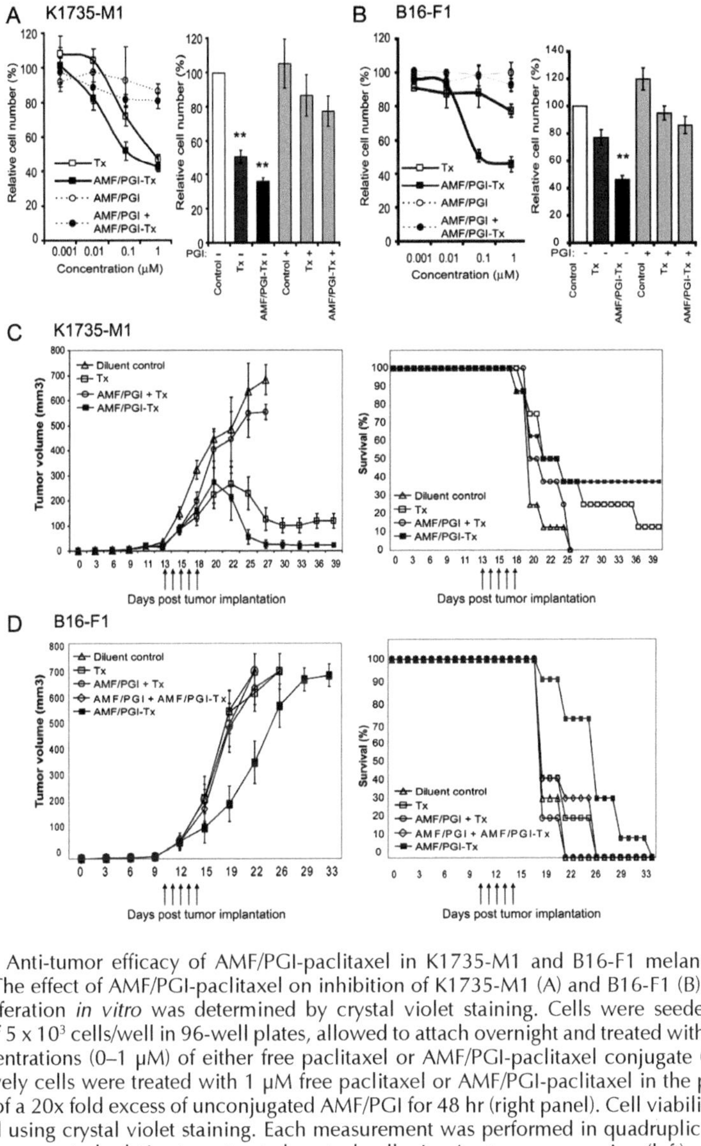

Figure 6. Anti-tumor efficacy of AMF/PGI-paclitaxel in K1735-M1 and B16-F1 melanoma tumor models. The effect of AMF/PGI-paclitaxel on inhibition of K1735-M1 (A) and B16-F1 (B) melanoma cell proliferation *in vitro* was determined by crystal violet staining. Cells were seeded at initial density of 5 x 10^3 cells/well in 96-well plates, allowed to attach overnight and treated with increasing log concentrations (0–1 μM) of either free paclitaxel or AMF/PGI-paclitaxel conjugate (left panel). Alternatively cells were treated with 1 μM free paclitaxel or AMF/PGI-paclitaxel in the presence or absence of a 20x fold excess of unconjugated AMF/PGI for 48 hr (right panel). Cell viability was then measured using crystal violet staining. Each measurement was performed in quadruplicate and the results are presented relative to untreated control cells. *In vivo* tumor regression (left) and survival (right) in mice bearing K1735-M1 (C) or B16-F1 (D) melanoma s.c. tumors were measured after i.t. treatment with AMF/PGI-paclitaxel. The K1735-M1 (C) or B16-F1 (D) melanoma cells were injected s.c. into the flank of C3H or C57/BL6 mice, respectively, and tumor volumes measured every other day. As indicated, mice were injected i.t. for five consecutive days with paclitaxel (Tx, □), AMF/PGI and paclitaxel (AMF/PGI + Tx, ○), AMF/PGI-paclitaxel conjugate (AMF/PGI-Tx, ■) and, for B16-F1 tumors, AMF/PGI and AMF/PGI-paclitaxel conjugate (AMF/PGI + AMF/PGI-Tx, ◊). Control mice (□) received injections of diluent (sterile PBS). Results show means ± S.E. for AMF/PGI-paclitaxel group versus free paclitaxel and control groups: K1735-M1 (tumor regression: $P \leq 0.001$; survival: $P \leq 0.05$); B16-F1 (tumor regression: $P \leq 0.05$; $P \leq 0.05$). In K1735-M1 tumors, complete regression of tumor growth was observed in three out of 16 tumors after treatment with five consecutive daily i.t. injections of AMF/PGI-paclitaxel.

0.05). The MST of this group was 27 days (17–39 days), and three of eight mice were still alive after 39 days, not having tumor relapse and exhibiting tumor regression of 90%. This efficacy was not associated with measurable physical and behavioral changes (weight loss, sickness, aggressiveness, or decreased physical activity), suggesting that the short-term treatment with AMF/PGI-paclitaxel was efficacious and without detrimental side effects.

Results obtained from the B16-F1 melanoma model show that neither paclitaxel alone nor paclitaxel plus AMF/PGI affected B16-F1 tumor growth. While paclitaxel alone did not impact on tumor size, AMF/PGI-paclitaxel significantly ($p < 0.05$) suppressed tumor growth of B16-F1 tumors (Figure 6D, left panel). The MST of AMF/PGI-paclitaxel treated mice was 29 (19–32) days compared to 20 (19–22) days for untreated and 21 (19–24) days for taxol treated mice, and significantly prolonged survival ($p < 0.05$). (Figure 6D, right panel). The AMF/PGI-paclitaxel therefore suppresses tumor growth and extends the survival time of mice bearing primary B16-F1 tumors more effectively than an equimolar dose of free paclitaxel.

Mice receiving combinatorial treatment with AMF/PGI-paclitaxel and free AMF/PGI had no effect on tumor growth regression or MST compared to control treatments in both the K1735-M1 and B16-F1 primary melanoma tumor models (Figures 6C, D). Free AMF/PGI also effectively abrogated the anti-tumor effect of free paclitaxel in the K1735-M1 model suggesting that AMF/PGI may exhibit a pro-survival, anti-chemotherapeutic activity *in vivo*.

Selective Targeting of Tumor and Not Normal Immune Cells Upon Systemic Delivery of AMF/PGI

The AMF/PGI exhibits lymphokine activity and is a maturation factor for cells of immune lineage (Gurney et al., 1986; Xu et al., 1996). We therefore assessed gp78/AMFR expression in lymphoid tissues from adult immunocompetent mice. Immunohistochemical labeling of spleen and thymus tissue sections was performed using the anti-gp78/AMFR mAb. Tissue sections of early neonatal mouse brain and HCT116 colon tumor were included as positive controls. Strong positive gp78/AMFR staining was detected in 20-day-old HCT116 colon tumor sections as well as in 5-day old mouse brain, as previously reported in developing rat brain (Leclerc et al., 2000). Immunoreactivity in the brain and tumor sections was localized to both the cytoplasm and the cell surface. However anti-gp78/AMFR labeling was not detected in adult spleen and thymus sections (Figure 7A).

We then used flow cytometry to evaluate gp78/AMFR surface expression and AMF/PGI uptake in single cell suspensions prepared from spleens and thymuses, as well as in an enriched population of spleen macrophages. Relative to MDA-435 cells, included as a positive control (Kojic et al., 2007), both gp78/AMFR cell surface staining and AMF/PGI-FITC uptake were dramatically lower (40-fold) in the primary immune cells (Figure 7B). Only 2% of splenic cells and thymocytes were gp78/AMFR positive. Surface gp78/AMFR expression was slightly higher in the enriched population of splenic macrophages but AMF/PGI-FITC uptake was not increased (Figure 7B). Both gp78/AMFR surface expression and AMF/PGI uptake are therefore significantly lower in normal immune cells relative to tumor cells.

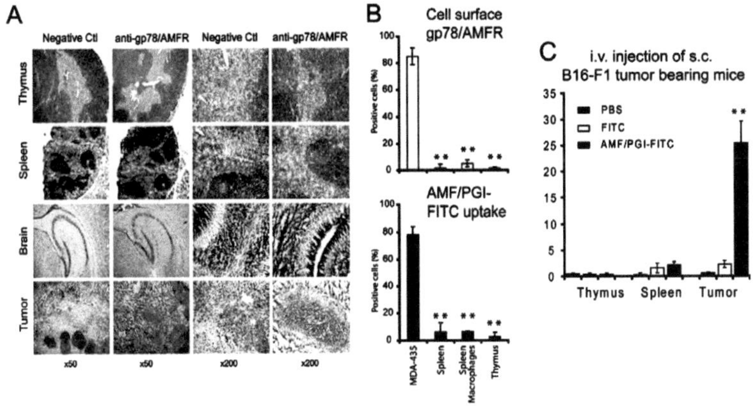

Figure 7. The Gp78/AMFR expression and AMF/PGI uptake in normal mouse immune tissue and cells. (A) Immunohistochemical labeling of tissue sections showed no gp78/AMFR reactivity in normal mouse spleen and thymus. However, strong positive gp78/AMFR staining was detected in 5-day-old mouse brain tissue and in 20 day old HCT116 s.c. tumor sections. A representative experiment of eight is shown (original magnification, x50 and x200). (B) Cell surface gp78/AMFR expression (top panel) and AMF/PGI-FITC uptake (bottom panel) of single cell suspensions prepared from mouse spleen and thymus, an enriched population of spleen macrophages as well as MDA-435 cells were assessed by flow cytometry and the percentage of positive cells is presented. The data represent the average of three separate experiments (mean ± SEM; **, $P \leq 0.001$).). (C) The B16-F1 melanoma tumors were established s.c. in C57/BL6 mice and after 12 days, mice were injected i.v. with PBS, 250 μg/ml AMF/PGI-FITC or an equivalent concentration of free FITC. After 2 hr, spleen, thymus and B16-F1 s.c. tumors were mechanically dissociated, treated with pronase, and analyzed for FITC positivity by flow cytometry. The data represent the average of six different tumors (mean ± SEM; **, $P \leq 0.001$, relative to PBS injected mice).

To assess whether systemic delivery of AMF/PGI could selectively target tumor cells, mice bearing s.c. B16-F1 melanoma tumors were injected i.v. with AMF/PGI-FITC, free FITC or PBS alone. Two hours following i.v. injection, we performed flow cytometry on single cell suspensions prepared from spleen, thymus, and tumor tissues (Figure 7C). We detected no significant fluorescence in cells from all three sources following injection of PBS or free FITC. However, we were able to detect selective uptake of AMF/PGI-FITC in approximately 25% of the tumor cells and essentially no uptake in spleen or thymus cells. This suggests that systemic i.v. administration is potentially a valid and selective delivery route for AMF/PGI-conjugated molecules to tumor cells.

KEYWORDS

- **Autocrine motility factor/phosphoglucose isomerase**
- **Intraperitoneal**
- **Intratumoral**
- **Intravenous**
- **Metastasis**
- **Subcutaneous**

AUTHORS' CONTRIBUTIONS

Conceived and designed the experiments: Liliana D. Kojic, Sam M. Wiseman, and Ivan R. Nabi. Performed the experiments: Liliana D. Kojic, Fariba Ghaidi, and Bharat Joshi. Analyzed the data: Liliana D. Kojic, Sam M. Wiseman, Bharat Joshi, and Ivan R. Nabi. Contributed reagents/materials/analysis tools: Hinyu Nedev and H. Uri Saragovi. Wrote the chapter: Liliana D. Kojic, Sam M. Wiseman, H. Uri Saragovi, and Ivan R. Nabi. Prepared reagents: Hinyu Nedev and H. Uri Saragovi.

ACKNOWLEDGMENTS

The authors thank Majid Alimohammadi and Patrick Lajoie for their assistance with certain elements of the study and Pamela Austin, Caylib Durand, and Robyn Lett for their help with the obtention of mouse tissues and tumors.

Chapter 13

Adenovirus Dodecahedron, as a Drug Delivery Vector

Monika Zochowska, Agnieszka Paca, Guy Schoehn, Jean-Pierre Andrieu, Jadwiga Chroboczek, Bernard Dublet, and Ewa Szolajska

INTRODUCTION

Bleomycin (BLM) is an anticancer antibiotic used in many cancer regimens. Its utility is limited by systemic toxicity and dose-dependent pneumonitis able to progress to lung fibrosis. The latter can affect up to nearly 50% of the total patient population, out of which 3% will die. We propose to improve BLM delivery by tethering it to an efficient delivery vector. Adenovirus (Ad) dodecahedron base (DB) is a particulate vector composed of 12 copies of a pentameric viral protein responsible for virus penetration. The vector efficiently penetrates the plasma membrane, is liberated in the cytoplasm and has a propensity to concentrate around the nucleus; up to 300,000 particles can be observed in one cell *in vitro*.

Dodecahedron (Dd) structure is preserved at up to about 50°C at pH 7–8 and during dialysis, freezing and drying in the speed-vac in the presence of 150 mM ammonium sulfate, as well as during lyophilization in the presence of cryoprotectants. The vector is also stable in human serum for 2 hr at 37°C. We prepared a Dd-BLM conjugate which upon penetration induced death of transformed cells. Similarly to free BLM, Dd-BLM caused dsDNA breaks. Significantly, effective cytotoxic concentration of BLM delivered with Dd was 100 times lower than that of free BLM.

Stability studies show that Dds can be conveniently stored and transported, and can potentially be used for therapeutic purposes under various climates. Successful BLM delivery by Ad Dds demonstrates that the use of virus like particle (VLP) results in significantly improved drug bioavailability. These experiments open new vistas for delivery of non-permeant labile drugs.

The Ad penton, a non-covalent complex of two oligomeric proteins, fiber, and penton base, localized at 12 vertices of the icosahedral virion is responsible for virus entry. The trimeric antenna-like fiber protein attaches the virus to the primary receptor on the host cell plasma membrane while the pentameric penton base, through interaction of its Arg-Gly-Asp containing (RGD) motif with host cell αv integrins, is involved in virus endocytosis. In certain Ad serotypes pentons self-assemble into a VLP called the Dd that is built of 12 pentons, thereby comprising 12 penton bases and 12 fibers (Norrby, 1968). We expressed the penton components of Ad serotype 3 in the baculovirus system, which resulted in spontaneous formation of Ad3 dodecahedra in insect cells (Fender et. al., 1997). In addition, expression under similar conditions of penton base (Pb) alone led to formation of a dodecahedric particle made of 12 bases (DB), which demonstrated that dodecahedron is assembled independently of the fiber protein through interaction of only the Pbs. This chapter describes the properties of DB, for which both terms, the Dd and DB will be used. The term Dd will be used throughout this work to describe Ad DB.

Working with the recombinant Dd of serotype 3 (Ad3), our group has shown that Dd components that are responsible for Ad cell entry retain these functions in the virus-like particle, which exhibits very efficient internalization and has a propensity to concentrate around the cell nucleus (Fender et al., 1997). Since the recombinant wild type Dd harbors no genetic information, it is a safe alternative to Ad in gene transfer. In addition, we have recently shown that Dd enters the cell through a heparan sulfate pathway, not used by the virus of origin (Vives et al., 2004). This allows Dd to penetrate a wider range of cells than can the Ad, the most efficient vector known to date. Finally, studies in our group have demonstrated that Dd is able to translocate DNA to cells, resulting in gene expression (Fender et al., 1997), as well as to transfer proteins directly, with the transferred protein remaining active inside the transduced cells (Garcel et al., 2006).

To date, VLPs have been produced for more than 30 different viruses (for review see Noad and Roy, 2003). This includes viruses with single or multiple capsid proteins as well as those with and without lipid envelopes. The Ad is a non-enveloped virus with a dsDNA genome, and among this type of viruses the VLPs have been described for various human papillomavirus (HPV) serotypes, polyomavirus simian virus serotype 40 (SV40), and John Cunningham virus (JC). However, usually these VLPs retain the virions' size and mimic their organization, whereas Ad, Dd is forming VLPs much smaller than the virion itself and with different intra-particle interactions. Therefore, data on Dd stability cannot be inferred from those obtained for Ad virions (for example, those described by Rexroad and coworkers, 2006).

In order to employ the remarkable cell entry properties of Dd for drug delivery, we needed data concerning the vectors' stability. Hence, the stability of Dd was studied under various conditions of salt concentration, pH and temperature. We optimized conditions for vector stability and storage, and analyzed its integrity in cell culture and in human serum. Finally, we used Dd as a vector for delivery of the lipophilic, non-permeant, and labile anticancer antibiotic BLM, which resulted in significant increase in BLM bioavailability.

MATERIALS AND METHODS

Cells

The HeLa cells were cultured in EMEM (Lonza, Basel, Switzerland) supplemented with 10% fetal calf serum (FBS) (Invitrogen, Carlsbad CA, USA), penicillin (50 IU/ml), and streptomycin (50 μg/ml) (Invitrogen) at 37°C, in 5% CO_2 atmosphere.

Protein Electrophoresis, Antibodies, and Immunological Analyses

Proteins were separated on SDS–PAGE, and stained with Coomassie Brilliant Blue (CBB) or analyzed by Western blotting. The assembly status of purified Dds was analyzed by native agarose gel electrophoresis. Protein samples were mixed with loading buffer (3 mM Tris-HCl, pH 8.0, containing 6 mM NH4Cl, 3 mM magnesium acetate, 14 mM potassium acetate, 10% glycerol, and 0.005% bromophenol blue) and subjected to electrophoresis in 0.8% agarose gels containing 50 mM Tris and 200 mM glycine, pH 8 at 75 V at 4°C (Gallegos and Patton, 1989). After electrophoresis proteins were stained with CBB or blotted onto Immobilon-P transfer membrane in 20 mM Tris buffer pH 7.5, containing 150 mM NaCl and 2 mM EDTA.

For Western blot analysis, the rabbit anti-Ad3 Dd (prepared in the laboratory) at 1:40,000 and as the secondary antibody anti-rabbit-horseradish peroxidase (Sigma) at 1:1,60,000 dilution were used. The ECL detection system (Amersham Biosciences, Piscataway NJ, USA) was used throughout this work.

For immunofluorescent microscopy the following antibodies were used: anti-Dd at 1:1,000; anti-tubulin MAb (Sigma, St Louis MO, USA) at 1:400; and anti-γ-H2AX (polyclonal, Calbiochem, Darmstadt, Germany) at 1:100 dilution. The secondary Abs were goat anti-rabbit FIlabeled (Santa Cruz Biotechnology, Santa Cruz CA, USA) (1:200; 1 hr at room temperature), sheep anti-rabbit Texas Red-labeled (Jackson, ImmunoResearch Laboratories, West Grove PA, USA 1:250; 1 hr at 37°C), FITC-conjugated goat anti-mouse (Jackson, 1:250; 1 hr at 37°C).

Dd Expression and Purification

Full-length human Ad3 penton base gene was cloned and expressed in the baculovirus system (Fender et al., 1997). Virus amplification was performed in monolayers of Spodoptera frugiperda (Sf21) cells maintained in TC100 medium supplemented with 5% (v/v) fetal calf serum (both from Invitrogen). For Dd expression Trichoplusia ni (High-Five, HF) cells, grown in suspension, in Express Five SFM medium (*Invitrogen*) with gentamycin (50 mg/l) and amphotericin B (0.25 mg/l), were infected with the recombinant baculovirus at multiplicity of infection of 4 pfu/cell. After 48 hr cells were collected and lysed by three rounds of freezing and thawing. Clarified lysates were fractionated on 15–40% sucrose density gradients as previously described (Fender et al., 1997). Gradients were analyzed by SDS-PAGE with CBB staining.

Heavy sucrose density gradient fractions containing DB were pooled, dialyzed against 20 mM Tris, pH 7.5, containing 2 mM EDTA, 5% glycerol and protease inhibitors (Roche, Indianapolis IN, USA), and subjected to ion-exchange chromatography on a Q-Sepharose column (2 or 5-ml Econo-Pac High Q Cartridge, Bio-Rad, Hercules CA, USA) equilibrated with dialysis buffer. Proteins were eluted at 4°C with NaCl gradient in dialysis buffer. Purified proteins were stored at 4°C in the purification buffer (dialysis buffer containing 280 or 370 mM NaCl). Peak fractions were pooled, and when necessary, concentrated by ultrafiltration in a Microcon unit (cutoff 10,000, Millipore, Billerica MA, USA). The purity of protein preparations was assessed by 12% SDS-PAGE. The assembly status of purified recombinant penton base protein was analyzed on native agarose gels and by negative stain EM.

N-terminal Amino Acid Sequence Determination

Aliquots of purified proteins were subjected to SDS-PAGE and electrotransferred onto Immobilon-P PVDF membrane. Amino acid determination based on Edman degradation was performed using an Applied Biosystems gas-phase sequencer model 492 (s/n: 9510287J). Phenylthiohydantoin amino acid derivatives generated at each sequencing cycle were identified and quantified online with an Applied Biosystems Model 140C HPLC system using the data analysis system for Applied Biosystems Model 610A (software version 2.1). The PTH-amino acid standard kit (Perkin-Elmer, Waltham MA, USA) was used and reconstituted according to the manufacturer's instructions. The reagents used to identify and quantify the derivatized amino acids were removed at each sequencing cycle. Retention times and integration values of peaks were compared to the chromatographic profile obtained for a standard mixture of derivatized amino acids.

Thermal Stability Studies

Samples of purified Dds were dialyzed at 4°C for 24 hr against buffers of different pH and ionic strengths, with three changes of each. The samples were stored at 4°C or were subjected to different temperature treatments by incubation in water bath. Some samples were centrifuged for 30 min at 13,000 rpm in the Eppendorf centrifuge. The dialyzed proteins and those in the supernatants recovered after centrifugation were analyzed on non-denaturing agarose gels.

Denaturation curves were obtained for Dd and Dd-BLM conjugate as a function of temperature and pH, by the DLS technique. Protein samples (0.2 μg/μl) were dialyzed against pre-filtered (0.45 μm-pore-size filter) buffer solutions. Samples were placed in a reduced-volume cuvette (45 μl, Greiner, Frickenhausen, Germany). Automated measurements were collected with a Zetasizer Nano ZS (Malvern, Worcestershire, UK), using a 2°C incremental temperature ramp, from 12 to 65°C, and a 2 min equilibrium time at each measurement temperature. The data were adjusted using the cumulant method.

Kinetics of Dd Penetration

The HeLa cells were attached to the wells of 96-wells plastic dishes (2×10^4 cells). The medium was removed, the purified Dds (4 μg/100 μl, 10.8 nM) were applied to cells in EMEM medium without FBS, and the dishes were returned to the incubator. Three hours after Dds application the medium was enriched with FBS to 10% final concentration. Cells were collected at the indicated periods (1–96 hr, see Figure 4), lysed in Laemmli solution or suspended in hypotonic buffer. Samples containing half of cells in each well were run on SDS-PAGE or native agarose gels, and analyzed by Western blot using anti-Dd antibody.

Electron Microscopy

Samples at approximately 0.1 mg protein/ml were applied to the clean side of carbon on mica (carbon/mica interface) and negatively stained with 1% sodium silicotungstate, pH 7.0. Micrographs were taken under low-dose conditions with a Jeol 1200 EX II microscope (Tokyo, Japan) at 100 kV and a nominal magnification of 40,000.

Bleomycin Cross-Linking to Dd

Bleomycin A_5 hydrochloride (Hangzhou Xiangyuan Co., Ltd., China) was chemically cross-linked to purified Dd during a two step conjugation procedure using 1-ethyl-(3-dimethylaminopropyl) carbodiimide hydrochloride (EDC) (Pierce, Rockford IL, USA) and N-hydroxysulfosuccinimide (sulfo-NHS) (Pierce). The Dd (27 nM) was activated in 0.1 M MES buffer pH 6.0, 0.5 M NaCl, in the presence of 0.31 mM EDC and 5 mM Sulfo-NHS. Cross-linking with BLM A_5 (23 mM) was performed during 2 hr incubation with mixing at room temperature. After quenching the reaction by addition of hydroxylamine to a final concentration of 10 mM, chemical reagents and free BLM were removed from the preparation by dialysis (24 hr, four changes of 20 mM Tris pH 7,5, 150 mM NaCl, 5% glycerol). The amount of BLM cross-linked to Dd was evaluated by ms analysis.

Matrix-assisted Laser Desorption Ionization Time-of-flight (MALDI-TOF) Mass Spectrometry Analysis

Laser desorption/ionization mass spectrometric analysis was performed with a Perseptive Biosystems (Framingham, MA) Voyager EliteXL time-of-flight mass spectrometer with delayed extraction, operating with a pulsed nitrogen laser at 337 nm. Positive ion mass spectra were acquired using a linear, delayed extraction mode with an accelerating potential of 25 kV, a 93% grid potential, a 0.2% guide wire voltage, and a delay time of 1,000 ns. Each spectrum represents the results from 100 averaged laser pulses. Samples were concentrated with ZipTipC4 (Millipore) as described by the manufacturer using a saturated solution of sinapinic acid (Fluka) prepared in an 80% (v/v) of acetonitril/0.3% trifluoroacetic acid for elution. The elution mixture was placed on a stainless steel plate and air-dried prior to analysis. External calibration was performed with bovine albumin (Applied Biosystems) using the m/z value of 66,431 Da for the mono-charged ion and 33,216 Da for the di-charged ion. The values expressed are average mass and correspond to the $(M+H)^+$ ion.

Bleomycin Cytotoxicity

Cytotoxic activity of Dd-BLM preparation was tested *in vitro* using MTT (3-(4,5-dimethylthiazol-2-yl)2,5-diphenyltetrazolium bromide) assay, based on the ability of viable cells to reduce a soluble yellow tetrazolium salt (MTT) to blue formazan crystals. The HeLa cells grown in a 96-multiwell plate at 10^4 cells per well were incubated for 3 hr at 37°C in 100 μl of EMEM medium without FBS containing different amounts of Dd (where 1 μg amounts to 2.7 nM), BLM-Dd (where 1 μg amounts to 2.7 nM of Dd and 0.08 μM of BLM), or free BLM (0.13, 1 and 8 μM). Then FBS was added to a final concentration of 10%. After various times of incubation at 37°C the culture medium was removed and 100 μl EMEM medium containing 0.5 mg/ml MTT (Sigma) was added to each well. The plates were incubated, developed and read according to manufacturer's instructions, in Synergy HTi plate reader (Biotek, Winooski VT, USA). The number of viable cells was calculated as described by Mosmann (1983).

Confocal Microscopy

The HeLa cells (5×10^4) were grown overnight on coverslips. Different amounts of Dd, Dd-BLM conjugate or free BLM were applied on cells in EMEM without serum. After 3 hr incubation FBS was added to a final concentration of 10% and cells were grown at 37°C. At indicated time points cells were rinsed with cold PBS and fixed in 100% cold methanol for 10 min. Fixed cells were incubated for 1 hr with the following primary Abs: rabbit polyclonal anti-Dd, at room temperature, anti β-tubulin MAb (Sigma) at 37°C and rabbit polyclonal anti γ-H2AX (Calbiochem) at 37°C, rinsed with PBS and incubated with the secondary Abs: goat anti-rabbit Texas Red-labeled (Jackson), FITC-conjugated goat anti-mouse (Jackson), and finally with DAPI (Applichem, 1 μg/μl solution, 5 min RT). Antibodies dilutions are given earlier. Images were collected with EZ-C1 Nikon CLSM attached to a inverted microscope Eclipse TE2000 E (Nikon) using oil immersion objective ×60, Plan Apo 1.4 NA (Nikon). DAPI, FITC and Texas Red fluorescence was excited at 408, 488, and 543 nm, and emission was measured at 430–465, 500–530, and 565–640 nm, respectively. Images show a single confocal scans averaged 4 times with 10 μs pixel dwell. All images were collected with 512 × 512 resolution and zoom 2.0. Figures were processed with EZ-C1 Viewer and Photoshop 6.0.

FACScan Analysis

Non-synchronized HeLa cells were treated with different amounts of purified Dd in EMEM without serum. After 1 hr incubation the floating cells were recovered and combined with attached cells harvested by treatment with 2 mM EDTA in PBS. Pooled cells were rinsed with cold PBS and fixed in 100% cold methanol overnight. Fixed cells were pelleted, resuspended in PBS and incubated with the primary anti-Dd antibody (1:1,000; 1 hr at room temperature), washed with PBS and then incubated with goat anti-rabbit secondary FITC-labeled antibody (Santa Cruz) (1:200; 1 hr at room temperature). After several PBS washes, portions of approximately 10,000 cells were analyzed by flow cytometry on a FACSCalibur (Beckton Dickinson).

DISCUSSION

Dodecahedra composed of 12 Ad3 pentons are produced in human cells upon Ad3 infection (Norrby, 1968). They are synthesized abundantly in Ad3-infected cells in culture, resulting in 5.5 × 106 Dds produced per one infectious virus (Fender et al., 2005). The Ad Dd is significantly smaller than the original virus. This is unlike some other known VLPs of non-enveloped viruses such as HPV or Norwalk (Caliciviridae) VLPs, whose VLPs morphologically mimic native virions (Jiang et al., 1992; Lenz et al., 2001). In contrast, Ad base dodecahedron, composed of pentameric penton bases normally capping the vertices of the icosahedral virion, is significantly smaller than the complete virus, measuring 280 Å versus approximately 900–1,000 Å for the fiberless virions (Fabry et al., 2005). Lacking several structural components of virions this type of VLP exhibits functional and structural properties different from those of the virus capsid. For example, we have shown that when both primary and secondary receptors are blocked, Ad still infects the cells, but now through interaction of the major virion protein, the hexon, with plasma membrane lipids (Balakireva et al., 2003). Dodecahedra, which do not contain Ad hexons, will be not able to employ this entry mechanism. In contrast, Dd is able to attach to and penetrate cells through interaction with heparan sulfate, a pathway not used by the virus of origin, Ad3 (Fender et al., 2008; Vives et al., 2004). Since heparan sulfates recognize patches of basic amino acids, this gain-of-function most probably stems from decreased distances between groups of basic residues of neighboring penton bases in Dd, versus more distant, separated by hexons, penton bases in Ad virions.

Through expression in the baculovirus system we are able to produce DFs and also Dds built of bases alone (DB). Both kinds of Dds very efficiently penetrate cells in culture (Fender et al., 1997; Garcel et al., 2006). The Dds assemble in the absence of any viral scaffolding proteins and do not require nucleic acid for assembling. When these dodecahedral particles are isolated from insect cells, they are contaminated with host (insect) cell nucleic acid. The latter can be removed on an ion-exchange column without loss of particle integrity, suggesting its external attachment. This is different, for example, from VLPs of human BK polyomavirus, which seem to pack DNA internally upon assembly (Li et al., 2003).

The yield of recombinant Dd production in the baculovirus system is about 10 mg from 100 ml (8×10^7) of cultured insect cells, which is comparable with a very efficient bacterial system (Song et al., 2008). The purification protocol consists of a simple two-step procedure, yielding non-tagged Dds. However, the particles in the absence of salt have a tendency to aggregate, similarly to papillomavirus VLPs (Shi et al., 2005). The Ad2 virions have been observed to be rather stable under mildly acidic conditions (Rexroad et al., 2006). In contrast, DB seems to be more stable in the pH range 7–8, with about 10°C difference in Tm between pH 5 and 7 (Figure 3), similarly as described for the VLPs of papilloma virus type 11 and of polyoma virus (Brady et al., 1977; McCarthy et al., 1998).

Our physicochemical and functional analyses have shown that Ad3 Dds exhibit remarkable stability. These particles are stable for long periods of storage at 4°C and even at room temperature. In the presence of 150 mM NaCl they can be stored at temperatures up to 40°C at pH 4–5 and up to 50°C at pH 6–8. Moreover, at increased ionic strength they withstand temperatures up to 60°C (Figure 3C). Dodecahedra can be frozen and lyophilized in the presence of cryoprotectants, without losing their integrity upon thawing and reconstitution with water. Finally, Dds retain their particulate integrity during incubation in human serum at 37°C for at least 2 hr (Figure 4B). These data show that Dds can be conveniently stored and transported, and can potentially be used for therapeutic purposes under various climates.

We have taken advantage of the remarkable penetration properties of Dds to improve cell delivery of the anticancer antibiotic BLM. Since their discovery, BLMs have been used in a number of combination anticancer regimens. They are interesting therapeutics as they exert selective tumor cytotoxicity and exhibit low myelo- and immunosuppression (Chen and Stubbe, 2005; Lehane et al., 1975). However, despite the fact that as few as 500 BLM molecules introduced into the cytosol are able to kill the cell (Poddevin et al., 1991), high BLM doses have to be used in clinical treatment.

BLM not only crosses poorly plasma membranes which have very few receptors for BLM (Pron et al., 1999), but in addition, cell-internalized BLM is inactivated in the cytosol by neutral cysteine aminopeptidase called BML hydrolase (Sebti et al., 1991). Hence, only a fraction of applied BLM reaches the cell nucleus where it cleaves the DNA (Hecht, 2000). As a result of the high-dose treatment requirements, BLM utility is limited by the systemic toxicity and the dose-dependent pneumonitis, able to progress to lung fibrosis. The latter can affect nearly 50% of total patient population, out of which 3% will die (Sleijfer, 2001). It is therefore important to be able to decrease the effective dose of BLM.

The Dd on its own is only weakly cytotoxic and the cytotoxicity is observed only after prolonged treatment (50 hr). Since the largest cytotoxic effect for the Dd-BLM conjugate is seen after the first 10 hr of treatment (Figure 5C), the weak Dd toxicity will not be important in Dd-BLM applications. Moreover, results presented in Figure 6 show rather normal appearance of Dd-treated cells (row Dd), even at 30 and 50 hr.

Ad dodecahedron, similarly to other nanoparticles, possesses a large surface area which can be exploited for multiple ligand presentation. Clustering the ligands on the VLP surface allows multiple ligand-receptor interaction or multivalency. The collective binding between multiple ligands and receptors results in increased affinity. This is even more true for the conjugate of Dd-BLM since not only does one Dd particle bring multiple copies of BLM but, in addition, several types of receptors are in play. The Dd recognizes two types of receptors. It has an affinity for the omnipresent heparan sulfates (Fender et al., 2008; Vives et al., 2004), and in this respect it is not very specific for tumor cells (with the possible exception of hepatic cancers). In addition, Dd retains the affinity of its building blocks, penton bases, for av integrins (Wickham et al., 1993). These integrins are highly expressed on activated endothelial cells and tumor cells but are not present in resting endothelial cells and most normal organ systems; in particular their expression on the neoplastic blood vessels is known to be upgraded (Eliceiri and Cheresh, 1999; Pasqualini et al., 1997). Affinity for av integrins suggests tumor-tropicity of Dd. In addition the Dd-BLM conjugate will be able to recognize the third type of receptors, specific for BLM (Pron et al., 1999). Thus, BLM-Dd conjugate represents a case of a monovalent ligand attached to the polyvalent carrier, together able to recognize the three cellular receptors.

The BLM is a multifunctional molecule composed of three active parts. It was thus possible that its function would be impaired by the cross-linking reaction. However, DLS analysis of Dd-BLM conjugate suggested that the chemical treatment did not introduce gross changes in Dd structure. Application of the Dd-BLM conjugate resulted in cell death, further suggesting that neither the transducing properties of Dd nor BLM cytotoxicity were compromised by the cross-linking reaction. Importantly, the specific DNA-damaging activity of free BLM resulting in dsDNA breaks was retained also by BLM delivered with the dodecahedric vector. Moreover, the bioavailability of BLM delivered with the aid of Dd was 100 times higher than that of free BLM. This is an important result because it shows that BLM delivery can be significantly improved and its cytotoxic effect can possibly be attenuated by attaching it to a suitable vector, conceivably resulting in diminished side effects of BLM therapy. For comparison, when

BLM was delivered by electroporation, the bioavailability was improved only 2 to 10-fold (Horiuchi et al., 2000; Yanai et al., 2002), whereas the use of bleomycin-loaded microspheres did not improve the drug bioavailability when compared to free BLM (Wang et al., 2008). Ultrasound application improved BLM bioavailability 8-fold, and the effect was enhanced 33 times when microbubbles were included in the treatment (Sonoda et al., 2007). Finally, the use of liposomes for BLM delivery brought about 20 to 40-fold increase in bioavailability (Gabizon et al., 1990), resulting in a significant decrease in BLM-induced lung injury (Arndt et al., 2001).

Induction of giant cells upon Dd-BLM treatment is due to the presence of the antibiotic since cells treated with Dd alone did not exhibit such a phenotype (Figures 6 and 7). This phenotype resembles the one observed for cells treated with other cell-cycle arresting chemotherapy drugs, where response to treatment quite often results in induction of polyploid giant cells. Drugs interacting with DNA activate several signal transduction pathways, which culminate in the induction of apoptosis. Mitotic or reproductive death after G2 stage arrest is induced by DNA damaging agents and produces enlarged cells containing multiple nuclear fragments, readily distinguished from apoptotic nuclear fragments. After a prolonged incubation, multinucleated cells lose attachment to the tissue culture plate and undergo apoptosis (Demarcq et al., 1994; Lock et al., 1994). This has been shown for both transformed cells treated with cisplatin, doxorubicin, or etoposide and for established tumors treated with cisplatin (Lock and Stribinskiene, 1996; Puig et al., 2008; Sliwinska et al., 2008).

Different physicochemical approaches such as photochemical internalization, electroporation, and ultrasounds, as well as the use of liposomes have been attempted to improve BLM cell entry, its release from endosomes and passage through the cytoplasm (Arndt et al., 2001; Berg et al., 2005; Larkin et al., 2008; Sersa et al., 2008). We propose attaching BLM to a vector that carries out all these functions, namely efficiently penetrates the plasma membrane, is quickly liberated in the cytoplasm and has a propensity to concentrate around the nucleus (Fender et al., 1997). Our data on the kinetics of Dd inside transduced cells suggest that the intracellular vector undergoes slow proteolysis, liberating BLM peptides. These small BML conjugates are probably able to easily translocate to the nucleus, where BLM exerts its cytotoxic effect.

It should not be forgotten, however, that we describe here a protein-based system, and therefore the host immune response might pose a major problem in medical application. On the other hand, we wish to apply the Dd-BLM conjugate locally in the glioblastoma animal model, and the nervous tissues are thought to enjoy a conditionally privileged immune status: they are normally unreachable for self-reactive T and B cells, lack lymphatic drainage and are deficient in local antigen-presenting cells. Moreover, it has long been considered that administration of foreign antigens into the brain can lead to a state of tolerance rather than immunization (see (Cobbold et al., 2006) and references therein).

In conclusion, it is possible to deliver BLM with the aid of a VLP, Ad Dd, in order to significantly improve drug bioavailability. These experiments open new vistas for improved delivery of impermeant labile drugs, bringing us closer to *in vivo* use of Ad dodecahedron as a delivery vector.

RESULTS

Db Expression and Purification

Ad penton base polypeptides upon expression in human and insect cells oligomerize into pentamers. For Ad3, the majority of pentameric Pbs assemble into symmetrical particles called dodecahedra base (or dodecahedra), of 3.6 MDa, which are made up of 12 pentameric Pbs. In the first step of purification from insect cells the dodecahedric VLPs were isolated from 15 to 40% sucrose gradient, where they sedimented in 30–40% sucrose, with free pentameric Pbs recovered from lighter sucrose (Fender et al., 1997).

Since sucrose fractions containing particles were contaminated with cellular proteins and nucleic acids (Figure 1A, left panel), final Dds purification was achieved by ion exchange chromatography on a Q-Sepharose column. The Pbs containing material was eluted in two peaks: at 280 mM and 380 mM NaCl (P1 and P2 in Figure 1A), while the third peak observed at 630 mM NaCl contained insect cell DNA (see Figure 1B, middle panel). Proteins in peaks 1 and 2 migrated with different velocity on native agarose gel (Figure 1B, right panel). Negative stain electron microscopy (EM) analysis showed non-assembled free base pentamers in peak 1 (Figure 1C, left panel), whereas the material in peak 2 consisted of dodecahedra bases (Figure 1C, right panel). It is possible that in sucrose density gradient some Pbs sedimented with the bulk of DBs due to their assembly into larger structures on cellular DNA. Cell penetration assay showed that gradient-purified preparation contained mixed material of varying penetration ability, while Dds obtained from the Q-Sepharose column contained more uniformly penetrating particles (Figure 1D).

Up to 25% of Dds obtained after sucrose density gradient did not bind to the Q-Sepharose column. Although both pools of unattached and column-purified Dds were able to penetrate cells in culture to a similar extent, the former was unstable upon storage, probably due to proteolysis. DB expression in the baculovirus system was remarkably high, reaching 1 mg of purified particles per about 8×10^6 insect cells. The N-terminal analysis of numerous batches of purified DB showed that it consists of a mixture of N-terminally truncated penton base polypeptides. Cleavage at glycine 9 accounted for approximately 42% of free N-termini, while that at Ala 38, Pro 230, and Val 317 for 13, 7, and 7%, respectively. Interpolating from the data on atomic structure of Ad2 dodecahedron (Zubieta et al., 2005), it appears that Val 317 is located in the flexible RGD loop whereas Pro 230 is in an exposed loop near the top of the molecule. The RGD loop is involved in Pb interaction with integrins during Ad cell entry, while the second loop is involved in fiber binding and in interactions with the adjacent Pb monomer (Zubieta et al., 2005). It is conceivable that a proteolytic attack on these two exposed loops results in a small portion of dodecahedra being impaired in their penetration ability. Similar proteolysis was observed for simultaneously expressed Ad3 Pb. Our attempts to inhibit proteolysis during the purification process were unsuccessful because the Pb had already been cleaved during expression in insect cells (results not shown).

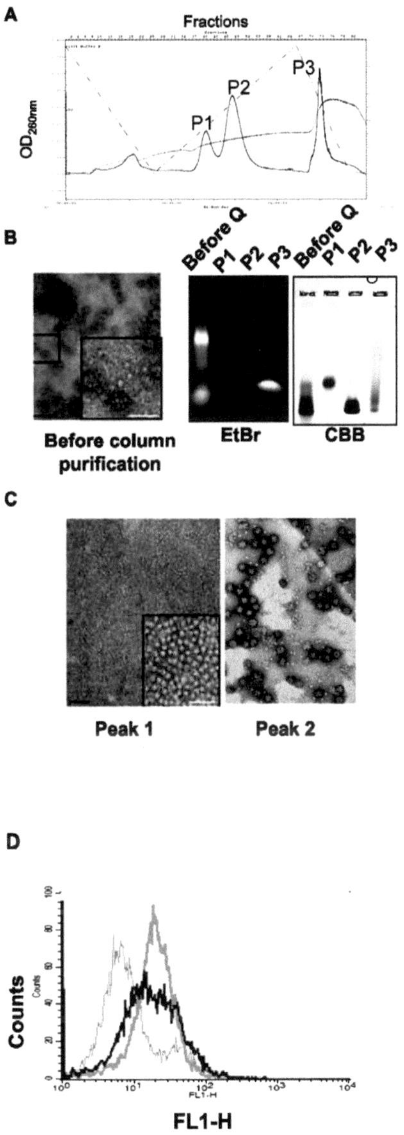

Figure 1. Purification of recombinant Ad3 DB expressed in the baculovirus system.
(A) Dodecahedra initially purified on sucrose density gradient were fractionated on a Q-Sepharose column in 20 mM Tris buffer, pH 7.5, using NaCl gradient. (B) Analysis of purified Dds. Left panel-negative stain electron microscopy (EM) of Dds purified on sucrose density gradient. Middle and right panels-non-denaturing agarose gel electrophoresis of fractions recovered from the Q-Sepharose column with detection with ethidium bromide (EtBr, middle panel) followed by Commassie Brilliant Blue (CBB) staining (right panel). (C) Negative stain EM showing free pentameric bases recovered in peak 1 (left panel) and complete dodecahedra in peak 2 (right panel) of the Q-Sepharose column (P1 and P2 in A). Scale bar equals 100 nm. (D) Flow cytometry analysis of HeLa cells transduced with Dd (see Materials and Methods). Sucrose density gradient-purified Dds–purple curve, Q-Sepharosepurified Dds—green curve. Blue curve shows the antibody background in the absence of Dd.

Studies on DB Stability

VLP of SV40 is stabilized by calcium ions and the disulfide bond at Cys 9 prevents SV40 VLPs dissociation, probably by increasing binding of calcium ion (Ishizu et al., 2001). Similarly, the disulfide bonds play an important role in maintaining the integrity of JC virus VLPs by protecting calcium ions from chelation (Chen et al., 2001). In contrast, disulfide bonds alone stabilize HPV11, and cation chelation does not affect the stability of HPV11 VLPs (McCarthy et al., 1998). Not much is known about factors involved in Ad3 Dd stability, but preliminary data obtained for Ad3 DB crystals at 3.8 Å resolution showed a metal ion that is almost certainly calcium in the region of contact between subunits (personal communication, Dr. S. Cusack). This led us to test the effect of metal-ion chelators on Dd stability. However, Dd retained its structure in the presence of 100 mM EDTA or EGTA (results not shown), suggesting that divalent ions are not involved in maintaining its integrity.

We tested the stability and solubility of purified DB particles over a pH range from 4 to 10.9. For this purpose ion exchange-purified Dds were dialyzed overnight at 4°C against various buffers and subsequently incubated at 30 or 37°C. Following incubation, some preparations were subjected to centrifugation to separate the soluble fraction from the aggregated particles. The assembly status of proteins in the supernatants was analyzed by native agarose gel electrophoresis.

The DB particles were readily soluble at 4°C in all the buffers used, but remained in solution only in the presence of 150 mM NaCl (Figure 2A, four leftside lanes). Without NaCl DB remained in solution in a rather unstable manner, disappearing from the supernatants and pelleting upon centrifugation (Figure 2A, left panel, four rightside lanes). Clearly, NaCl at a physiological concentration protects DB from precipitation. A protective effect of NaCl was observed also during incubation at 30°C (Figure 2A, right panel).

For pH values above 8 we used 100 mM sodium carbonate buffer, which up to pH 10.9 did not cause visible protein aggregation, even during incubation at 37°C. However, at pH 10.4 Dds dissociated to free pentameric Pbs, and an increase in temperature to 37°C (30 min incubation) resulted in nearly total DB dissociation already at pH 9.6 (Figure 2B).

To probe Dd stability upon prolonged temperature treatment, we performed 24 hr dialysis at 37°C against buffers of different ionic strength (Figure 2C). The presence of 370 mM or 1 M NaCl in the purification buffer was sufficient to prevent protein aggregation, but dissociation to free pentameric Pbs was observed under conditions of prolonged temperature treatment. However, the presence of ammonium sulfate significantly stabilized Dd, preventing its dissociation to free pentameric Pbs (Figure 2C, lanes AS).

In order to apply a more general approach to the question of Dd thermal denaturation, we used dynamic light scattering technique (DLS), which allows monitoring of protein denaturation or unfolding. When denaturation occurs, the size of the protein is increased to a value consistent with a random coil polymer of the same mass. In the absence of aggregation-prohibiting agents, interpolymer hydrophobic interactions can quickly lead to non-specific aggregation of the denatured polypeptide chains. The protein melting point temperature (T_m), obtained during DLS analysis is indicative of the thermal stability of a protein. A positive shift in Tm indicates stabilization of the protein by an increase in structural order and a reduction in conformational flexibility, while a negative shift in Tm indicates destabilization. The change in mean particle size that accompanies DB denaturation was measured at different pH and ionic conditions, applying a thermal gradient from 12 to 65°C.

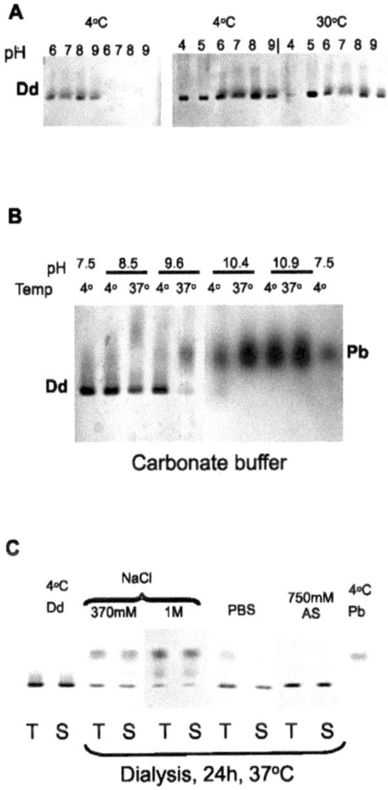

Figure 2. Dd stability under different conditions of temperature, pH and ionic strength, analyzed by native gel electrophoresis. Purified Dds were dialyzed overnight at 4°C (A, B) or for 24 hr at 37°C (C) against different buffers at the indicated pH. (A) Effect of pH on Dd solubility. The Dd was dialyzed against the following 50 mM buffers: MES, pH 6; Hepes, pH 7; Tris, pH 8, and CAPS, pH 9. Left panel: samples were prepared in duplicates and after dialysis the second batch was centrifuged at 13000 rpm for 30 min. The first four lanes contain the dialyzed samples; the next lanes contain the supernatants after centrifugation. Right panel: samples were dialyzed against the same buffers as described for the left panel and also against citric acid, pH 4, and acetic acid, pH 5, but all buffers contained 150 mM NaCl. Samples were prepared in duplicates and one batch was kept at 4°C while the second one was incubated for 20 min at 30°C. Soluble proteins contained in the supernatants obtained by 30 min centrifugation at 13000 rpm were applied on agarose gel. (B) The Dd stability in carbonate buffer. Carbonate buffer (100 mM) was prepared at the indicated pH and used for Dds dialysis. Some samples were incubated at 37°C for 20 min. All samples were centrifuged as above and the supernatants were electrophoresed on native agarose gel. First and last lanes, control Dd and Pb preparations, respectively. (C) Effect of ionic conditions on Dd thermal stability. The Dds were dialyzed for 24 hr at 37°C against the purification buffer containing NaCl or $(NH_4)_2SO_4$ (AS) at indicated concentrations or against PBS, pH 7.5. Non-treated samples (T for total) or supernatants after centrifugation at 13000 rpm for 30 min (S) were analyzed on the agarose gel. The first two lanes contain control Dd while the last lane contains Pb preparations, all in purification buffer.

Figure 3A shows the temperature dependent Z-average diameter measurements for DB. At temperatures up to 40°C the particle size was constant at pH 4–9, suggesting a stable structure. Above this temperature the particle size increased exponentially with temperature, indicating the presence of denatured aggregates. The Dd denaturation/aggregation started at approximately 10°C lower temperature at pH 4–5 than at pH 7–8. At pH 9 (CAPS) and 10 (carbonate buffer) only small changes in particle size were observed, in particular at pH 10. Native gel analysis of Dd treated with the same temperature gradient as the one applied during DLS analysis (Figure 3B) showed that

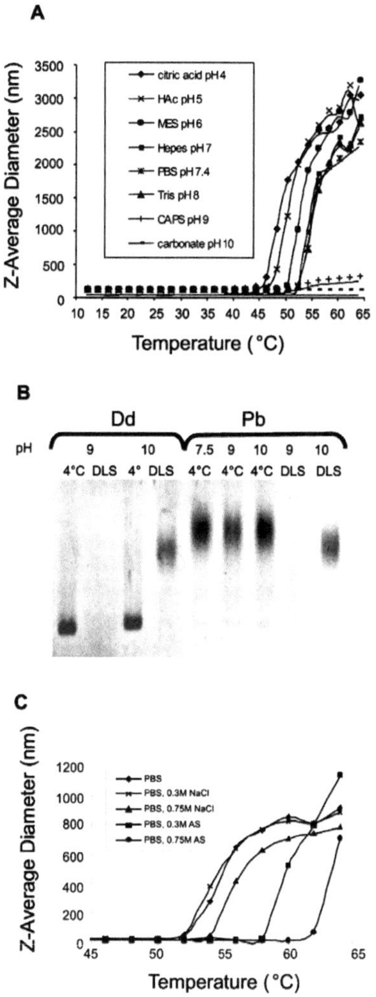

Figure 3. Thermal Dd stability as a function of pH and ionic strength. (A) Dd was analyzed by dynamic light scattering (DLS) at different pH in the presence of 150 mM NaCl as a function of temperature, as described in Materials and Methods. (B) Native gel analysis of Dds and Pbs, in CAPS pH 9, and carbonate buffer, pH 10. Some samples were subjected to temperature treatment imitating DLS temperature gradient (marked DLS). (C) The DLS analysis carried out on Dds in PBS under different ionic strength conditions. Mean values of three apparatus readings are shown.

while at pH 10 Dd dissociates to free bases, at pH 9 (CAPS buffer) the protein disappears, suggesting aggregate formation. Similar DLS-imitating temperature treatment of free pentameric bases confirmed aggregation of this protein at pH 9 (Figure 3B, lanes Pb/DLS). Of note, CAPS is an organic buffer that may have a propensity to interact with hydrophobic patches on the protein surface, which can induce protein aggregation. It seems that a temperature increase at pH 4–8 led to rapid Dd aggregation, while at pH 9 Dd first dissociated to free pentameric bases which then underwent aggregation. Addition of 750 mM NaCl to PBS caused a positive shift in the T_m of Dd suggesting structure stabilization (Figure 3C). But the most significant increase in T_m values was caused by addition of ammonium sulfate (positive shift of about 12°C, Figure 3C), which confirmed the stabilizing effect of this salt observed during Dd dialysis at 37°C (Figure 2C).

Prolonged Dodecahedron Stability in Cultured Cells and in Human Serum *In Vitro*

In order to be able to store the vector we tested the effect of freezing and thawing on Dd integrity. After dialysis to water Dd aggregated even in the presence of the cryoprotectants, which was to be expected as it precipitates in the absence of salt (see Figure 2A). The Dd survived freezing at −80°C in 150 mM ammonium sulfate, and then subsequent thawing at room temperature. The Dd structure was preserved upon dialysis, freezing and drying in the speed-vac in the presence of 150 mM ammonium sulfate (Figure 4A). Although during lyophilization of Dd in 150 mM aqueous ammonium sulfate Dd integrity was not maintained, it was preserved in the presence of the cryoprotectants such as 0.4% sucrose and 0.4% mannitol (Figure 4A, compare the last two lanes).

Intracellular vector survival was tested by Western blotting performed on HeLa cell extracts, which were prepared at different periods following Dd application and resolved on native agarose gels. The amount of intracellular Dd increased significantly up to 32 hr post transduction, with noticeable Pb proteolysis resulting in only a fraction of intracellular Pb remaining after 4 days (Figure 4B, left panel). Native agarose gel analysis showed that 96 hr post penetration the majority of intracellular material was running between bona fide Dd and Pb (Figure 4B, right panel, marked with a dot), suggesting the removal of external loops from Dd, albeit with some degree of particle integrity remaining. It is relevant that the anti-Dd antibody recognized proteolyzed Dd forms better than the original ones on native Western blots.

We also tested the integrity of Dd under conditions imitating its potential situation *in vivo*. In freshly prepared human serum the vector seemed to be stable for at least 2 hr at 37°C (Figure 4C).

Bleomycin Delivery by Dd

Bleomycin is a family of metal-binding glycopeptide antibiotics with antimicrobial, antiviral, and antitumor properties (Takeshita et al., 1978). The BLM is an extremely cytotoxic agent once inside the cell nucleus, where it cleaves the DNA (Hecht, 1994; Poddevin et al., 1991). However, BLM cytotoxicity is limited by its inability to freely diffuse through membranes (Mir et al., 1996) and by its cleavage by intracellular proteases (Sebti and Lazo, 1988). In consequence, high doses of BLM have to be used in therapeutic treatment, which in turn leads to serious side effects like non-specific cytotoxicity, including acute lung fibrosis (Chen and Stubbe, 2005).

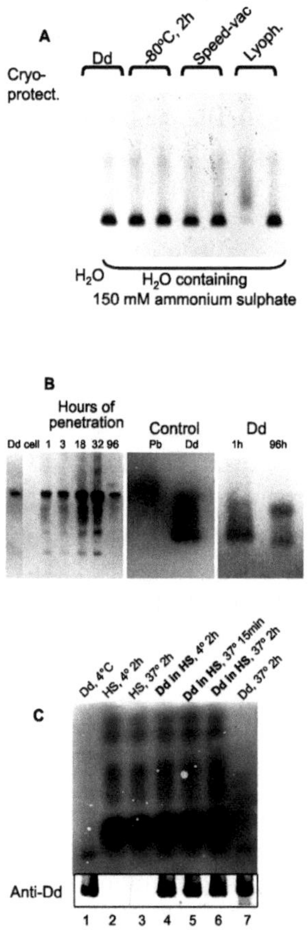

Figure 4. The Dd stability upon lyophilization, inside HeLa cells and in human serum. (A) Purified Dds were dialyzed overnight at 4°C against water or 150 mM $(NH_4)_2SO_4$ in water. Mannitol (0.4%) and sucrose (0.4%) were added to samples marked "Cryoprotect. +". The Dd samples were frozen at –80°C, dried in speed-vac or lyophilized (marked Lyoph. +). Dry samples were reconstituted in the starting volume of water. All preparations were centrifuged for 30 min at 13000 rpm and the supernatants were applied onto native agarose gel. (B) Stability of Dd after application to HeLa cells. Purified Dds (2 μg in 100 μl) were applied to 2 x 10^4 portions of HeLa cells. After indicated periods of penetration cell lysates were analyzed on SDS-PAGE (left panel) or on native agarose gel (two right panels). Control Dd samples contained 30 ng protein, while control Pb sample contained 10 ng protein. (C) Stability of Dd upon incubation in human serum. Samples of Dd concentrated by ultrafiltration in Microcon unit (Millipore) (5 μg each) were incubated in human serum (HS) at 4°C for 2 hr (lane 4) and at 37°C for 15 min or for 2 hr (lanes 5 and 6, respectively). Samples were resolved by native agarose gel electrophoresis and analyzed by Western blot performed with anti-Dd serum. The upper part shows CBB stained gel with proteins remaining after transfer, and the lower part the developed Western blot. Lanes 1 and 7 show Dd non-treated or incubated for 2 hr at 37°C, respectively, in the absence of serum. Lanes 2 and 3 show human serum after 2 hr incubation at 4 and 37°C, respectively. The Dd samples incubated with the serum are denoted in bold.

We attached BLM to Dd chemically, which resulted in a Dd-BLM conjugate with each penton base monomer carrying between 0 and two BLM molecules (BLM molecular mass is 1,400), with a clear predominance of the species with one BLM moiety attached, as shown by mass spectroscopy analysis (Figure 5A). These data suggest that one Dd particle carries on the average 60 BLM molecules. The DLS analysis showed the melting profile of the conjugate to be quite similar to that of untreated Dd (Figure 5B). Preliminary experiments with cytotoxic concentrations of free BLM revealed that the antibiotic must remain in the culture medium all the time; its removal 3 hr after application did not result in cell deaths. Since the amount of intracellular Dd increased significantly up to 32 hr post transduction (Figure 4B, left panel), we analyzed the kinetics of cell survival with Dd-BLM conjugate, which showed that at 14 hr application about 40% of cells survived while at 48 hr application the survival was below 20% cells (results not shown).Therefore, both, BLM and Dd-BLM (as well as Dd alone) were left in the medium throughout the experiment.

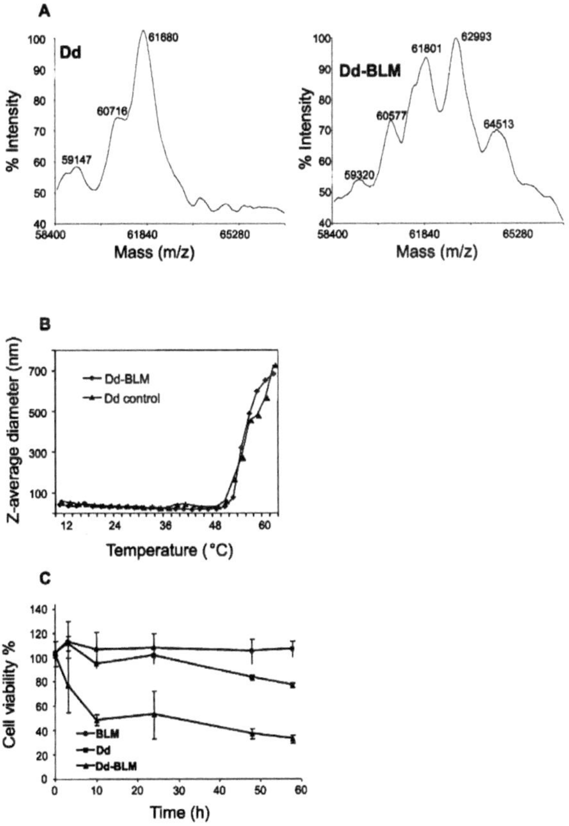

Figure 5. Cell toxicity of bleomycin (BLM) delivered with the aid of Dd. The BLM was chemically attached to Dds as described in Materials and Methods. (A) Characterization of Dd-BLM conjugate by mass spectrometry analysis (Maldi). (B) The DLS analysis of the BLM conjugate. (C) The MTT assay of cell toxicity. The HeLa cells were treated with free BLM (0.13 μM), Dd (1 μg), and Dd-BLM (1 μg delivering 0.08 μM BLM), as described in Materials and Methods.

The Dd-BLM preparations containing on average 0.08 μM BLM showed significant cytotoxic activity while application of comparable amounts of BLM in the free form did not affect cell growth (Figure 5C). A comparable level of cell death was observed when at least 8 μM solution of free BLM was used (results not shown).

The next step involved observation by confocal microscopy. Fascan analysis showed that the entry potential of Dd is not affected by the chemical treatment during conjugate preparation as both free vector particles and the Dd-BML conjugate had similar entry capacity (Figure 6A). Since the anti-BLM serum appropriate for confocal microscopy is not available, the presence of Dd-BLM conjugate was demonstrated using the anti-Dd

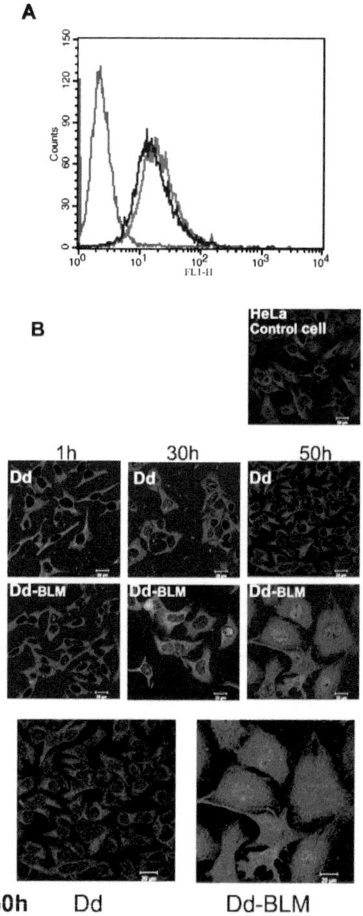

Figure 6. Effect of Dd and Dd-BLM conjugate on HeLa cells. (A) Flow cytometry analysis of Dd (green curve) and Dd-BLM (pink curve) cell entry. Cells were treated with appropriate vector for 1 hr at 37°C as described in Materials and Methods. The blue curve shows the antibody background in the absence of Dd. (B) Cells were treated with 1 μg Dd or Dd-BLM for indicated times and analyzed with anti-Dd serum (in red) by confocal microscopy, as described in Materials and Methods. Nuclei were stained blue with DAPI. Last row shows the 50 hour-treatment without nuclear staining. Scale bar equals 20 μm.

antibody. Remarkably, 1 hr after Dd application all cells were found to be transduced with Dd, whose presence was clearly seen in the cytoplasm of each cell (Figure 6, 1 hr, Dd). At 50 hr post application with free Dd, the amount of intracellular Dd significantly diminished with the red signal still limited to the cytoplasm (Figure 6, 50 hr, Dd), suggesting destruction of free Dds and their removal from cells. A 1 hr post application cells treated with Dd-BLM exhibited similar image as cells treated with Dd alone at this timepoint (Figure 6, 1 hr). However, at 30 hr post application, cells treated with Dd-BLM conjugate appeared somewhat bigger (Figure 6, 30 hr, Dd-BLM). Finally, at 50 hr post application Dd-BLM caused the appearance of giant cells with intense red Dd signal in the entire cell, suggesting a collapse of the nuclear membrane (Figure 6, compare 50 hr with Dd versus Dd-BLM, last row, nuclear stain removed).

The mechanism of the cytotoxic activity of BLM is based on host DNA cleavage (Mir et al., 1996). One of the well-characterized DNA-damage-responsive chromatin modification events is the phosphorylation of the C-terminal tail of histone H2A or the H2AX variant in higher eukaryotes (Kinner et al., 2008). Therefore, we used the antibody recognizing the phosphorylated form of the H2AX histone for monitoring DNA damage in HeLa cells. Control as well as Dd-treated cells did not show DNA damage as judged by nearly total absence of cells stained red with anti-γ-H2AX (Figure 7, rows of HeLa and Dd). Similarly, no DNA damage was observed upon application of free BLM up to approximately 8 μM concentration (not shown). However, at 8 μM free BLM there was significant DNA cleavage at all analyzed timepoints, accompanied by an increase in cell size starting from 30 hr post application (Figure 7, BLM row). Similar though even more pronounced symptoms were observed upon application of Dd-BLM conjugate, delivering 100 times less BLM (Figure 7, Dd-BLM).

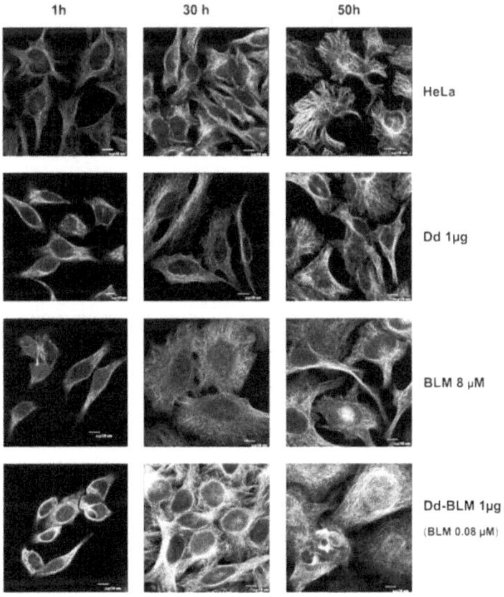

Figure 7. Kinetics of Dds DNA breaks as jugded by induction of γ-H2AX foci. The HeLa cells were treated either with Dd, with free BLM or Dd-BLM for indicated periods and analyzed with anti-γ-H2AX Ab (in red) and with anti-tubulin Ab (in green) by confocal microscopy, as described in Materials and Methods. Scale bar equals 10 μm.

KEYWORDS

- **Adenovirus**
- **Bleomycin**
- **Coomassie Brilliant Blue**
- **Dodecahedron base**
- **Human papilloma virus**
- **Virus-like particle**

AUTHORS' CONTRIBUTIONS

Conceived and designed the experiments: Jadwiga Chroboczek and Ewa Szolajska. Performed the experiments: Monika Zochowska, Agnieszka Paca, Guy Schoehn, Jean-Pierre Andrieu, Bernard Dublet, and Ewa Szolajska. Analyzed the data: Guy Schoehn Jadwiga, Chroboczek, and Ewa Szolajska. Contributed reagents/materials/analysis tools: Ewa Szolajska. Wrote the chapter: Jadwiga Chroboczek and Ewa Szolajska.

ACKNOWLEDGMENTS

We acknowledge the technical assistance of Elzbieta Malinska in part of this work. We thank Iwona Cymerman (International Institute of Molecular and Cell Biology, Warsaw) and Anna Anielska (IBB, Warsaw) for instructions on FACScan and confocal microscopy analysis. We are indebted to Maxim Balakirev, Sebastian Launois (CEA-French Atomic Energy Commission, Grenoble) and Igor Andreyev (Institute of Molecular Biology and Genetics, Kiev) for discussion on cross-linking reaction, for help with DLS analysis and with native Western blot analysis, respectively.

Chapter 14

Exon Skipping Oligonucleotides and Concomitant Dystrophin Expression in Skeletal Muscle of mdx Mice

Jason H. Williams, Rebecca C. Schray, Shashank R. Sirsi, and Gordon J. Lutz

INTRODUCTION

Exon skipping oligonucleotides (ESOs) of 2'O-Methyl (2'OMe) and morpholino chemistry have been shown to restore dystrophin expression in muscle fibers from the mdx mouse, and are currently being tested in Phase I clinical trials for Duchenne muscular dystrophy (DMD). However, ESOs remain limited in their effectiveness because of an inadequate delivery profile. Synthetic cationic copolymers of poly(ethylene imine) (PEI) and poly(ethylene glycol) (PEG) are regarded as effective agents for enhanced delivery of nucleic acids in various applications.

We examined whether PEG-PEI copolymers can facilitate ESO-mediated dystrophin expression after intramuscular injections into tibialis anterior (TA) muscles of mdx mice. We utilized a set of PEG-PEI copolymers containing 2 kDa PEI and either 550 Da or 5 kDa PEG, both of which bind 2'OMe ESOs with high affinity and form stable nanoparticulates with a relatively low surface charge. Three weekly intramuscular injections of 5 μg of ESO complexed with PEI2K-PEG550 copolymers resulted in about 500 dystrophin-positive fibers and about 12% of normal levels of dystrophin expression at 3 weeks after the initial injection, which is significantly greater than for injections of ESO alone, which are known to be almost completely ineffective. In an effort to enhance biocompatibility and cellular uptake, the PEI2K-PEG550 and PEI2K-PEG5K copolymers were functionalized by covalent conjugation with nanogold (NG) or adsorbtion of colloidal gold (CG), respectively. Surprisingly, using the same injection and dosing regimen, we found no significant difference in dystrophin expression by Western blot between the NG-PEI2K-PEG550, CG-PEI2K-PEG5K, and non-functionalized PEI2K-PEG550 copolymers. Dose-response experiments using the CG-PEI2K-PEG5K copolymer with total ESO ranging from 3–60 μg yielded a maximum of about 15% dystrophin expression. Further improvements in dystrophin expression up to 20% of normal levels were found at 6 weeks after 10 twice-weekly injections of the NG-PEI2K-PEG550 copolymer complexed with 5 μg of ESO per injection. This injection and dosing regimen showed over 1000 dystrophin-positive fibers. The H&E staining of all treated muscle groups revealed no overt signs of cytotoxicity.

We conclude that PEGylated PEI2K copolymers are efficient carriers for local delivery of 2'OMe ESOs and warrant further development as potential therapeutics for treatment of DMD.

Steric block oligomers such as of 2'OMe and phosphorodiamidate morpholino (PMO) oligonucleotides possess high affinity for their complementary pre-mRNA targets and can modulate alternative splicing, correct aberrant splicing, and induce skipping or inclusion of specific exons (for reviews see (Kole et al., 2004; Garcia-Blanco et al. 2004)). These splice modulating oligonucleotides (SMOs) represent a powerful class of compounds with broad utility for basic and translational research and are poised to show rapid growth as pharmaceuticals. However, for many *in vivo* applications, SMOs administered alone show an inadequate delivery profile for reaching target cell nuclei, necessitating the use of carriers. Indeed, inefficient delivery of SMOs remains the foremost limitation to their usefulness as pharmaceuticals.

The DMD is a fatal x-linked disease caused by mutations in the gene encoding the 427 kDa membrane-associated cytoskeletal protein dystrophin, resulting in progressive body-wide muscle weakening and death usually in the early to mid third decade of life. The DMD mutations are most often comprised of insertions and deletions that alter the dystrophin reading frame or encode premature stop codons (Aartsma-Rus et al., 2006a). These types of mutations result in production of truncated and non-functional dystrophin that is rapidly degraded.

Steric block ESOs have been shown in cultured mouse, canine, and human cells to cause skipping of targeted dystrophin exons, resulting in production of full-length dystrophin mRNA (minus only the skipped exons), and restoration of the reading frame (Aartsma-Rus et al., 2003, 2004, 2006b, 2007; Gebski et al., 2003; Mann et al., 2001; McClorey et al., 2006). The classical animal model for DMD, the mdx mouse, has a point mutation in dystrophin exon 23 that produces a premature stop codon. ESOs have been shown to promote skipping of exon 23 and concomitant dystrophin expression in skeletal muscles of mdx mice after both local and systemic delivery (Alter et al., 2006; Fletcher et al., 2005, 2007; Lu et al., 2003c, 2005; Mann et al., 2001; Wilton et al., 1999; Williams et al., 2006), and this technology in the context of therapy for DMD has been recently reviewed (Aartsma-Rus and van Ommen, 2007; Wilton and Fletcher, 2006). However, the efficiency of 2'OMe ESO delivery, and level of concomitant dystrophin expression in the mdx mouse remains relatively modest (Lu et al., 2003c, 2005; Williams et al., 2006). Despite the fact that ESOs without a carrier have progressed to Phase I clinical trials, improved carriers must be developed before the ESO approach can be considered as a viable therapeutic for improving health and longevity in DMD patients.

The amine-rich cationic polymer PEI is a well-studied compound that is effective at condensing large plasmid DNA, enabling improved cellular uptake (Bieber et al., 2002; Kichler, 2004; Petersen et al., 2002a, 2002b; Suh et al., 2003; Thomas and Klibanov, 2003b). Although most often applied to plasmid delivery, recent studies have also documented PEI-enhanced delivery of small nucleic acid agents such as oligonucleotides and siRNA (Brus et al., 2004; Fischer et al., 2004; Jeong et al., 2003; Kunath et al., 2004; Schiffelers et al., 2004; Vinogradov et al., 1998, 1999, 2003). The positive surface charge of PEI-nucleic acid polyplexes interacts with negatively charged elements on the cell membrane, stimulating non-specific receptor-mediated endocytotic uptake (Bieber et al., 2002; Boussif et al., 1995; Godbey et al., 1999; Kichler, 2004; Suh et al., 2003; Thomas and Klibanov, 2003b). Once internalized, the "proton sponge effect" enabled by PEI's buffering capacity induces the rupturing of the endosomal compartment due to osmotic lysis (Akinc et al., 2005; Boussif et al., 1995; Sonawane et al., 2003; Thomas and Klibanov, 2002). While the intracellular dynamics of PEI-nucleotide complexes once released from the endosome are unknown, oligonucleotides must dissociate from PEI to reach the nucleus, as the nuclear envelope is likely impermeable to PEI. Using dual-fluorescence tracking we recently showed PEG-PEI copolymers enhanced SMO delivery to myonuclei of cultured mdx myofibers, while the copolymers were mainly excluded from entering the nuclei (Sirsi et al., 2005).

The functionality and biocompatibility of PEI is greatly improved by incorporation of the nonionic linear polymer PEG into PEG-PEI copolymers (Kichler, 2004; Petersen et al., 2002a). The macromolecular properties of PEG-PEI-oligonucleotide polyplexes are greatly influenced by the molecular weight of PEI and nature of PEGylation, which in-turn effects transfection capacity (Petersen et al., 2002a, 2002b; Sung et al., 2003). We recently showed that PEG-PEI copolymers made of low MW PEI2K significantly improved delivery of ESOs to myofibers of mdx mice after intramuscular injections compared to high MW PEI25K copolymers (Williams et al., 2006). We attributed the superior efficacy of the PEI2K-based copolymers to the low surface charge and high stability of the nanoparticles formed during complexation with ESOs (Glodde et al., 2006). Although intramuscular injection of these PEG-PEI-ESO polyplexes produced significantly more dystrophin-positive fibers than ESO alone, the level of dystrophin expression by Western blot reached only 2–5% of the normal level in TA muscles. Therefore, in this report we evaluated whether new injection regimens and further functionalization of PEG-PEI copolymers with gold nanoparticles might improve dystrophin expression. Our results show that repeat injections of small amounts of PEG-PEI-ESO are very effective at transducing dystrophin expression, reaching up to 20% of normal levels under the most favorable formulation and injection regimen.

MATERIALS AND METHODS

Animals

Male mdx mice (C57BL/10ScSn-Dmd^{mdx}/J) and age-matched 6–9 week old normal mice (C57BL/10SnJ) were obtained from Jackson Laboratories (Bar Harbor, ME). All animals were housed according to NIH and University guidelines (Drexel University College of Medicine, ULAR facility, Philadelphia, PA).

Nanopolymer Synthesis

The synthesis and physiochemical characterization of the PEI2K(PEG550)$_{10}$ and PEI2K(PEG5K)$_{10}$ copolymers were previously described (Glodde et al., 2006; Lutz et al., 2007). Copolymers are designated using a nomenclature where the subscript indicates the number of PEG chains grafted per molecule of PEI. For example, PEI2K(PEG550)$_{10}$ indicates 10 PEG chains of 550 Daltons grafted to each 2 kDa

PEI molecule. Nanogold (NG) particles were conjugated to PEI primary amine groups on PEI2K(PEG550)10 coploymers using the Sulfo-N- Hydroxy-Succinimido Nanogold labeling reagent (Nanoprobes, Yaphank, NY). In this reaction, 75 nmols of PEI2K$(PEG550)_{10}$ was mixed with 6 nmols of NHS-nanogold in 780 μl of sterile water (pH = 8.0). The solution was incubated for 24 hr on ice, frozen, and subsequently freeze-dried and stored at 20°C. Adsorption of CG to PEI2K$(PEG5K)_{10}$ was performed by mixing 300 μl of 5 nM CG particles (Sigma-Aldrich) with 30 mg of PEI2K$(PEG5K)_{10}$ (in 1 ml DI H20) and incubating at 4°C overnight. The polymer solution was subsequently freeze-dried and stored at 20°C. The NG and CG labeled copolymers are designated as NG-PEI2K$(PEG550)_{10}$ and CG-PEI2K$(PEG5K)_{10}$, respectively.

Preparation of PEG-PEI-ESO Polyplexes

The ESO used in all experiments was a 20-mer oligoribonucleotide (5'-GGCCAAAC-CUCGGCUUACCU-3') previously shown to cause skipping of dystrophin exon 23 in mdx mice (Lu et al., 2003c, 2005; Mann et al., 2002). During synthesis (Trilink, San Diego, CA) each base was phosphorothioated and contained a methoxy group at the 2' carbon. PEG-PEI-ESO polyplexes were prepared at a nitrogen to phosphate ratio of 5 (N:P = 5); where N represents moles of amine on PEI, and P represents moles of phosphate on ESO. Polyplexes were formed by the addition of the PEG-PEI copolymer solution to the ESO solution (in sterile saline). Polyplex solutions were vortexed briefly, sonicated for 30 min using a bath sonicator, incubated on ice for 30 min, and used immediately.

Intramuscular Injections of PEG-PEI-ESO Polyplexes

Male mdx mice (6–9 weeks of age) were anesthetized with ketamine/xylazine and shaved for visualization of hindlimb muscles. A 15 μl volume of PEG-PEI-ESO polyplex solution at various concentrations was injected bi-laterally into the mid-belly portion of TA muscles using a 31 gauge insulin syringe. After recovery from anesthesia, mice were returned to normal cage activity.

We used both a 3 weeks and 6 weeks polyplex injection schedule as follows. For the 3 weeks groups, mice were injected on days 0, 7, and 14; and were harvested on day 21. In one series of experiments muscles were injected with 5 μg of ESO (15 μg total) complexed with either the PEI2K$(PEG550)_{10}$, NG-PEI2K$(PEG550)_{10}$, or CG-PEI2K$(PEG5K)_{10}$ copolymers. For dose-response analysis of a single polyplex, muscles were injected with 1, 5, 10, or 20 μg of ESO (3, 15, 30, and 60 μg total) complexed with the CG-PEI2K$(PEG5K)_{10}$ copolymer. For the 6 weeks groups, mice were injected on days 0, 4, 8, 12, 16, 20, 24, 28, 32, and 36; and were harvested on day 42. For this experiment, muscles were injected with either 1 or 5 μg of ESO per injection (10 and 50 μg total) complexed with the NG-PEI2K$(PEG550)_{10}$ copolymer. For all groups, two mice (N = 4 muscles) were analyzed.

Muscle Harvest, Immunohistochemistry, Histology, and Fiber Counts

At designated time points mice were killed and TA muscles were removed, pinned to parafilm-covered cork, snap frozen in liquid N_2-cooled isopentane, and stored at 80°C.

Control muscles were harvested from uninjected age-matched mdx and normal mice. Transverse frozen sections (10 μm) were cut from the belly of each TA muscle using a cryostat (Leica CM 3050 S, Bannockburn, IL) and melted onto slides for immunohistochemistry and histochemistry. Thick (60 μm) transverse sections, immediately adjacent to the thin sections were cut in the cryostat and placed in 1.5 ml centrifuge tubes on dry ice, and stored at –80°C for subsequent western analysis.

For immunolabeling, muscle sections were blocked with 10% normal goat serum in 1% BSA/PBS for 1 hr and then incubated for 1 hr in rabbit polyclonal anti-dystrophin (1:200; Abcam, Cambridge, MA) or anti-nNOS (1:125; Invitrogen, Carlsbad, CA). The secondary antibody was Cy3-Anti-Rabbit IgG (1:500; Jackson Immunoresearch, West Grove, PA). Slides were coverslipped with Vectashield mounting medium with DAPI (Vector Laboratories, Burlingame, CA) and imaged (4/10/20× objective; Olympus, AX70, Melville, NY). Composite images of entire transverse sections were constructed from overlapping low magnification images using Adobe Photoshop (Adobe, San Jose, CA). Fiber counts of dystrophin-positive fibers were obtained using the cell counter function of ImageJ software (rsb.info.nih.gov/ij/plugins/cell-counter.html).

Western Analysis of Dystrophin Expression

Sections of frozen TA muscles (60 μm) were extracted in 1.5 ml centrifuge tubes by pipetting up and down in 50 μl of protein extraction buffer containing 125 mM Tris (pH 6.8), 4% SDS, 2 M Urea, 5% 2-mercaptoethanol, 10% glycerol, 5 μl of protease inhibitor cocktail (Sigma, St. Louis, MO) and protease inhibitors calpeptin (100 nM; Calbiochem, San Diego, CA), and calpain inhibitor I (25 μM; Calbiochem, San Diego, CA). The extract was incubated on ice (15 min), boiled (5 min), and centrifuged (4,000 × g for 5 min), and the supernatant was transferred to a clean tube. Protein concentration was measured in extracts using the Coomassie assay (Pierce, Rockford, IL) and an equal volume of SDS-PAGE sample buffer (125 mM Tris (pH 6.8), 4% SDS, 5% 2-mercaptoethanol, 10% glycerol, and 0.05% bromophenol blue) was added to the extract. Samples containing 25 μg of total protein were loaded onto pre-cast SDS-PAGE gels (3% stacking: 7.5% resolving; Bio-Rad, Hercules, CA) and run at 150 V for 75 min. Gels were transferred to nitrocellulose at 30 V for 16 hr and membranes were stained with Ponceau S (Sigma, St. Louis, MO) to visualize proper transfer and even loading. Membranes were cut to allow separate immunoblotting of dystrophin and vinculin and blocked in Odyssey blocking buffer (LI-COR Biosciences, Lincoln, NE) for 1 hr. Membranes were incubated for 1 hr in mouse monoclonal anti-dystrophin (MANDYS8; Sigma, St. Louis, MO) and anti-vinculin (VIN1; Sigma, St. Louis, MO) at dilutions of 1:400 and 1:2,000, respectively. Donkey anti-mouse IRDye 800 CW secondary antibody (LI-COR Biosciences, Lincoln, NE) was applied for 1 hr and membranes were scanned on an Odyssey Infrared Imaging System following multiple TBS-T/TBS washes. Odyssey imaging software was used for densitometry and the integrated intensity of sample bands was used for calculating the percentage of dystrophin expression as compared to the normal muscles. For each muscle, 2–3 separate 60 μm sections were extracted and used in western analysis.

Statistical Analysis

All data are reported as mean values ± SEM. Statistical differences between treatment groups were evaluated by ANOVA (Statview; SAS Institute, Cary, NC).

DISCUSSION

The growing opinion that ESOs are on the path to becoming a viable therapeutic option for DMD is well supported by cell culture and animal data showing specific skipping of various targeted exons and resultant induction of nearly full-length dystrophin (Aartsma-Rus et al., 2002, 2003, 2004a, 2004b; Alter et al., 2006; Fletcher et al., 2005, 2007; Gebski et al., 2003; Lu et al., 2003c, 2005; McClorey et al., 2006; Williams et al., 2006). However, there is vigorous debate as to which ESO chemistry may work best, and what type of carrier compound will provide adequate delivery to body musculature. The ESOs of phosphorothioate 2'OMe and PMO chemistry have been the best studied in animal models for DMD and both are currently being tested in Phase I clinical safety trials (Foster et al., 2006). Both 2'OMe and PMO ESOs function by sterically blocking pre-mRNA target sequences, and it is thought that they may be used interchangeably once an optimal sequence (for a single chemistry) has been empirically determined (Adams et al., 2007). However, fundamental differences in 2'OMe and PMO backbone chemistry preclude the use of a universal carrier for efficient delivery. Specifically, PMOs are synthetic compounds that are extraordinarily resistant to chemical degradation, but they are also charge neutral which limits cell surface interactions and cellular uptake. The non-degradable nature of PMOs also raises concerns over their safety after extended applications In contrast, 2'OMe ESOs are anionic RNA, and despite improved stability due to their phosphorothioate backbone, remain somewhat susceptible to degradation, while the negative charge hinders biodistribution and cellular uptake.

In this study we showed that PEG-PEI copolymers formulated with low MW PEI2K function as effective carriers for delivery of 2'OMe ESOs to myofibers of mdx mice after intramuscular injections, resulting in improved levels of dystrophin expression. Specifically, 3 weekly intramuscular injections of only 5 μg of ESO complexed with the PEI2K(PEG550)$_{10}$ copolymer resulted in about 600 dystrophin-positive fibers and about 11% of the normal level of dystrophin expression at 3 weeks after the initial injection. Still higher levels of dystrophin expression were achieved using a twice-weekly injection regimen extended out to 6 weeks. Specifically, 10 consecutive injections of the NG-PEI2K(PEG550)$_{10}$ copolymer complexed with 5 μg of ESO produced over 1200 dystrophin positive fibers and 20% of normal levels of dystrophin expression. In regions with the most highly transfected fibers, we observed a concomitant increase in membrane-associated nNOS, specifically in dystrophin-positive fibers, in agreement with previous reports using this ESO (Lu et al., 2003c). Our lab, as well as other, have demonstrated that intramuscular injections of 2'OMe ESO alone, using very similar conditions as used herein, produced very few dystrophin-positive fibers and negligible levels of dystrophin on western blots (Williams et al., 2006; Wells et al., 2003). In addition, we previously showed that single injections of the PEI2K(PEG550)$_{10}$ copolymer complexed with 20 μg of ESO produced about 460 dystrophin-positive fibers at 3 weeks after the injection, but western blots showed dystrophin expression was only 2–5% of normal levels (Williams et al., 2006). Taken together, the current results suggest that PEG-PEI copolymers enhance dystrophin expression and that repeat injections are more effective at transfecting a greater number of muscle fibers than individual injections containing about the same amount of ESO.

Although the dystrophin expression levels shown in this report demonstrate the utility of PEG-PEI nanopolymers for delivery of ESOs, these compounds appear to be somewhat less effective than PMOs. Specifically, Alter et al., (2006) recently showed that single intramuscular injections of 10 μg of PMO resulted in up to 60% of the normal level of dystrophin expression, although this report appeared to provide only an estimate of efficacy and lacked statistical validation. Other recent studies of PMOs with conjugated peptide cell-targeting moieties showed impressive numbers of dystrophin-positive fibers, but did not provide a thorough evaluation of dystrophin expression by western blots (Fletcher et al., 2007).

The PEI2K$(PEG550)_{10}$ and PEI2K$(PEG5K)_{10}$ copolymers utilized in this study were previously shown to form exceptionally stable complexes when mixed with negatively charged ESO and the surface charge of the resultant nanoparticulates was relatively low (Glodde et al., 2006). We propose that the high stability and low surface charge of these polyplexes are two salient features that make them better suited for *in vivo* delivery of ESOs than high MW PEI25K-based copolymers. Specifically, the low polyplex surface charge favors biodistribution and reduces cytotoxicity, while the high stability allows the polyplex to remain associated during extracellular to intracellular trafficking.

Gold nanoparticles such as NG and CG have been shown to improve biocompatibility and enhance cellular uptake of various types of cargo in drug delivery applications (Hainfeld et al., 2000; Noh et al., 2007; Shukla et al., 2005; Thomas and Klibanov, 2003a). In particular, NG conjugated to low MW PEI2K showed at least an order of magnitude greater efficiency than PEI25K and was 12 times more potent than unmodified PEI2K for delivery of plasmid DNA in cell culture (Thomas and Klibanov, 2003a). Unexpectedly, our results showed that neither covalent conjugation of NG or electrostatic surface coating with CG of the PEG-PEI copolymers improved ESO delivery. Polyplex stability assays in PBS showed CG and NG caused only moderate weakening of polyplex stability (data not shown), making this an unlikely explanation for the lack of improved delivery. A possible explanation for the lack of improvement is that the CG coating was not stable enough to adhere to the copolymer during delivery. On the other hand, NG was covalently conjugated to PEG-PEI, and we postulate that its ineffectiveness was more likely due to the 1:10 NG to PEI2K ratio, which may have been too low to improve functionality.

The dystrophin expression achieved in the present study was accomplished with PEG-PEI carriers that did not appear to elicit any overt signs of cytotoxicity. This is in contrast to previous studies using non-PEGylated PEI25K as a carrier of 2'OMe ESOs, which was ineffective and resulted in significant damage following only a very limited number of injections (Bremmer-Bout et al., 2004; Lu et al., 2003b). Based on these results, it was concluded that cationic polymers are unsuitable for *in vivo* delivery of

AO in skeletal muscle (Lu et al., 2003a, 2003c). However, the PEI-nucleotide particles used in these previous studies undoubtedly had very high positive surface charges, because they did not contain PEG, which is known to provide steric shielding of the PEI surface charge. In addition, dispersion of the highly-charged particles after intramuscular injection is probably severely hindered by charge interactions between the PEI and negatively-charged elements within the extracellular environment. Therefore, it is not surprising that these previous muscle transfection studies with non-PEGylated PEI produced unsatisfactory results. We suggest that the combination of a low MW PEI and extensive PEGylation used presently provided a favorable formulation which was both effective and non-toxic. However, the lack of cytotoxicity observed does not preclude the possibility that some damage to muscle occurs immediately after injection, resulting in some level of degeneration-regeneration. This process may underlie to some extent the high number of dystrophin-positive fibers observed in our 6 weeks (10 injection) trials. Although not systematically evaluated, we have observed that short-term mechanical damage occurs in mdx muscles after intramuscular injections of various solutions (even saline) that does not occur in normal muscle. Because of the lack of dystrophin, mdx muscles are more susceptible to mechanical damage than normal muscle. This effect may be exacerbated to some extent by cationic particles, or for that matter, any type of carrier compound.

We suggest that the major limitation of the carrier-ESO formulations described in this report was inadequate carrier functionality, and not a lack of intrinsic potency of the ESO. The ESO used in the present study (designated in the literature as M23D(+02–18)) has been shown *in vitro* to predominantly produce skipping of exon 23, although some exon 22–23 double skipping does occur (Mann et al., 2002). Moreover, in this study we showed that under the most effective condition, about 50% of fibers were dystrophin-positive, resulting in about 20% of normal dystrophin expression. This indicates that on average dystrophin-positive fibers contained about 40% of the normal level of dystrophin. A similar calculation based on data reported by Lu et al. (2003c), and our recent study with TAT-conjugated copolymers (Sirsi et al., manuscript submitted) suggests that dystrophin per transfected fiber may reach 75% of normal levels. Thus, the main limitation with cationic carriers seems to be their poor diffusional distribution, as indicated by large regions in muscles with no apparent transfection. Thus, further improvements in carrier functionality will likely be required to enable their usage in a clinical setting for DMD. Our group recently showed that conjugation of multiple HIV-TAT epitopes to PEI2K(PEG5K)10 copolymers greatly improved ESO delivery, using a similar dosing and intramuscular injection regimen as reported here, resulting in up to 30% dystrophin expression (Sirsi et al., manuscript submitted). Various other types of cell targeting ligands, cell penetrating peptides, or fusogenic peptides may also be conjugated to PEI to improve functionality. Importantly, this type of peptide-PEI conjugate can likely be formulated for improved systemic delivery, which will be required to achieve meaningful therapeutic benefit. PMOs have already been shown to have limited efficacy after systemic delivery. For example, intraperitoneal injections into neonatal mdx mice of 5 mg/kg/week with PMO-peptide produced widespread dystrophin in diaphragm muscle, with low levels of expression observed in limb muscles (Fletcher et al., 2007; Moulton et al., 2007).

RESULTS

Induction of Dystrophin Expression Following Intramuscular Injection of PEG-PEI-ESOs

The goal of this study was to determine an effective PEG-PEI-ESO polyplex formulation and injection scheme for enhanced dystrophin expression after intramuscular injection into the TA muscle of 6–8 weeks old male mdx mice. The ESO for all experiments was a 2'OMe oligonucleotide that was previously shown to produce specific skipping of mouse dystrophin exon 23, thereby removing a point mutation that encodes a premature stop codon (Lu et al., 2003c; Mann et al., 2002). Mice were given 3 weekly intramuscular injections of 5 μg of ESO complexed with either PEI2K(PEG550)10, NG-PEI2K(PEG550)10, or CG-PEI2K(PEG5K)10 copolymers and were analyzed for dystrophin expression at one week after the third injection. Immunohistochemistry of transverse sections showed that all three copolymer formulations produced substantially greater expression of dystrophin-positive fibers compared to muscles from uninjected mdx mice (Figure 1). The H&E staining showed morphological integrity to be well preserved, with no overt signs of muscle necrosis or cytotoxic damage (Figure 1). Quantitative evaluation of whole muscle cross-sections showed that injections with the PEI2K(PEG550)10-ESO formulation produced 594 ± 120 dystrophin-positive fibers (Figure 2), which corresponds to roughly 30% of the approximately 2,000 fibers in the TA muscle (Lu et al., 2003c; Wells et al., 2003).

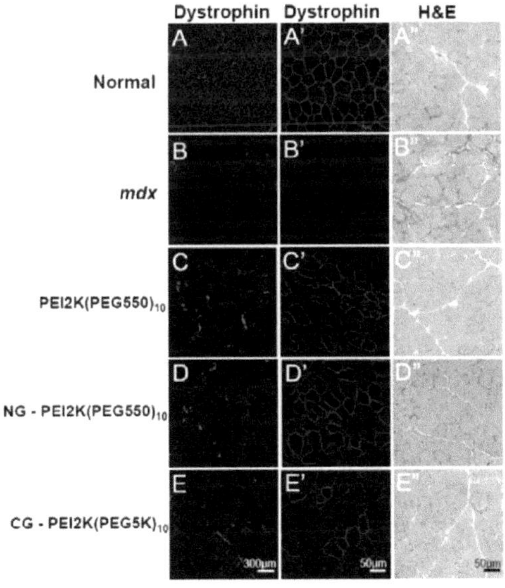

Figure 1. Dystrophin induction in limb musculature of mdx mice after intramuscular injections of 2'OMe ESO complexed with cationic nanopolymers. The TA muscles of mdx mice were given 3 weekly intramuscular injections of various PEG-PEI copolymers complexed with 5 μg of ESO and harvested 3 weeks after the first injection. Dystrophin immunolabeling (Hoechst dye counterstained) at two different magnifications and H&E staining of serial transverse sections from TA muscles from the following groups: (A-A") normal age-matched controls, (B-B") mdx untreated, (C-C") mdx injected with PEI2K(PEG550)10-ESO, (D-D") mdx injected with NG-PEI2K(PEG550)10-ESO, and (E-E") mdx injected with CG-PEI2K(PEG5K)10-ESO.

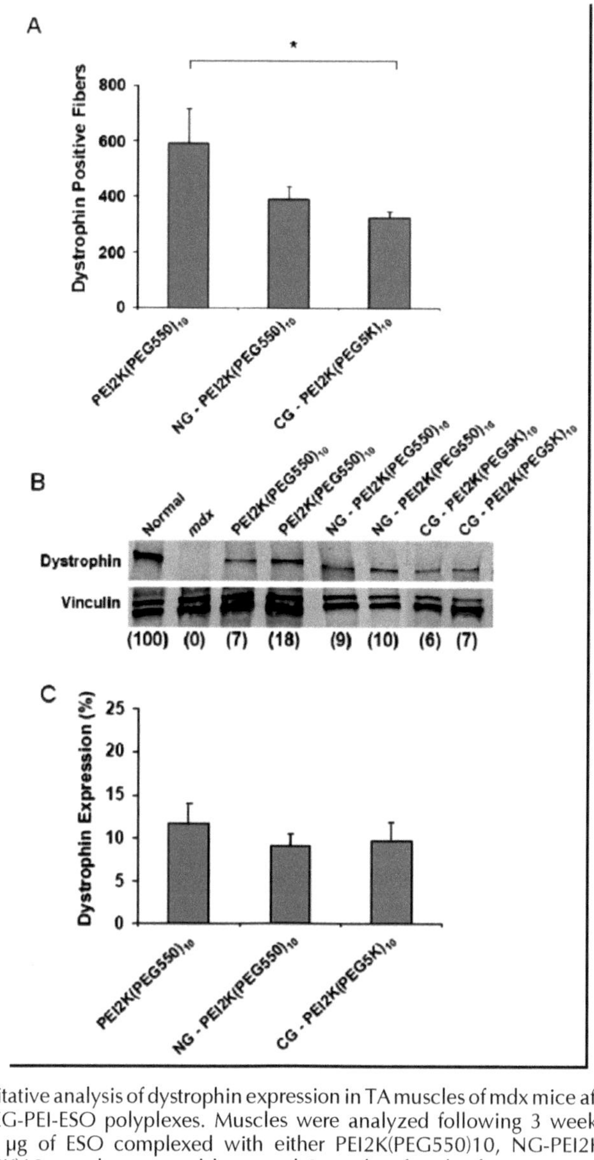

Figure 2. Quantitative analysis of dystrophin expression in TA muscles of mdx mice after intramuscular injections of PEG-PEI-ESO polyplexes. Muscles were analyzed following 3 weekly intramuscular injections of 5 μg of ESO complexed with either PEI2K(PEG550)10, NG-PEI2K(PEG550)10, or CG-PEI2K(PEG5K)10 copolymers, and harvested 3 weeks after the first injection. (A) Number of dystrophin-positive fibers for each treatment group was obtained from whole transverse sections that were immunolabeled for dystrophin. The number of dystrophin-positive fibers was significantly lower in muscles injected with NG-PEI2K(PEG550)10-ESO and CG-PEI2K(PEG5K)10-ESO polyplexes compared with the basic PEI2K(PEG550)10-ESO formulation ($P < 0.05$, $N = 4$ muscles per group). (B) Western blots show dystrophin expression in thick (60 μm) transverse cryosections taken directly adjacent to segments used for fiber counts in panel A. Images show blots of dystrophin (top) and vinculin (bottom) obtained from the same gel. All samples contained 25 μg of total protein, and dystrophin expression as a percent of normal is indicated in parentheses below each lane. (C) Quantitative western analysis of dystrophin expression as a percent of the level in age-matched normal mice for each of the three PEG-PEI-ESO polyplex formulations. No significant differences were observed between treatment groups ($P > 0.05$; $N = 4$ muscles per group).

In accordance with previous studies showing improved biocompatibility and enhanced cellular uptake of gold-conjugated nanoparticles (Shukla et al., 2005; Thomas and Klibanov, 2003a), we hypothesized that conjugation or adsorption of NG or CG to PEG-PEI copolymers would improve the potency of these carriers. Surprisingly, injections with NG-PEI2K(PEG550)$_{10}$-ESO and CG-PEI2K(PEG5K)$_{10}$-ESO resulted in only 380 ± 36 and 322 ± 24 dystrophin-positive fibers, respectively, both of which were significantly less than found with the unconjugated PEI2K(PEG550)$_{10}$ copolymer (Figure 2A; $P < 0.05$).

To quantify dystrophin expression, Western blots were performed on whole muscle transverse sections directly serial to those on which fiber counts were obtained. Dystrophin expression following 3 weekly injections of the PEI2K(PEG550)$_{10}$-ESO polyplex (5 μg ESO per injection) reached 11.2 ± 2.4% of the level found in normal muscles (Figure 2B, C). As expected, dystrophin expression in control mdx muscles was not detectable, and was likely less than 1% of normal. The NG-PEI2K(PEG550)$_{10}$-ESO and CG-PEI2K(PEG5K)$_{10}$-ESO formulations resulted in 7.6 ± 1.0% and 9.8 ± 2.1% of the normal level of dystrophin expression, neither of which was statistically different than the unconjugated copolymer (Figure 2B, C). Although we did not perform injections of ESO without polymers in this study, we have shown in other studies that injections of 2'OMe ESO alone, under very similar dosing and injection regimens as used herein, produced very low numbers of dystrophin-positive fibers, and showed no detectable dystrophin on Western blots ((Williams et al., 2006) and Sirsi et al., manuscript submitted). Similarly, a previous study using this ESO delivered without a carrier showed no improvement in the number of dystrophin positive fibers over mdx control muscles (Wells et al., 2003). The ineptitude of 2'OMe ESO delivery without a carrier in the mdx mouse has led to omitting ESO alone in other studies examining dystrophin induction following local and systemic delivery (Lu et al., 2003c, 2005).

Dose-Response Profile of PEG-PEI-ESO Polyplexes

Using the same triple-injection regimen as above, the dose-response properties of CG-PEI2K(PEG5K)$_{10}$-ESO polyplexes was evaluated over a range from 3 to 60 μg of total ESO. Dystrophin-positive fibers were detected at all dosages (Figure 3), but muscles injected with the smallest test dosage of ESO (1 μg × 3 injections) expressed significantly fewer dystrophin-positive fibers than doses of 15, 30, or 60 μg (Figure 4A; $P < 0.05$). Western analysis showed that the highest level of dystrophin induction was achieved using 5 μg of ESO per injection, resulting in 14.2 ± 1.6% expression (Figure 4B, C), with apparent saturation at higher doses.

In an attempt to further improve dystrophin expression, we carried out longer term repeat injection experiments using the NG-PEI2K(PEG550)$_{10}$-ESO polyplexes. Mice were given 10 consecutive intramuscular injections of NG-PEI2K(PEG550)$_{10}$-ESO polyplexes (1 or 5 μg of ESO per injection), with 4 days between injections, and were harvested at 6 weeks after the first injection. Immunohistochemistry of whole transverse sections showed that this protocol resulted in marked improvement in ESO delivery to myofibers, producing extensive regions of intensely labeled dystrophin-positive fibers (Figure 5). On average, muscles injected with the 1 and 5 μg of ESO per injection (10 and 50 μg total ESO over 6 weeks) contained 832 ± 167 and 1,225 ±

343 dystrophin-positive fibers, respectively (Figure 6B). The number of dystrophin-positive fibers after delivery of 10 μg total ESO for 6 weeks was 2.2-fold greater than found after 15 μg of ESO for 3 weeks using the same NG-PEI2K(PEG550)10 copolymer. The H&E staining confirmed the increased dystrophin expression following repeated injections was not associated with any overt signs of cytotoxicity (Figure 6A).

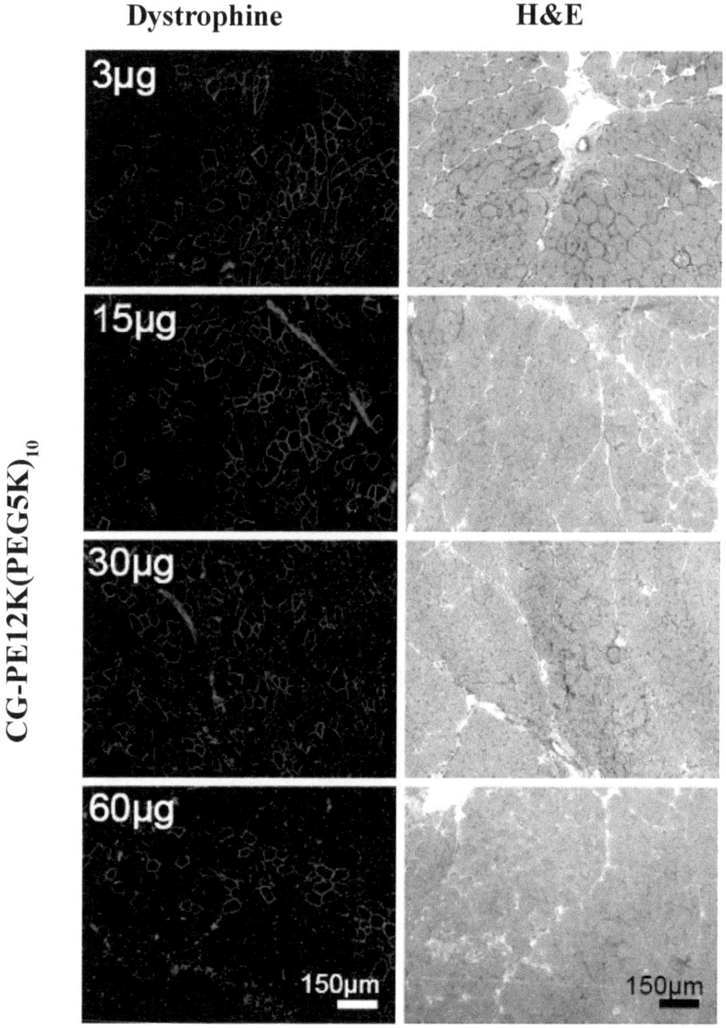

Figure 3. Dose-response profile of dystrophin expression after intramuscular injections of CG-PEI2K(PEG5K)$_{10}$-ESO polyplexes. The TA muscles of mdx mice were given 3 weekly intramuscular injections of CG-PEI2K(PEG5K)$_{10}$ copolymers complexed with 1, 5, 10, or 20 μg of ESO per injection (3, 15, 30, and 60 μg total) and harvested 3 weeks after the first injection. Images show dystrophin immunolabeling (Hoechst dye counterstained) and H&E staining of serial transverse sections from TA muscles for each of the 4 polyplex doses.

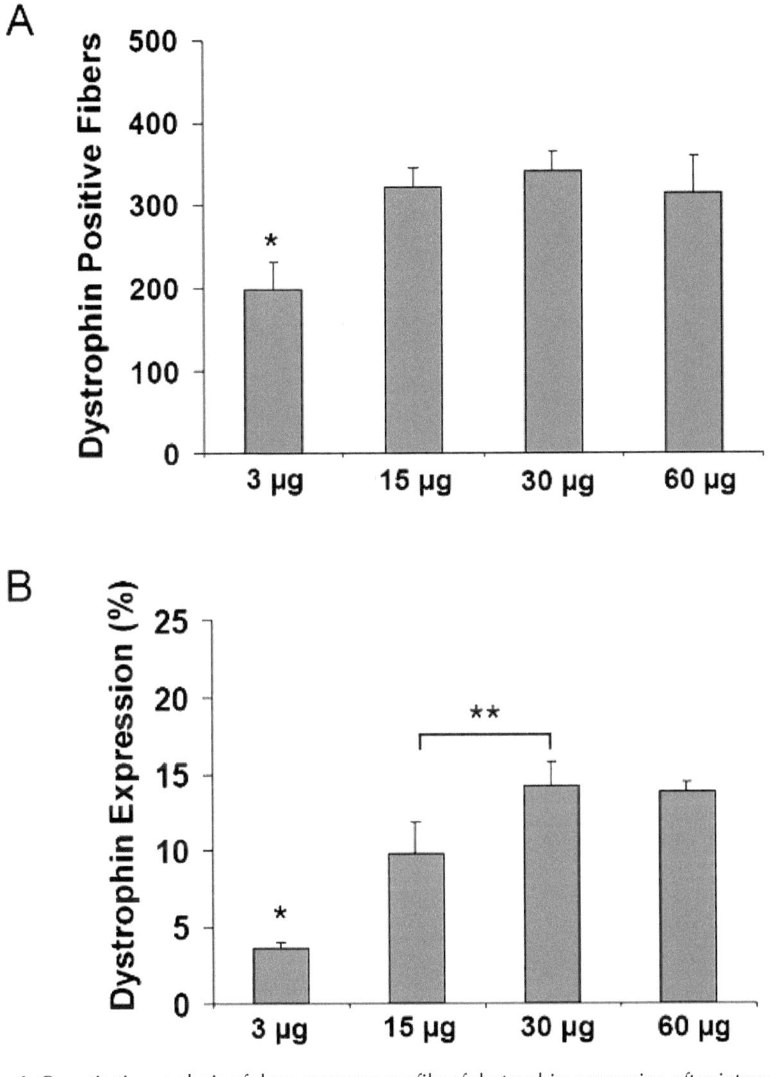

Figure 4. Quantitative analysis of dose-response profile of dystrophin expression after intramuscular injections of CG-PEI2K(PEG5K)$_{10}$-ESO polyplexes. Muscles were analyzed following 3 weekly intramuscular injections of 1, 5, 10, or 20 µg of ESO (3, 15, 30, and 60 µg total) complexed with CG-PEI2K(PEG5K)$_{10}$ copolymers, and harvested 3 weeks after the first injection. (A) Number of dystrophin-positive fibers for each dosage was obtained from whole transverse sections that were immunolabeled for dystrophin. Number of dystrophin-positive fibers was significantly lower for the 1 µg injections than for all other doses ($P < 0.05$, $N = 4$ muscles per group). (B) Quantification of dystrophin expression as a percentage of age-matched normal mice for each of the 4 polyplex dosages based on densitometry of western blots (not shown). Samples were prepared from thick (60 µm) transverse cryosections taken adjacent to segments used for the fiber counts. Each increase in dosage resulted in significantly greater level of dystrophin expression, except between the 30 µg and 60 µg dosages which reached a plateau. Longer term repeat ESO injections increase dystrophin expression.

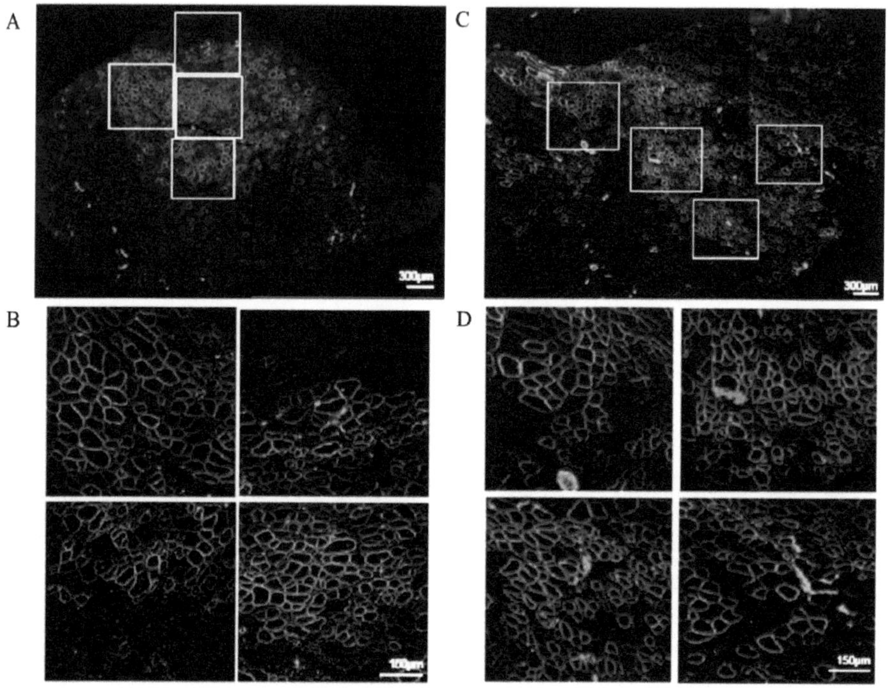

Figure 5. A 6 week, repeat intramuscular injection, regimen of PEG-PEI-ESO polyplexes produced widespread manifestation of dystrophin-positive fibers. Dystrophin immunolabeling of whole transverse sections of TA muscles of mdx mice is shown after 10 twice-weekly intramuscular injections of either 1 μg (A-B) or 5 μg (C-D) of ESO complexed with the NG-PEI2K(PEG550)$_{10}$ copolymer. Muscles were harvested at 6 weeks after the first of the 10 injections. High magnification views of four individual regions of each muscle section (boxed) are shown.

Western blots further established the potency of the 10-repeat injection regimen using the NG-PEI2K(PEG550)$_{10}$-ESO polyplexes (Figure 6C, D). On average, muscles injected with 50 μg of ESO expressed 19.1 ± 1.8% of the normal amount of dystrophin, a level which was previously shown to be sufficient for improvement in mdx muscle mechanical properties (Phelps et al., 1995; Wells et al., 1995, 2003). The dystrophin expression after 50 μg of ESO was significantly greater than the 8.1 ± 2.8% produced with 10 μg of ESO ($P < 0.05$). However, there was exceptionally high variability in dystrophin expression within the 10 μg group as the lowest and highest values ranged from 4 to 23%. The peak level of 23% dystrophin expression after only 10 μg ESO injected over 6 weeks demonstrates the effectiveness of the nanopolymer-ESO formulation coupled with a low dose-high frequency delivery schedule.

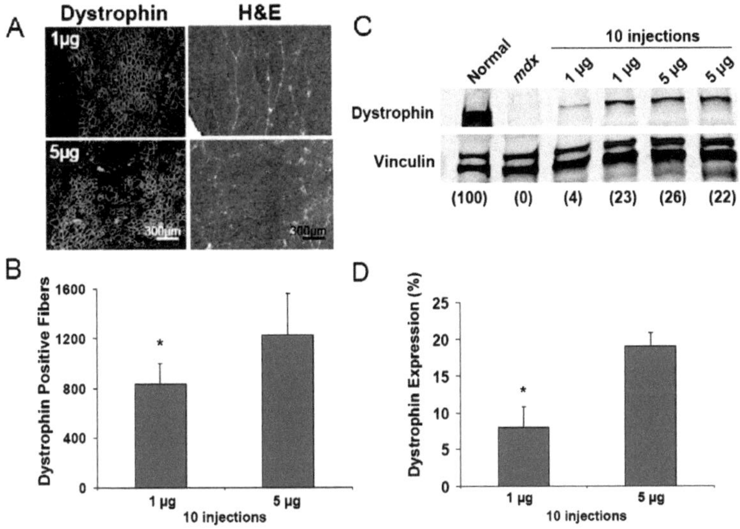

Figure 6. Quantitative analysis of dystrophin expression following a 6 weeks, repeat intramuscular injection regimen of NG-PEI2K(PEG550)$_{10}$ polyplexes. Tissues were analyzed following 10 twice-weekly intramuscular injections of either 1 or 5 μg of ESO complexed with NG-PEI2K(PEG550)$_{10}$ copolymers, and harvested 6 weeks after the first injection. (A) Dystrophin immunolabeling (Hoechst dye counterstained) and H&E staining of serial transverse sections from TA muscles from the 10 μg (1 μg x 10 injections) and 50 μg (5 μg x 10 injections) groups. (B) Number of dystrophin-positive fibers, obtained from whole transverse sections immunolabeled for dystrophin, was significantly lower in muscles injected with 10 μg ESO compared with the 50 μg group ($P < 0.001$, $N = 4$ muscles per group). (C) Western blots showing dystrophin expression in thick (60 μm) transverse cryosections taken adjacent to segments used for the fiber counts in panel B. Images show blots of dystrophin (top) and vinculin (bottom) obtained from the same gel. All samples contained 25 μg of total protein, and dystrophin expression as a percent of normal is indicated in parentheses below each lane. (D) Dystrophin expression determined from Western blots reached 20% of normal levels in muscles injected with NG-PEI2K(PEG550)$_{10}$-ESO containing 50 μg ESO, which was significantly greater than the 10 μg group ($P < 0.001$, $N = 4$ muscles per group).

Expression of nNOS in Mdx Muscles Treated with PEG-PEI-ESOs

Muscles from polyplex-treated mdx mice were analyzed for nNOS expression as evidence for expression of functional dystrophin with an intact N-terminal binding domain. It was previously shown that nNOS expression is absent from muscles of mdx mice (Wells et al., 2003) and may be upregulated following exon-skipping restoration of dystrophin expression (Lu et al., 2003c). Therefore, we asked whether the current strategy for restoring dystrophin expression increased the level of nNOS protein localized at the myofiber membrane, where it serves to maintain normal cellular function in close association with dystrophin. Serial sections immunolabeled for dystrophin and nNOS showed a very tight correlation between dystrophin- and nNOS-positive fibers (Figure 7). Specifically, membrane-associated nNOS appeared to be expressed only in the mdx muscle cells that also showed enhanced dystrophin expression, indicating that ESO-expressed dystrophin was functionally intact. As expected, nNOS expression was absent from mdx un-injected control muscles.

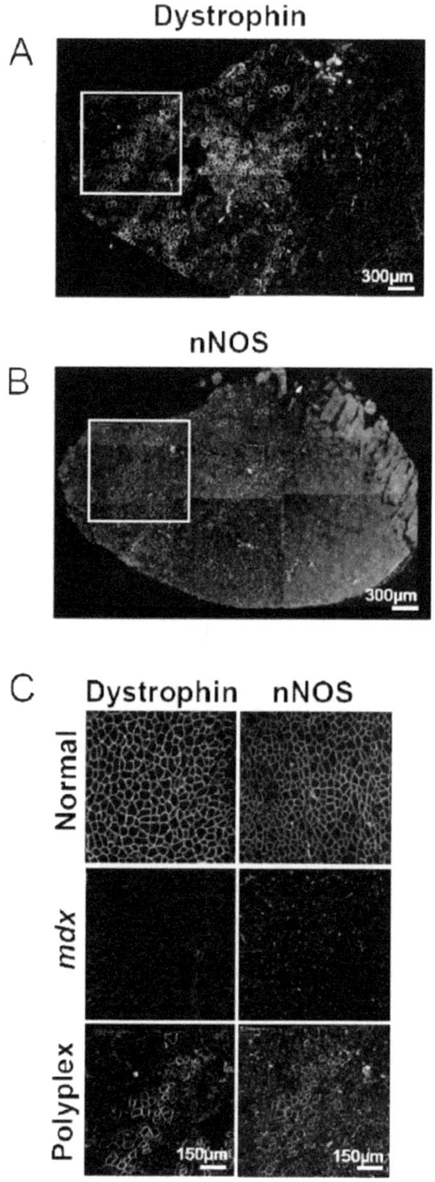

Figure 7. The nNOS expression in mdx mice after treatment with PEG-PEI-ESO. Membrane-associated nNOS expression is upregulated in PEG-PEI-ESO treated mdx muscles in regions highly positive for dystrophin expression. The TA muscles were given 10 twice-weekly intramuscular injections of 5 µg of ESO complexed with the NG-PEI2K(PEG550)$_{10}$ copolymer, and harvested 6 weeks after the first injection. (A-B) Images of serial whole transverse sections immunolabeled for dystrophin (A) and nNOS (B) show the correlation in ESO-mediated upregulation of these two membrane-associated proteins. (C) Higher magnification images of specific regions from panels A and B show clearly the concomitant (co-localized) upregulation of both dystrophin and nNOS in the same set of fibers of the polyplex-injected muscles. As expected nNOS expression in untreated mdx controls was negligible.

CONCLUSION

In this chapter, we show that PEGylated amine-rich branched cationic nanopolymers comprised of low MW PEI2K are effective carriers for delivery of ESOs to myofibers of mdx mice after intramuscular injections. Our results indicate that high frequency, low-dosage, long-term injection regimens using these carrier-ESO compounds provide the most favorable outcome in terms of dystrophin expression. While other studies have shown improvements utilizing gold nanoparticles, we showed no enhancement when conjugated to the current PEG-PEI formulations. Despite the lack of improvement using these novel conjugations, PEGylated PEI2K copolymers remain as one of the most efficient carriers for local delivery of 2'OMe ESOs and warrant further development as potential therapeutics for treatment of DMD.

KEYWORDS

- **Duchenne muscular dystrophy**
- **PEG-PEI copolymers**
- **TAT-conjugated copolymers**

AUTHORS' CONTRIBUTIONS

Jason H. Williams carried out western and immunoflourescence analysis, assisted with harvesting of muscle tissue, participated in the design of the study and drafted the manuscript. Rebecca C. Schray maintained animal colonies, carried out injections and harvesting of tissues and participated in design of the study. Shashank R. Sirsi carried out chemical synthesis and functionalization of copolymers and contributed to the conception of the study. Gordon J. Lutz conceived the study, drafted the final manuscript and participated in all stages of the work. All authors read and approved the final manuscript.

ACKNOWLEDGMENTS

We thank Michelle Erney for assistance with the immunofluorescence and Nilo Pebdani and Elisa McDaniel for assistance with the Western blotting. This work was supported by a grant from the Muscular Dystrophy Association (USA).

COMPETING INTERESTS

The author(s) declare that they have no competing interests.

Chapter 15

In Vitro Drug Release Behavior

Chang Yang Gong, Shuai Shi, Peng Wei Dong, Xiu Ling Zheng, Shao Zhi Fu, Gang Guo, Jing Liang Yang, Yu Quan Wei, and Zhi Yong Qian

INTRODUCTION

Most conventional methods for delivering chemotherapeutic agents fail to achieve therapeutic concentrations of drugs, despite reaching toxic systemic levels. Novel controlled drug delivery systems (DDSs) are designed to deliver drugs at predetermined rates for predefined periods at the target organ and overcome the shortcomings of conventional drug formulations therefore could diminish the side effects and improve the life quality of the patients. Thus, a suitable controlled DDS is extremely important for chemotherapy.

A novel biodegradable thermosensitive composite hydrogel, based on poly(ethylene glycol)-poly(ε-caprolactone)-poly(ethylene glycol) (PEG-PCL-PEG, PECE) and Pluronic F127 copolymer, was successfully prepared in this work, which underwent thermosensitive sol-gel-sol transition. And it was flowing sol at ambient temperature but became non-flowing gel at body temperature. By varying the composition, sol-gel-sol transition and *in vitro* drug release behavior of the composite hydrogel could be adjusted. Cytotoxicity of the composite hydrogel was conducted by cell viability assay using human HEK293 cells. The 293 cell viability of composite hydrogel copolymers were yet higher than 71.4%, even when the input copolymers were 500 μg per well. Vitamin B_{12} (VB_{12}), honokiol (HK), and bovine serum albumin (BSA) were used as model drugs to investigate the *in vitro* release behavior of hydrophilic small molecular drug, hydrophobic small molecular drug, and protein drug from the composite hydrogel respectively. All the above-mentioned drugs in this work could be released slowly from composite hydrogel in an extended period. Chemical composition of composite hydrogel, initial drug loading, and hydrogel concentration substantially affected the drug release behavior. The higher Pluronic F127 content, lower initial drug loading amount, or lower hydrogel concentration resulted in higher cumulative release rate.

The results showed that composite hydrogel prepared in this chapter were biocompatible with low cell cytotoxicity, and the drugs in this work could be released slowly from composite hydrogel in an extended period, which suggested that the composite hydrogel might have great potential applications in biomedical fields.

Cancer is a major public health problem in the world, which causes millions of death each year. Approximately 1.5 million new cancer cases and more than 500,000 deaths from cancer are projected to occur in 2008 in USA (Jemal et al., 2008). Now, one in four deaths in USA is due to cancer. As conventional therapy for cancer, chemotherapy has wide applications in clinical, which has been proven to be effective.

Although chemotherapeutic agents may prolong the survival time of the patients, unfortunately most of them have severe side toxic effects, which would decline the life quality of patients. Most conventional methods for delivering chemotherapeutic agents, such as intravenous injection or oral ingestion, fail to achieve therapeutic concentrations of drugs, despite reaching toxic systemic levels. Novel controlled DDSs are designed to deliver drugs at predetermined rates for predefined periods at the target organ, which could be used to overcome the shortcomings of conventional drug formulations, therefore could diminish the side effects and improve the life quality of the patients (Hatefi and Amsden, 2002; Qiu and Park, 2001). Thus, a suitable controlled DDS is extremely important for chemotherapy.

Hydrogels are a special class of macromolecules, which could absorb much water while maintaining their integrity in water. Over the past decades, the stimuli-sensitive hydrogel has attracted increasing attention owing to their responsiveness to the environmental stimulus, including chemical substances and changes in temperature, pH, or electric field (Jeong et al., 1997; Lee and Mooney, 2001). The biodegradable thermosensitive physical crosslinked hydrogels have been extensively studied due to their great biodegradability, biocompatibility, and responsiveness to temperature. Therefore, biodegradable thermosensitive hydrogels have been investigated as *in situ* gel-forming system, such as controlled drug delivery, tissue repair, and cell encapsulation (Bromberg and Ron, 1998; Li et al., 2003).

Poly(ethylene glycol)-poly(propylene glycol)-poly(ethylene glycol) triblock copolymer (PEG-PPG-PEG), known as Pluronic or Poloxamer, has been extensively studied as a potential drug delivery vehicle due to their excellent biocompatibility and thermosensitivity (Gilbert et al., 1987; Xiong et al., 2003). These copolymers have been widely used as emulsifiers, wetting agents, and solubilizers (Rangelov et al., 2005). However, due to weak hydrophobicity of PPG block, the Pluronic F127 copolymer forms a fast-eroding gel and could persist a few hours *in vivo* at most, which greatly restricted its application as *in situ* gel-forming controlled DDS.

In our previous study, we prepared a new kind of biodegradable and injectable thermosensitive PECE hydrogel controlled DDS (Gong et al., 2009a). At low temperature, PECE hydrogel is injectable flowing sol, which could be easily mixed with pharmaceutical agent, and it forms non-flowing gel at body temperature as sustained drug delivery site *in vivo*. The PCL and PEG are biocompatible and have been widely used in several FDA approved products (Chung et al., 2002; Iza et al., 1998). The PCL is lack of toxicity and has great permeability (Zhou et al., 2003). Due to combination of great advantages of PEG and PCL, the PECE hydrogel might have great potential application in biomedical field.

In our last work (Gong et al., 2009b), we prepared a new biodegradable and injectable composite hydrogel based on PECE and Pluronic F127 copolymer. The composite hydrogel undergoes sol-gel-sol transition, which is free flowing sol at room temperature and becomes a non-flowing gel at body temperature. Our last work mainly focused on the synthesis, *in vivo* gel formation and degradation assay, and toxicity evaluation of the composite hydrogel. It is well known that Pluronic copolymer forms a fast-eroding hydrogel which could not persist longer than a few hours. And PECE hydrogel could persist 2 weeks *in vivo* (Gong et al., 2009a). According to our results, by simply altering the composition of PECE and Pluronic F127 copolymers, the *in vivo* sustained time of the composite hydrogel could be controlled, which could meet the different requirements of *in vivo* sustained time, therefore the composite hydrogel is very useful for its potential application as injectable *in situ* gel-forming DDS.

In the present study, cytotoxicity and *in vitro* drug release behavior of the composite hydrogel were studied in detail. Many factors affecting *in vitro* drug release behavior of the composite hydrogel were investigated, including different kinds of drugs, initial drug loading, concentration of composite hydrogel, and chemical composition of the composite hydrogel. By altering the composition of composite hydrogel, sol-gel-sol transition behavior and *in vitro* drug release behavior of the prepared composite hydrogel could be controlled, which was of great importance for their further application as injectable *in situ* gel-forming drug release system.

METERIALS AND METHODS

Poly(ethylene glycol) methyl ether (MPEG, Mn = 550, Aldrich, USA), ε-Caprolactone (ε-CL, Alfa Aesar, USA), Pluronic F127 (Fluka, USA), Hexamethylene diisocyanate (HMDI, Aldrich, USA), Stannous octoate (Sn(Oct)2, Sigma, USA), Dulbecco's modified Eagle's medium (DMEM, Sigma, USA), 3-(4,5-dimethylthiazol-2-yl)-2,5-diphenyl tetrazolium bromide (MTT, Sigma, USA), bovine serum albumin (BSA, BR, BoAo Co. Ltd, China), and VB_{12} (Sigma, USA) were used without further purification. The HK were isolated and purified in our lab (Chen et al., 2007). All the materials used in this chapter were analytic reagent (AR) grade and used as received.

Preparation of Composite Hydrogel

The PECE copolymer were synthesized and purified as reported previously (Gong et al., 2009a). Briefly, PEG-PCL diblock copolymers were prepared by ring opening polymerization of ε-CL initiated by MPEG using stannous octoate as catalyst; PECE triblock copolymers were synthesized by coupling PEG-PCL diblock copolymers using HMDI as coupling agent (Gong et al., 2007, 2009a). The just-obtained PECE triblock copolymers were dissolved in dichloromethane, and then reprecipitated from the filtrate using excess cold petroleum ether. Then, the mixture was filtered and vacuum dried to constant weight at room temperature. The purified copolymers were kept in air-tight bags before further use.

The obtained PECE copolymer was characterized by FTIR (Nicolet 200SXV, Nicolet, USA), ^{1}H-NMR (Varian 400 spectrometer, Varian, USA), and GPC (Agilent 110 HPLC, USA). The M_n and PEG/PCL ratio of PECE triblock copolymer calculated from ^{1}H-NMR spectra was 3408 and 960/2448 respectively. Macromolecular weight and macromolecular weight distribution (polydispersity, PDI, M_w/M_n) of PECE triblock copolymer determined by GPC were 4391 and 1.30 respectively (Gong et al., 2009a).

Preparation scheme of composite hydrogel was described in Figure 1. Aqueous PECE solutions were prepared by dissolving PECE copolymers in deionized water at a designated temperature then cooled to 4°C. Then, different amounts of Pluronic F127 were dissolved in icy cold deionized water to a transparent solution. Subsequently, the obtained two solutions were mixed together under mild agitation to obtain a homogeneous liquid solution. The final solution contained a given concentration and composition of the two copolymers to form the different composite hydrogel samples. The composite hydrogels prepared in this work were listed in Table 1.

Table 1. The composite hydrogels prepared in this work.

Code	PECE : Pluronic F127 (ww, %)	Phase Transition	The Concentration Region with Phase Transition behavior (Wt%)
S1	100 : 0	Sol-gel-sol	15% to 35%
S2	80 : 20	Sol-gel-sol	25% to 35%
S3	60 : 40	Sol-gel-sol	20% to 35%
S4	40 : 60	Sol-gel-sol	20% to 35%
S5	20 : 80	Sol-gel-sol	20% to 35%
S6	0 : 100	Sol-gel-sol	15% to 35%

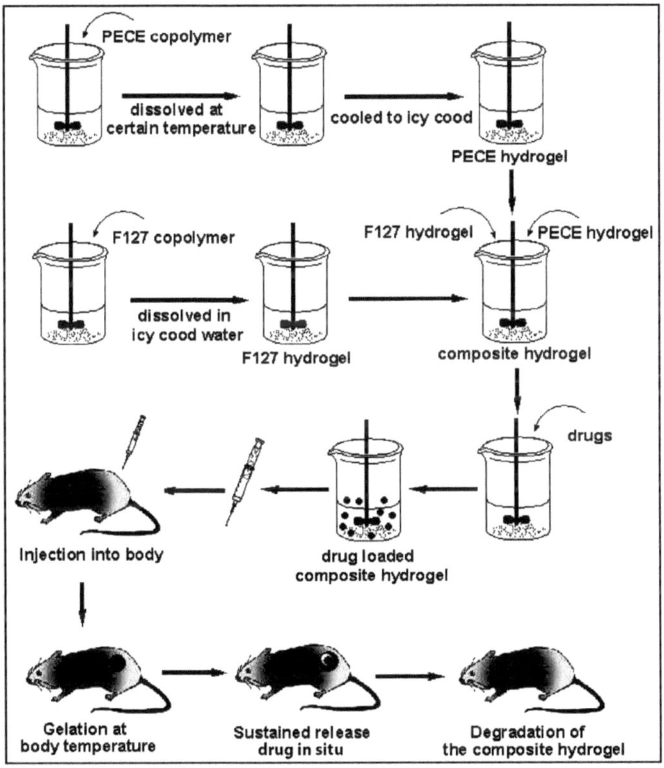

Figure 1. Preparation scheme of demonstrated injectable thermosensitive composite hydrogel. The PECE hydrogel solutions were prepared by dissolving PECE copolymers in deionized water at a designated temperature then cooled to 4°C. Then, Pluronic F127 were dissolved in icy cold deionized water to a transparent solution. Subsequently, the obtained two solutions were mixed together under mild agitation to obtain homogeneous liquid solution, and then drug were added into the composite hydrogel. The prepared hydrogel containing drug was inhaled into injector and injected into or around the focus of infection in animal. Thus, composite sol turned into gel state and acted as depots for sustained release of drug *in situ* when the cold sol is warmed to body temperature (37°C) *in vivo*. At last, for the degradation of the composite hydrogel, the introduced drug delivery system was gradually emanated from body.

Sol-Gel-Sol Phase Transition Behavior Study

Sol-gel-sol phase transition diagrams of composite hydrogels were recorded using test tube-inverting method (Gong et al., 2007, 2009a). The sol-gel-sol transition was visually observed by inverting the vials, and conditions of sol and gel were defined as "flowing" and "non-flowing" in 1 min, respectively.

In this work, the volume of the composite hydrogel solution was kept to 0.5 ml in total, regardless of the concentration. After incubated in water bath at 4°C for 20 min, the hydrogel samples were slowly heated at a rate of 0.5°C/min, from 4°C to the temperature when the sol states occurred again.

Cytotoxicity Assay of Composite Hydrogel

Cytotoxicity evaluation of composite hydrogel (Supplimentary movie S1, S3, S4, and S6) was performed by MTT assay using HEK293 cells, which were grown in DMEM with 10% of fetal bovine serum (FBS) and were cultured in a humidified atmosphere containing 5% CO_2 at 37°C. Cell suspensions were distributed in a 96-well plate at a density of 1 × 104 cells/well in DMEM medium with 10% of FBS for 24 hr. Then, the medium was replaced by 200 μl of fresh DMEM per well containing different amounts of composite hydrogel copolymers (the amount of PECE and Pluronic F127 copolymer, which do not contain water) from 50 to 2,500 μg/ml, respectively. After 48 hr, the cell cultures were washed with PBS solution and MTT assay was conducted. Untreated cells were taken as control with 100% viability. The cell cytotoxicity of composite hydrogel was defined as the relative viability (%) which correlates with amount of liable cells compared with cell control.

Preparation of Honokiol Micelles

The HK micelles were prepared and characterized in our previous work (Gou et al., 2008). Briefly, certain amount of HK was dissolved into Et Ac to form HK solution. Then, the prepared HK-Et Ac solution was introduced into 4 ml of F127 aqueous solution at the concentration of 5%w/w under extreme stirring by T10 (T10, IKA, German). About 10 min later, oil in water (O/W) emulsion well formed. Then, Et Ac was evaporated in rotator evaporator ((Büchi, Switzerland) and the HK micelles were obtained. The content of HK in the prepared HK micelles suspension was determined by high-performance liquid chromatography (HPLC). At last, the HK micelles slurry was lyophilized and the power was stored at 4°C before further use.

In Vitro Drug Release Behavior from the Composite Hydrogel

Release Behavior of Hydrophilic Small Molecular Drugs

The VB_{12} was used as model to determine the release behavior of hydrophilic small molecular drug from composite hydrogel *in vitro*. 200 μl of VB_{12} loaded composite hydrogel (30 wt% of S1 with 1 mg of VB_{12}, 30 wt% of S4 with 1 mg of VB_{12}, 30 wt% of S6 with 1 mg of VB_{12}, 30 wt% of S3 with 1 mg of VB_{12}, 30 wt% of S3 with 2 mg of VB_{12}, and 20 wt% of S3 with 1 mg of VB_{12}, respectively) were placed into 4 ml-Eppendorf (EP) tubes and allowed to gel in an incubator at 37°C for 12 hr. Then, the gels were immersed in 1 ml of PBS (pH = 7.4) and were shaken at 100 rpm at 37°C.

At specific time intervals, all the release media were removed and replaced by fresh release media. After centrifuged at 13000 rpm for 10 min, the supernatant of the removed release media were collected and stored at –20°C until analysis. The collected supernatants were detected on UV spectrophotometer at 362 nm to determine the concentration of VB_{12}. The accumulatively released VB_{12} was calculated according to the following equation (Gong et al., 2009a):

$$Q = C_n V_t + V_s \sum C_{n-1} \quad (1)$$

where Q was accumulatively released weight, and C_n was the VB_{12} concentration at time t. V_t was the volume of medium (V_t = 1 ml), and V_s was the volume of solution removed from supernatant (V_s = 1 ml).

Release Behavior of Hydrophobic Small Molecular Drugs

Freshly prepared HK micelles loaded composite hydrogel were used to assay *in vitro* release behavior of hydrophobic small molecular drugs. In detail, 200 µl of prepared HK micelles loaded composite hydrogel (30 wt% of S1 with 1 mg of HK, 30 wt% of S3 with 1 mg of HK, 30 wt% of S6 with 1 mg of HK, 30 wt% of S4 with 1 mg of HK, 30 wt% of S4 with 2 mg of HK, 20 wt% of S4 with 1 mg of HK, respectively) were transferred into 4 ml-EP tubes and allowed to gel in an incubator at 37°C for 12 hr. Then, the gels were immersed in 1 ml of PBS (pH = 7.4) and were shaken at 100 rpm at 37°C. At specific time intervals, all the release media were removed and replaced by fresh release media. After centrifuged at 13,000 rpm for 10 min, the supernatant of the removed release media were collected and stored at –20°C until analysis.

The concentration of HK was determined by HPLC Instrument (Waters Alliance 2695). Solvent delivery system equipped with a column heater and a plus autosampler. Detection was taken on a Waters 2996 detector. Chromatographic separations were performed on a reversed phase C18 column (4.6 × 150 mm–5 um, Sunfire Analysis column). And the column temperature was kept at 28°C. Acetonitrile/water (60/40, v/v) was used as eluent at a flow rate of 1 ml/min. The standard curve equation is: H = 105000*X + 4680 (H: The area of peak; X: The concentration of HK) and the correlation coefficient is 0.999994.

Release Behavior of Hydrophilic Macromolecular Protein Drugs

In vitro release behavior of BSA, which was used as the model protein or peptide drug, from BSA loaded composite hydrogel was studied in detail. The initial drug loading amount were 4 mg and 8 mg, respectively. The amount of BSA present in the supernatant was determined by bicinchoninic acid (BCA) assay using BCA™ Protein Assay Kit (PIERCE, USA). The SDS-polyacrylamide gel electrophoretic (SDS-PAGE) analysis was used to assay the stability of BSA in the supernatant.

All the release study experiments were repeated three times. All data are expressed as the mean ± S.D.

Scanning Electron Microscopy (SEM) of Composite Hydrogel

The SEM was employed to investigate morphology of composite hydrogel before and after drug release. The composite hydrogels (before drug release test and 8 hr after drug released) were quickly frozen in liquid nitrogen and lyophilized at –45°C for 72 hr. The composite hydrogels were sputtered with gold before observation. In this study, morphology of prepared composite hydrogels was examined on JEOL SEM (JSM-5900LV, JEOL, Japan).

DISCUSSIONS AND RESULTS

Synthesis of PECE Copolymers

The synthesis of PECE triblock copolymers has been reported in our previous work (Gong et al., 2007, 2009a). Briefly, ring-opening copolymerization of ε-CL onto MPEG was performed to synthesis PEG-PCL diblock copolymers, and stannous octoate was used as catalyst. The PEG-PCL diblock copolymers were then coupled using HMDI as coupling agent to produce the biodegradable PECE triblock copolymers.

Temperature-Dependent Sol-Gel-Sol Transition Behavior

The PECE and Pluronic F127 copolymers are both amphiphilic in nature, whose aqueous solution individually presented sol-gel-sol transition behavior. The composite hydrogel prepared in this work were composed of the two copolymers. As presented in Table 1, composite hydrogel based on PECE and Pluronic F127 copolymers from S1 to S6 all showed temperature-dependent reversible sol-gel-sol phase transition. The composite hydrogel flowed freely at lower temperature, but became a non-flowing gel at body temperature about 37°C (Figure 2). Figure 3 presented the sol-gel-sol phase transition diagrams of prepared composite hydrogel. When the copolymer concentrations are above the critical gelation concentration (CGC), aqueous solutions of composite hydrogel changed from "sol" phase to "gel" phase with increase in temperature to the lower critical gelation temperature (LCGT). With further increase of temperature to upper critical gelation temperature (UCGT), the sol phase occurs.

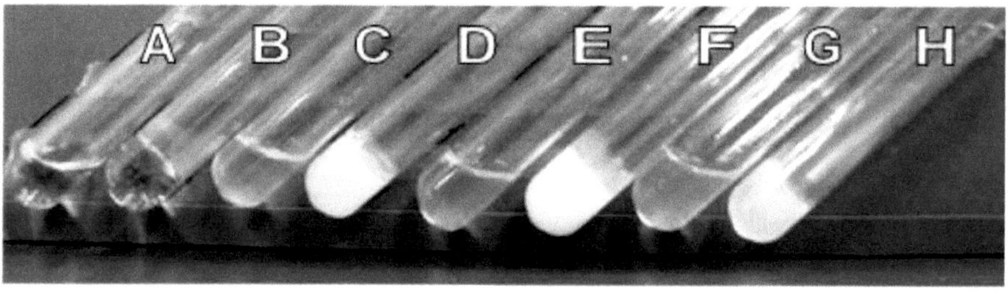

Figure 2. Photograph of composite hydrogel (30 wt%) at different temperature. S6 at 10°C (A) and 37°C (B); S4 at 10°C (C) and 37°C (D); S3 at 10°C (E) and 37°C (F); S1 at 10°C (G) and 37°C (H).

According to Figure 3, pure PECE hydrogel (S1) and pure Pluronic F127 hydrgel (S6) both have a CGC of approximately 15 wt%, but S6 have a much wider gelation window than that of S1. The UCGT of S6 at the concentration of 30 and 35% was not detected from 0°C to 100°C. The CGC of S2, S3, S4, and S5 were 25, 20, 20, and 20 wt%, respectively, which were much higher than that of two pure hydrogels. By mixing the two hydrogel together, the CGC of the composite hydrogel increased accordingly. CGC of S2 increased approximately 10 wt% than that of S1, whereas CGC of S5 increased approximately 5 wt% than that of S6. This phenomenon indicated that concerning CGC, the influence of Pluronic F127 hydrogel on PECE hydrogel was more dramatic than that of PECE hydrogel on Pluronic F127 hydrogel. As shown in Figure 3, with increase in PECE hydrogel content in composite hydrogel, the UCGT decreased significantly, whereas the LCGT increased slightly. The UCGT of S6 hydrogel at concentration of 30 and 35 wt% could not be detected from 0°C to 100°C, but the UCGT at concentration of 30 and 35 wt% were detected in S5 and S3 hydrogel, respectively, due to increase in PECE content.

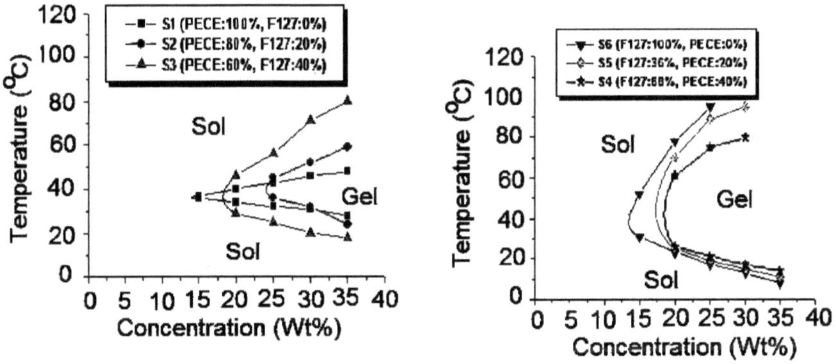

Figure 3. Sol-gel-sol transition phase diagram of composite hydrogel.

Therefore, it was obvious that sol-gel-sol transition behavior of composite hydrogel depended on the composition of the PECE and Pluronic F127 hydrogel. In fact, by altering the composition of composite hydrogel, the temperature range of sol-gel-sol phase transition could be broadened to a certain extent, which might be very useful for their further application as injectable *in situ* gel-forming DDS.

Cytotoxicity Study of Composite Hydrogel Copolymers

The cytotoxicity of the prepared composite hydrogels (S1, S3, S4, and S6) was evaluated by cell viability assay using HEK 293 cells. Figure 4 exhibited the HEK 293 cell viability of composite hydrogel copolymer with different concentration gradient. As shown in Figure 4, with increase of composite hydrogel copolymer amount, HEK 293 cell viability decreased accordingly. However, the 293 cell viability of S1, S3, S4, and S6 copolymers were yet higher than 72.5, 76.6, 78.0, and 71.4%, respectively, even when the input copolymers were 500 μg per well. According to Figure 4, the HEK 293 cell viability of composite hydrogel copolymer decreased as increase of composite hydrogel copolymers. Compared with S3 and S4 copolymers group, S1 copolymer has higher cell viability at 20 μg/well or lower, but cell viability decreased significantly at 50 μg/well or higher. Cell viability study implied that the composite hydrogel copolymers prepared in this chapter were biocompatible with low cell cytotoxicity. Therefore, composite hydrogel could be regarded as safe drug delivery carrier and is very promising for *in situ* gel-forming controlled DDS.

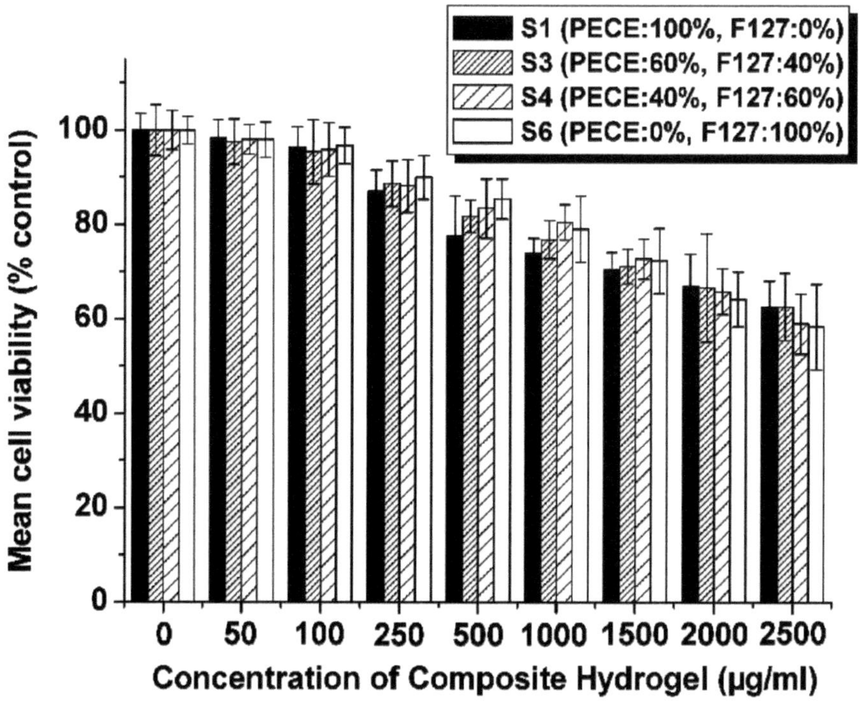

Figure 4. HEK 293 cell viability assay. Cell containing 1 x 10^4 cells in DMEM containing 10% FBS was incubated with S1, S3, S4, and S6 copolymers in 96-well in a humidified atmosphere containing 5% CO_2 at 37°C for 48 hr. Error bars represent the standard deviation (n = 6).

In Vitro Drug Release Profile of Composite Hydrogel

The VB_{12}, HK, and BSA were used as model drugs to investigate the release behavior of hydrophilic small molecular drug, hydrophobic small molecular drug, and protein drug from drug loaded composite hydrogels, respectively. Effect of the hydrogel composition, initial drug loading, and concentration of composite hydrogel on *in vitro* drug release behavior of the composite hydrogel were investigated in detail, which were discussed as follows.

Release Behavior of Hydrophilic Small Molecular Drug

In vitro release profile of VB_{12} from composite hydrogel in PBS was studied, and the results were shown in Figure 5. According to Figure 5, VB_{12} could be released in a sustained period. The hydrogel composition had great effect on VB_{12} release profile, and the results were shown in Figure 5A. The S6 hydrogel disappeared completely in 12 hr with a cumulative release rate of approximately 94.2%, whereas S1 and S4 hydrogel could maintain their integrity in the whole release period. The VB_{12} released faster and reached higher cumulative release rate (90.0%) from S3 hydrogel compared to S1 hydrogel (82.9%), which should be contributed to high composition (60 wt%) of fast-eroding Pluronic F127 in S3 hydrogel.

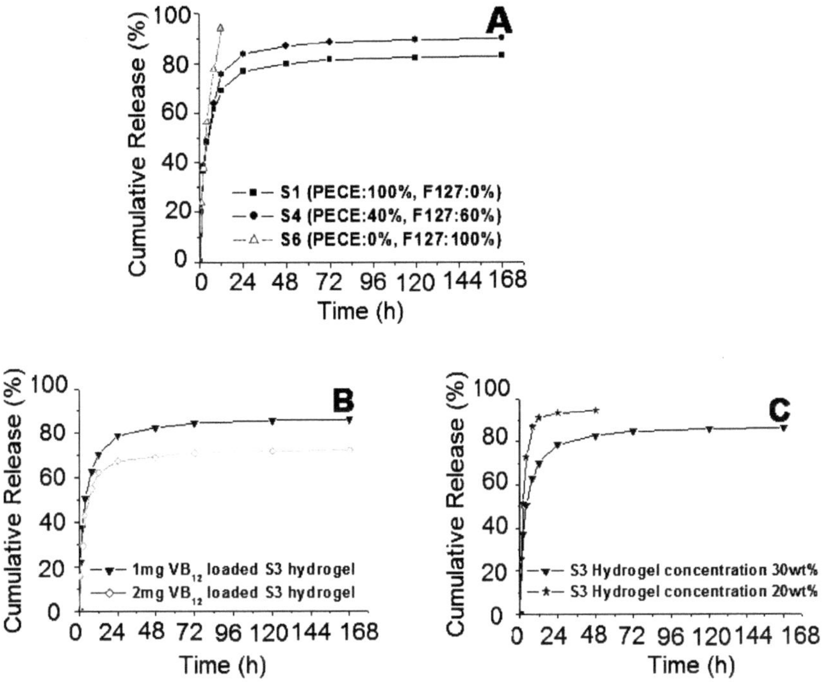

Figure 5. *In vitro* release behavior of VB_{12} from composite hydrogel. (A) Release behavior of S1, S4, an S6 hydrogel with the same hydrogel concentration (30 wt%) and initial drug loading amount (1 mg). (B) Release behavior of 30 wt% S3 hydrogel with different initial drug loading amount (1 mg and 2 mg). (C) Release behavior of 1 mg VB_{12} loaded S3 hydrogel with different hydrogel concentration (20 and 30 wt%). Error bars represent the standard deviation (n = 3).

Effect of initial drug loading amount on release profile of S3 hydrogel was investigated. As shown in Figure 5B, S3 hydrogel containing twice amount of VB_{12} result in a significant decrease of cumulative release rate from 86.3 to 72.4%, which was constant to our previous work. With the same initial drug loading amount but lower hydrogel concentration (20 wt%) of S3, VB_{12} released faster and reached higher cumulative release rate (96.7%) compared to 30 wt% concentration S3 hydrogel (86.3%). Due to the higher composition of fast-eroding Pluronic F127 copolymer and lower hydrogel concentration, the 20 wt% S3 hydrogel was completely eroded in 48 hr. In 20 wt% hydrogel, an initial burst release of 25.6% of loaded VB_{12} occurred in the first 1 hr, followed by release of 94.7% in 2 days, whereas, in 30 wt% hydrogel, the cumulative release rate of 1 hr, 2 days, and 7 days were 22.3, 82.5, and 86.3%, respectively.

Release Behavior of Hydrophobic Small Molecular Drug

The HK, as multi-functional drug, have great potential application in human disease therapy, especially in cancer therapy. Previously, a rapid separation approach to isolate and purify HK had been developed using high-capacity high-speed counter-current chromatography (high-capacity HSCCC) by Chen et al. in our lab (Chen et al., 2007).

For its great potential application and high hydrophobicity, HK was chosen for the hydrophobic model drug in this *in vitro* drug release study.

Due to high hydrophobicity, HK could not be well-disperse in the composite hydrogel to form homogeneous solution. The HK micelles were employed to solve above-mentioned problem. The obtained HK micelles with average particle size of 33.34 nm and polydisperse index (PDI) of 0.036 could be well-dispersed in water, and it was stable. Only Pluronic F127, a composition of composite hydrogel, was remained in the HK micelles, which would not affect *in vitro* release behavior of composite hydrogel.

The release behavior of HK from composite hydrogel was performed and the cumulative release profile was presented in Figure 6. In Figure 6A, with increase in content of Pluronic F127 copolymer from 0% (S1) to 100% (S6), cumulative release rate and burst release rate (in1 hr) increased from 37.1 to 86.5% and from 1.4 to 8.9%, respectively. According to Figure 6B, with increase of initial drug loading amount, the cumulative release rate of HK decreased dramatically from 62.1 to 51.0% in a 14-day period. As shown in Figure 6C, lower concentration of composite hydrogel led to higher cumulative release rate in a shorter time. Compared with VB_{12} release profile, cumulative release rate and burst release rate of HK were much lower, which should be contributed to the high hydrophobicity of HK.

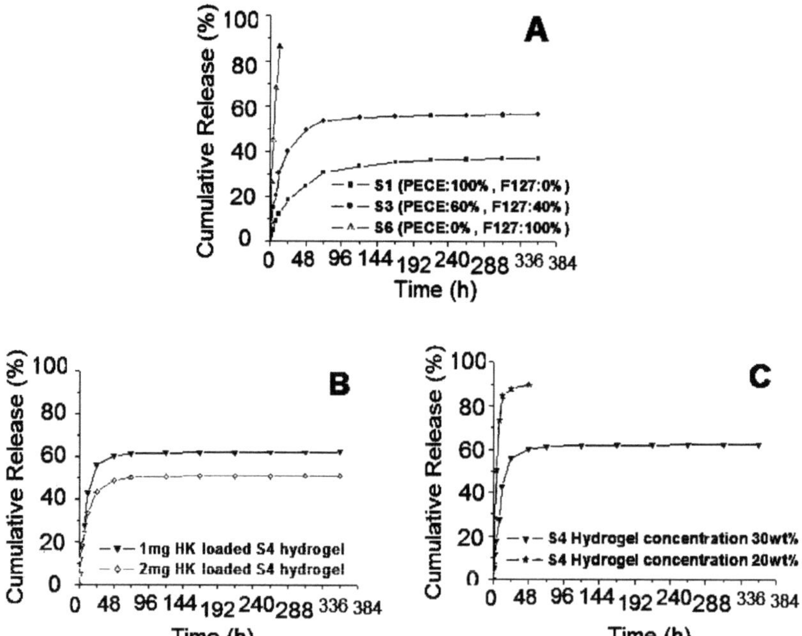

Figure 6. *In vitro* release behavior of HK from composite hydrogel. (A) Release behavior of S1, S3, an S6 hydrogel with the same hydrogel concentration (30 wt%) and initial drug loading amount (1 mg). (B) Release behavior of 30 wt% S4 hydrogel with different initial drug loading amount (1 and 2 mg). (C) Release behavior of 1 mg HK loaded S4 hydrogel with different hydrogel concentration (20 and 30 wt%). Error bars represent the standard deviation (n = 3).

Release Behavior of Hydrophilic Macromolecular Protein Drugs

In vitro release behavior of protein or peptide model drug from composite hydrogel was investigated, and the data were summarized in Figures 7A–C. The BSA could be released slowly from composite hydrogel in an extended period. As presented in Figures 7A–C, effects of hydrogel composition, initial drug loading amount, and hydrogel concentration on BSA release profile were investigated in detail. The results were similar to the influence of these factors on HK release profile. The SDS-PAGE was performed to evaluate the stability of BSA in the *in vitro* release period. According to Figure 7–D, the major band for BSA appeared at about 67 kD (lane2–lane10) according to the protein marker, which showed that BSA was stable in the experimental period.

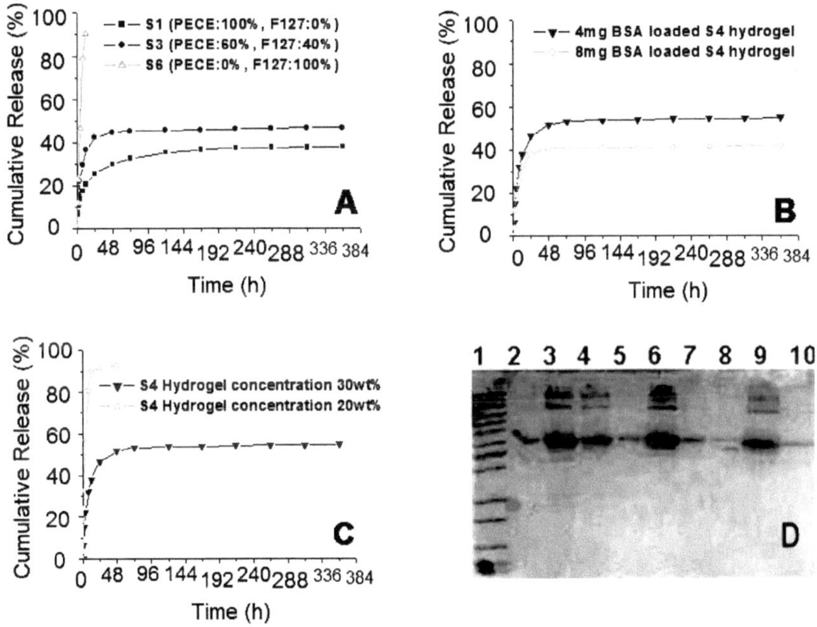

Figure 7. *In vitro* release behavior of BSA from composite hydrogel. (A) Release behavior of S1, S3, an S6 hydrogel with the same hydrogel concentration (30 wt%) and initial drug loading amount (4 mg). (B) Release behavior of 30 wt% S4 hydrogel with different initial drug loading amount (4 and 8 mg). (C) Release behavior of 4 mg BSA loaded S4 hydrogel with different hydrogel concentration (20 and 30 wt%). (D) SDS-PAGE results of BSA *in vitro* release profile; Lane 1: Marker; Lane 2: BSA standard; Lane 3: S1 at 24th hr; Lane 4: S1 at 168th hr; Lane 5: S1 at 360th hr; Lane 6: S3 at 24th hr; Lane 7: S3 at 168th hr; Lane 8: S3 at 360th hr; Lane 6: S3 at 12th hr; Lane 10: S3 at 48th hr. Error bars represent the standard deviation (n = 3).

Thus, composition of composite hydrogel, initial drug loading amount, and hydrogel concentration substantially affected the drug release behavior of composite hydrogel, where higher Pluronic F127 content, lower initial drug loading amount, or lower hydrogel concentration resulted in higher cumulative release rate, which means drug release rate of composite hydrogel could be controlled by simply altering the composition of PECE and Pluronic F127 copolymers. It is obvious that the influence of above-mentioned three factors is more dramatic on HK and BSA than VB_{12}. Due to the great water solubility, VB_{12} was released very fast from the composite hydrogel, which could weaken the influence of the factors.

Besides the factors mentioned above, physical and chemical property of the drugs played an important role in their release behavior. According to Figures 5–7, compared with hydrophobic small molecular drug, hydrophilic small molecular drug reached a higher cumulative release rate in a shorter period. In addition, cumulative release rate of hydrophilic small molecular drug was much higher than that of hydrophilic large molecular drugs.

Morphology of Composite Hydrogel

Interior morphology of composite hydrogel before and 8 hr after drug released was investigated by SEM. The composite hydrogels were frozen in liquid nitrogen and lyophilized for 72 hr before the test. According to Figure 8, all the hydrogel samples showed porous three-dimension structure, but the shape and mesh size of pores in the hydrogel were different. As shown in Figure 8A, S1 hydrogel before drug release presented approximately spherical pore with small mesh size. The S3 hydrogel (Figure 8C), composed of 60% PECE hydrogel and 40% Pluronic F127 hydrogel, also showed spherical pores, but have larger mesh size compared to S1 hydrogel. The morphology of S1 and S3 hydrogel suggested that the composition of composite hydrogel have great influence on their interior structure, which dramatically affected the drug release behavior of composite hydrogel. Eight hours after drug released, S1 hydrogel could maintain its integrity, but the hydrogel surface eroded (Figure 8B). In Figure 8D, S3 hydrogel after immersed in PBS for 8 hr showed large pores and cracks, due to the fast-eroding of Pluronic F127 from the composite hydrogel.

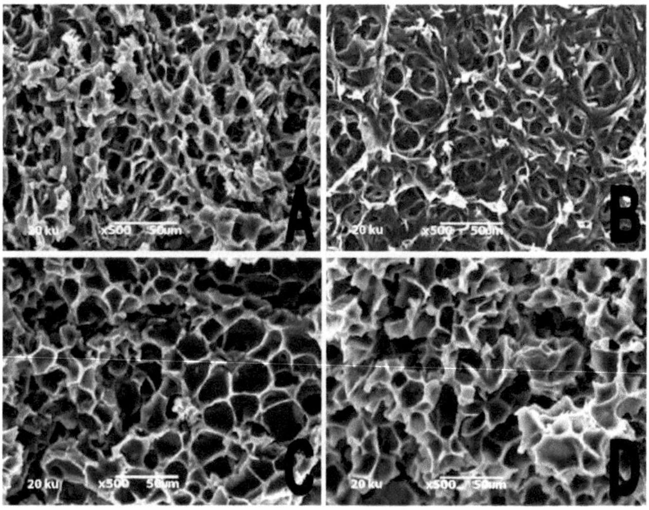

Figure 8. The SEM photograph of composite hydrogel before and after drug release. S1 hydrogel before (A) and after (B) drug release for 8 hr. S3 hydrogel before (C) and after (D) drug release for 8 hr.

CONCLUSION

A series of novel biodegradable and thermosensitive composite hydrogel were successfully prepared in this work. The obtained composite hydrogel underwent sol-gel-sol transition with increase in temperature, which was flowing sol at ambient temperature and became non-flowing gel at body temperature. By varying the composition of PECE and Pluronic F127 copolymers, sol-gel-sol transition behavior and *in vitro* drug release profile of composite hydrogel could be adjusted, which was very useful for its potential applications as *in situ* gel-forming controlled DDS.

KEYWORDS

- **Copolymer**
- **Hydrogel**
- **Pluronic F127**
- **Poly(ethylene glycol)-poly(ε-caprolactone)-poly(ethylene glycol)**
- **Sol-gel**

AUTHORS' CONTRIBUTIONS

Zhi Yong Qian, Yu Quan Wei, and Chang Yang Gong designed the experiments. And the research funds were supported by Zhi Yong Qian and Yu Quan Wei. Chang Yang Gong carried out experiments, analyzed the data, and wrote the manuscript; Zhi Yong Qian corrected the manuscript. Shuai Shi and Jing Liang Yang participated in the MTT cytotoxicity study of the hydrogels. Xiu Ling Zheng participated in the *in vitro* release study from the composite hydrogels. Peng Wei Dong, Gang Guo, and Shao Zhi Fu participated in synthesizing hydrogel and analyzing the data. All authors approved and read the final manuscript.

ACKNOWLEDGMENTS

We thank Ms. J. Zheng (Library of Chengdu University of Information Technology) for her kindly help during preparation and English editing of the manuscript. And this work was financially supported by National 863 Project (2007AA021902), National Natural Science Foundation (NSFC20704027), Specialized Research Fund for the Doctoral Program of Higher Education (SRFDP 200806100065), Sichuan Prominent Young Talents Program (07ZQ026-033), Sichuan Key Project of Science and Technology (2007SGY019), and Chinese Key Basic Research Program (2004CB518807).

COMPETING INTERESTS

The authors declare that they have no competing interests.

Chapter 16

Pharmaceutical Induction of ApoE Secretion

Suzanne Zeitouni, Brian S. Ford, Sean M. Harris, Mandolin J. Whitney, Carl A. Gregory, and Darwin J. Prockop

INTRODUCTION

Apolipoprotein E (ApoE) is a molecular scavenger in the blood and brain. Aberrant function of the molecule causes formation of protein and lipid deposits or "plaques" that characterize Alzheimer's disease (AD) and atherosclerosis. There are three human isoforms of ApoE designated ε2, ε3, and ε4. Each isoform differentially affects the structure and function of the protein and thus the development of disease. Homozygosity for ApoE ε4 is associated with atherosclerosis and AD whereas ApoE ε2 and ε3 tend to be protective. Furthermore, the ε2 form may cause forms of hyperlipoproteinemia. Therefore, introduction of ApoE ε3 may be beneficial to patients that are susceptible to or suffering from these diseases. Mesenchymal stem cells or multipotent mesenchymal stromal cells (MSCs) are adult progenitor cells found in numerous tissues. They are easily expanded in culture and engraft into host tissues when administered appropriately. Furthermore, MSCs are immunosuppressive and have been reported to engraft as allogeneic transplants. In our previous study, mouse MSCs (mMSCs) were implanted into the brains of ApoE null mice, resulting in production of small amounts of ApoE in the brain and attenuation of cognitive deficits. Therefore human MSCs (hMSCs) are a promising vector for the administration of ApoE ε3 in humans.

Unlike mMSCs, hMSCs were found not to express ApoE in culture; therefore a molecular screen was performed for compounds that induce expression. The PPARγ agonists, neural stem cell conditioned medium, osteo-inductive media, dexamethasone, and adipo-inductive media (AIM) were tested. Of the conditions tested, only AIM or dexamethasone induced sustained secretion of ApoE in MSCs and the duration of secretion was only limited by the length of time MSCs could be sustained in culture. Upon withdrawal of the inductive stimuli, the ApoE secretion persisted for a further 14 days.

The data demonstrated that pre-treatment and perhaps co-administration of MSCs homozygous for ApoE ε3 and dexamethasone may represent a novel therapy for severe instances of AD, atherosclerosis, and other ApoE-related diseases.

The ApoE is a 34 kDa secreted lipoprotein, first discovered by Shore and Shore in 1973, see Horejsi and Ceska, (2000). Like other apolipoproteins, its primary function is to scavenge cholesterol, associated lipids, and proteins for transport to the liver for processing. In healthy individuals, a plasma concentration of approximately 5 mg/dl is sufficient to maintain systemic lipid homeostasis (Mahley, 1988). Although primarily expressed in liver (Horejsi and Ceska, 2000), The ApoE contrasts with the other apolipoproteins in that it is also expressed in the spleen, lungs, kidneys, myoblasts, and macrophages (Cedazo-Minguez, 2007; Mahley, 1988). The ApoE is also highly expressed in the brain, by microglia and astrocytes (Bales et al., 2002; Cedazo-Minguez, 2007) and there have also been reports of ApoE production by neurons (Cedazo-Minguez, 2007). Although poorly understood, the role of ApoE in the central nervous system is thought to be comparable to its role in plasma, sequestering cholesterol, lipids, and other macromolecular debris from neural tissue (Hatters et al., 2006).

The effectiveness of ApoE as a lipid scavenger is closely related to the ApoE isoform. ApoE polymorphism is thought to be uniquely exhibited by humans (Cedazo-Minguez, 2007) in that it consists of three isoforms, ApoE ε2, ε3, and ε4. Although the isoforms vary only at two amino acid residues, the changes are sufficient to profoundly alter the tertiary structure and affect lipid binding properties of the protein (Cedazo-Minguez, 2007; Hatters et al., 2006). The ApoE polymorphism occurs at residues 112 and 158, ApoEε2 has two cysteines, ApoEε3 had a cysteine and an arginine and ApoEε4 has two arginines at these positions. The ApoE ε3 is the most common isoform with an incidence of approximately 77% in the population (Bales et al., 2002; Cedazo-Minguez, 2007; Horejsi and Ceska, 2000), followed by ε4 in approximately 15%, and then ε2 at approximately 7%.

Due to the profound effects on the functional and structural properties of the protein, different isoforms of ApoE are associated with different diseases such as stroke, multiple sclerosis, Parkinson's disease, alcoholic cirrhosis of the liver, and type 2 diabetes (Cedazo-Minguez, 2007; Hernandez-Nazaraet et al., in press; Kantarci, 2008; Lei et al., 2008). The role that ApoE isoforms play in disease development seems to be closely associated with different affinities of the various isoforms for the low density lipoprotein-receptor and lipids themselves. For instance in the case of AD, individuals that are homozygous or heterozygous for ApoE ε4, have a significantly increased risk of developing the disease with an earlier onset (Cedazo-Minguez, 2007) compared with individuals with the most common ApoE ε3/ε3 genotype (Bales et al., 2002; Cedazo-Minguez, 2007; Dodart et al., 2005; Horejsi and Ceska, 2000; Lusis et al., 2004; Peskind et al., 2001). Likewise, individuals homozygous for Apo ε2 or with an ApoE ε2/ε3 genotype also have normal susceptibility for AD. Although ApoE4 is not an absolute determinant of the disease 40–65% of AD patients have at least one copy of the four allele. However, the role of ApoE isoforms is complex with additional reports also implicating ApoE ε2 with hyperlipidaemia and ApoE ε4 with hypercholesterolaemia. (Lusis et al., 2004; Utermann, 1988). In consideration of the putative association of ApoE ε2 and ε4 with disease it is reasonable to assume that safe administration of ApoE ε3 could provide beneficial effects for some individuals.

The MSC, also known as marrow stromal cells or mesenchymal stem cells, are a heterogeneous population of non-hematopoietic cells representing 0.01–0.001% of the total bone marrow (Uccelli et al., 2006). The *in vivo* function of MSCs remains controversial, but they are generally regarded as hematopoietic support cells and also a source of progenitors for structural tissues (Prockop, 1997).

The existence of such cells was first suggested by Cohneheim in the 1870s (Prockop, 1997) but Friedenstein and his colleagues were the first to isolate and culture MSCs in the 1970s (Friedenstein et al., 1970, 1974a, 1974b, 1987; Owen and Friedenstein, 1988), followed by Caplan and colleagues (Haynesworth et al., 1992a, 1992b) who were the first to propose the phrase "mesenchymal stem cells." These cells are adherent to plastic and are known to differentiate to osteoblasts, chondrocytes, and adipocytes *in vitro* and *in vivo* (Gregory et al., 2005; Prockop, 1997; Prockop et al., 2003; Uccelli et al., 2006). However, more recent findings suggest that MSCs may differentiate to additional cell types (Prockop et al., 2003). Another remarkable characteristic of MSCs are their immunosuppressive qualities, suggesting that they may survive and engraft in allogeneic recipients (Uccelli et al., 2006). Because MSCs are easily expanded in culture, readily engraft into host tissues, and may locally modulate the immune response, they represent ideal candidates for cytotherapy. Specifically, MSCs represent an extremely useful tool for the treatment of deficits in ApoE function if harboring the ApoE ε3 isoform.

In a previous study we demonstrated that murine MSCs (mMSCs) injected into the lateral ventricles of 4-day-old ApoE null mice secreted small amounts of ApoE into the tissue (Peister et al., 2006). As ApoE null mice mature, the animals develop cognitive impairment, but upon behavioral analysis, the presence of mMSCs resulted in improved cognitive behavioral testing compared to the control groups (Peister et al., 2006). Therefore, hMSCs seemed a promising vector for the administration of ApoE ε3 in human diseases. In contrast to mMSCs, unmanipulated hMSCs do not synthesize ApoE mRNA *in vitro*, but expression could be observed after 7 days of adipocyte differentiation (Sekiya et al., 2004). Pharmaceutical induction of ApoE secretion has been demonstrated in macrophages, hepatocytes, adipocytes, and other cell types by a variety of agents. In two studies employing rat hepatocytes, ApoE secretion was stimulated using dexamathasone, insulin, or a combination of both (Lin, 1988; Martin-Sanz et al., 1990). In macrophages, secretion of ApoE was induced by treatment with TGFβ and dexamethasone (Zuckerman et al., 1993). Expression of ApoE mRNA by adipocytes was increased by pioglitazone and ciglitazone, neither of which affected the ApoE secretion of macrophages (Yue et al., 2004).

This study examined pharmaceutical induction of endogenous ApoE expression by hMSCs. We demonstrate here that dexamethasone alone or AIM containing dexamethasone, indomethacin and isobutylmethylxanthine resulted in the expression of high levels of ApoE by hMSCs *in vitro*. Maximal expression could be attained after approximately 5–10 days of dexamethasone or AIM treatment depending on the donor source of the cells. We found no correlation between the ApoE expression levels and the degree of cell expansion prior to the assay, nor did we find any correlation between sex or age and ApoE secretion kinetics. The maximal rate of secretion ranged between 0.004 and 0.006 ng $cell^{-1}$ day^{-1}. After withdrawal of the stimulus, ApoE expression remained approximately 14 days, but sometimes much longer, depending on the donor. These *in vitro* results demonstrate that ApoE expression by hMSCs is entirely possible through pharmaceutical induction without the necessity for genetic manipulation. Therefore, MSCs may represent a safe and feasible strategy for treatment of diseases that result from a functional deficit of ApoE.

MATERIALS AND METHODS

Culture of Human Multipotent Stromal Cells

Mutlipotent stromal cells were acquired from the Tulane University adult stem cell distribution facility. In accordance with institutional review board approved protocols, the cells were prepared from 2 ml posterior iliac crest bone marrow aspirates derived from seven males and one female between 25 and 34 yr of age. After a brief interval of monolayer culture to exclude non-adherent hematopoietic cells, hMSCs were expanded to 70% confluency prior to passage or use in experiments. Cells were cultured according to standard MSC culture conditions in complete culture medium (CCM), consisting of alpha minimal essential medium (GIBCO, Invitrogen, Carlsbad, CA) containing 20% (v/v) FBS (Hyclone, Logan, UT and Altanta Biologicals, Norcross, GA), 2 mM L-glutamine and 100 units ml^{-1} penicillin and 100 $\mu g\ ml^{-1}$ streptomycin (GIBCO, Invitrogen) (Gregory and Prockop, 2007; Gregory et al., 2003).

Differentiation of Human Multipotent Stromal Cells

To confirm that the cell preparations from the mononuclear layer were multipotent, a panel of differentiation assays were performed.

Osteogenic Differentiation and Alizarin Red S Staining

For osteogenic differentiation, confluent monolayers of hMSCs were incubated in CCM supplemented with 10^{-8} M dexamethasone, 50 $\mu g\ ml^{-1}$ ascorbic acid and 5 mM β-glycerol phosphate (Sigma, Poole, UK) for 21 days with changes of medium every 2 days. The monolayers were then stained with 40 mM Alizarin Red S pH 4.0 (Sigma) for 30 min and washed four times with distilled water. Micrographs were taken using an inverted microscope (Nikon Eclipse, TE200).

Adipogenic Differentiation and Oil Red O Staining

All reagents were purchased from Sigma. Confluent monolayers of hMSCs in six well plates (10 cm^2 per well) were incubated in AIM consisting of CCM containing 0.5 μM dexamethasone, 5×10^{-8} M isobutylmethylxanthine, and 5×10^{-7} M indomethacin (Sigma). Media was changed every 2–3 days. After 21 days, the adipogenic cultures are fixed in 10% formalin for 15 min and stained with fresh Oil Red-O solution 0.5 (w/v) (Sigma) in 30% (v/v) isopropanol in phosphate buffered saline (PBS) for 20 min. The dishes were washed three times with excess PBS and visualized using an inverted microscope (Nikon Eclipse, TE200).

Chondrogenic Differentiation and Processing

Micromass pellet chondrogenic differentiation was carried out in accordance with the protocol of Sekiya et al. on 200,000 pelleted cells (Sekiya et al., 2002). After 21 days of differentiation, the chondroid pellets were washed in PBS and fixed in 4% paraformaldehyde. The pellets were then embedded in paraffin, sectioned, then stained with toluidine blue to visualize sulphated proteoglycans and chondrocyte lacunae (Gregory and Prockop, 2007).

ELISA Detection of ApoE

Sample Preparation for ELISA

The hMSCs were plated in each well of a six well plate at 1,000 cells per cm^2 and grown to 70% confluency. The media was then changed to the appropriate conditions and maintained for the appropriate duration with changes every 2–3 days. All experiments were performed in triplicate. Media samples were taken at intervals defined in the results and stored for ELISAs at –20°C. Dexamethasone and dimethyl sulphoxide (vehicle) were purchased from Sigma and diluted into CCM from a 1000× stock solution. AIM and osteogenic media were prepared as described above and the individual components were added to CCM from stocks. For production of NSC conditioned medium, a frozen vial of murine neural stem cells (NSCs, a gift from Dr. Jeffrey Spees, Department of Medicine, Cardiovascular Research Institute, University of Vermont) was employed. The NSC conditioned medium was produced by incubation of the NSCs in NSC media (neurobasal alpha medium containing B27 supplement, L-glutamine, penicillin, streptomycin (Invitrogen), 10 ng ml^{-1} epidermal growth factor, 10 ng ml^{-1}, fibroblast growth factor (Sigma)) for 2 days. The NSC conditioned medium was mixed 1:1 with CCM prior to addition to the hMSCs. Ciglitazone was purchased from Tocris Biochemical (Bristol, UK) and troglitazone was purchased from Cayman Chemical (Ann Arbor, MI). The drugs were added to CCM from a stock dissolved in DMSO. All assays were conducted in parallel with vehicle, or unconditioned media controls.

Human ApoE Sandwich ELISA

A polyclonal goat-anti-human ApoE antibody (Academy Biomedical, Houston, TX) was diluted in PBS at 1:1000. Each well of a high binding microtiter plate (Fisher Lifesciences) was coated with 100 μl of the antibody solution for 15 hr at 4°C. The coating solution was then removed followed 3 × 5 min washes with 150 μl PBS. Wells were then blocked by addition of PBS containing 0.1% (v/v) Tween20 (Fisher Lifesciences) and 5% (w/v) bovine serum albumin (Sigma) for 2hr at room temperature. Block solution removed and the wells were washed for 3 × 5 min in PBS containing 0.1% (v/v) Tween20 (PBST). Media samples (100 μl) were added to the wells in triplicate. Standard solutions of recombinant human ApoE (Calbiochem, Gibbstown, NJ) were diluted in PBST. Samples were incubated in the microtiter plates for 15hr at 4°C. Plates were then washed for 3× for 5 min in PBST, and the detection antibody (100 μl) was added consisting of a 1:2000 dilution of HRP conjugated goat anti human ApoE IgG (Academy Biomedical) in PBST at room temperature. After 2hr, the wells were washed in PBST and developed by addition of 100 μl TMB (Pierce, Rockford IL).

After approximately 5 min, the reactions were stopped with the addition of 50 μl 2 N sulphuric acid (Fisher Lifesciences) and the resultant yellow substrate was measured by absorbance (450 nm) on a 96 well plate reader (Fluostar Optima, BMG).

Cell Number Evaluation

Cells were counted using a DNA intercalating dye that fluoresces upon incorporation (CyQuant dye, Invitrogen). Briefly, monolayers were recovered by trypsinization, washed in PBS, then resuspended in lysis buffer (PBS containing 0.1% Triton ×100, 1 mM $MgCl_2$) containing a 400 fold dilution of the CyQuant dye. At various dilutions, the labeling suspensions were aliquoted into a microtiter plate and fluorescence was measured at 480/525 nm on a 96 well plate reader (Fluostar Optima) using opaque black plates (Fisher Scientific). Fluorescence was proportional to DNA content, and thus cell number, when compared to known cell standards.

ApoE Detection by Western Blotting

Sample Preparation

The MSCs were plated on 15 cm plates at 100 cells per cm^2 and grown to 70% confluency. The cells were then maintained under experimental conditions for 21 days and recovered by scraping. The media was collected for ELISAs. Cells were washed in PBS, flash frozen in liquid nitrogen and then stored at –80°C for protein extraction. The proteins were solubilized using an extraction solution consisting of PBS containing 1 mM $MgCl_2$, 1% (w/v) SDS (Sigma), 0.1% Triton X-100 (Fisher Lifesciences) and 10 fold protease inhibitor cocktail (Roche Diagnostics, Nutley, NJ). Protein yield and quality was evaluated by gel electrophoresis (Novex electrophoresis system, Invitrogen) followed by silver staining (Invitrogen).

Western Blot Assay

Approximately 30 μg of protein were added to the appropriate volume of 2 × LDS-PAGE sample buffer (Invitrogen) containing 1 mM β-mercaptoethanol and 2 M urea (Sigma Aldrich). The samples were heated at 95°C for 5 min and electrophoresed on a 10% NuPage bis-Tris gel using the MOPS buffering system followed by transferral to PVDF for 7 min (iBlot, Invitrogen). Filters were blocked in PBS-T containing 5% (w/v) powdered milk (Santa Cruz Biotechnology, Santa Cruz, CA) for 2hr. For detection of ApoE the blots were incubated overnight in an HRP conjugated goat anti human ApoE (Academy Biomedical) at 1:500 in block buffer. For detection of GAPDH, blots were probed with a monoclonal antibody at a dilution of 1:1000 (clone 6C5, Chemicon, Temecula, CA). For secondary detection, a rabbit anti-mouse IgG antibody coupled to horse radish peroxidase was used at a dilution of 1:1500 (Sigma). The blots were developed in peroxidase substrate (100 mM Tris pH 8.0 containing 75 μM paracoumaric acid, 500 μM luminol and 0.006% (v/v) hydrogen peroxide, Sigma) for 5 min prior to exposure to photographic film (Pierce).

VLDL Binding Assay

The MSCs were transferred to serum free CCM containing Dex or vehicle. After 2 days, the conditioned medium was filtered through a 0.2 μm membrane. One milliliter of the conditioned medium was added to 50 μg of biotinylated human VLDL solution (Intracel, Fredrick, MD). The mixture was incubated for 4 hr with rotation, and large VLDL aggregates were removed by centrifugation at 15,000 g for 15 min. The mixture was then depleted of biotinylated components by four sequential 30 min incubations in wells of a streptavidin coated microtiter plate (Streptawell High Bind, Roche Diagnostics). The supernatant was then subjected to ELISA assay.

Production and Characterization of Lipid Micelles Containing Labeled Cholesterol Ester, Cholesterol, and MSC Derived ApoE

Conditioned serum free medium containing 50–100 ng ml^{-1} ApoE was incubated in 50 μg ml^{-1} 4,4-difluoro-5-(2-pyrrolyl)-4-bora-3a,4a-diaza-s-indacene-3-undecanoate (cholesteryl BODIPY 576/589 C11, Invitrogen), and 5 μg ml^{-1} 25-(N-((7-nitro-2-1,3-benzoxadiazol-4-yl)methyl)amino)-27-norcholesterol (NBD cholesterol). Cholesteryl BODIPY 576/589 C_{11} is a blue cholesteryl ester and NBD cholesterol consists of a cholesterol moiety covalently conjugated to a green fluorophore 460/534. Lipids were allowed to self-assemble at 21°C with slow mixing. In some cases, the micelles were recovered by centrifugation, washed in ice cold PBS and assayed for ApoE content by western blotting. For cell binding studies, Huh-7 hepatocytes (a gift from Srikanta Dash, Tulane Health Sciences Center) were expanded in six well plates containing standard media at 37°C with 5% (v/v) CO_2. Upon initiation of the experiment, 2 ml of micelle-containing serum free medium was added to the cultures and at hourly intervals, cultures were washed in warm PBS, then the medium was replaced by serum free medium without lipid. Cells were visualized by epifluorescent and phase microscopy. Kinetics of the uptake of NBD cholesterol was compared between ApoE containing and vehicle containing control media.

Statistical Analyses

Measurements were performed in triplicate for each media sample taken and measurements were considered acceptable when the variation was less than 5% of the value. For each condition tested, three to six replicate cultures were prepared and assayed. Data were presented as the mean of the measurements from replicate cultures with standard deviations. Representative data are presented from one donor in figures, but multiple donors were assayed yielding the same results.

DISCUSSION

There are a number of reports where ApoE has been successfully administered via direct gene delivery or virally in a variety of disease models including AD (Dodart et al., 2005), hypercholesterolemia (Athanasopoulos et al., 2000; Rinaldi et al., 2000; Signori et al., 2007; Stevenson et al., 1995), hyperlipidemia (Harris et al., 2006), atherosclerosis (Harris et al., 2006; Hasty et al., 1999; Kashyap et al., 1995), experimental stroke (McColl et al., 2007), and hematopoietic diseases (Gough and Raines, 2003). Direct gene introduction or direct viral therapy can be efficient and sustainable in some cases, but it is associated with safety concerns. To circumvent some of these problems, ApoE has been administered through hematopoietic stem cells (HSCs) in rodent models (Boisvert et al., 1995; Sakai et al., 2002; van Eck et al., 1997). The HSCs are administered to radioablated animal models and long term hematopoietic stem cells reconstitute the bone marrow compartment. In some studies, ApoE is introduced to the HSCs virally, and in others, the inherent ApoE is utilized mostly through expression by resultant macrophages. These studies suggest that bone marrow transplantation is a promising vector for cytotherapeutic ApoE administration but the process of radioablation in humans is a dangerous procedure, and graft versus host disease is a common problem with allogeneic recipients. Viral integration, especially with long term repopulating HSCs is also a source of concern for these strategies.

In consideration of all of these caveats, a safer cytotherapeutic vector would be beneficial. The MSCs are safely recovered from humans via a simple iliac crest aspirate and can be expanded by the million (Gregory and Prockop, 2007; Gregory et al., 2005). Their characteristics suggest that they would be an excellent delivery tool for ApoE; for instance, when administered into animal models, they survive for long periods in the brain (up to 6 months) and subcutaneously (Gregory et al., 2006; Isakova et al., 2007; Kopen et al., 1999; Peister et al., 2006; Phinney et al., 2006). When in the brain, hMSCs secrete trophic factors that stimulate neural stem cell proliferation and probably their own survival (Munoz et al., 2005). Upon subcutaneous implantation, the hMSCs distribute themselves close to capillary beds suggesting that they have the capacity to secrete proteins into the blood (Gregory et al., 2006). The MSCs are also immunomodulatory, with the capacity to suppress a variety of rejection mechanisms (Dodart et al., 2005), reducing the possibility of graft versus host complications, and improving the probability of allogeneic transplant. Finally, transplanted hMSCs do not rapidly proliferate in adult tissues in the same way repopulating HSCs do, suggesting that they may also be safer for accommodating viral transgenes.

In our previous study (Peister et al., 2006), mMSCs were administered to the lateral ventricles of ApoE null mice. As they age, untreated ApoE null mice develop cognitive deficits that resemble AD in addition to profound atherosclerotic pathogenesis. Remarkably, upon administration of the murine MSCs, the mice exhibited signs of improvement in some of the behavioral tests. When the brains of the experimental animals were examined, a small amount of murine ApoE could be detected. Although the presence of other mMSC derived factors could have contributed to functional recovery, the presence of ApoE 6 months after MSC administration strongly suggested that the functional deficit of ApoE in the null mice had been attenuated. We therefore hypothesized that hMSCs may provide a promising vector for administration of the ApoE3 isoform for the treatment of AD and possibly atherosclerosis.

We could not detect ApoE expression *in vitro*, when cultured under standard conditions, nor could we detect expression when cultured in murine neural conditioned medium. This was surprising, since administration of murine MSCs *in vivo*, stimulated expression. We hypothesize that the ApoE null environment may have been sufficient to stimulate expression or more likely, the hMSCs required contact with the neural cells to initiate expression. Due to the limited availability of human neural tissue, and in view of potential inter-species incompatibility, we decided to attempt induction of expression using commonly available pharmaceuticals. This approach has been utilized with a variety of cell lines and a variety of reagents (Lin, 1988; Martin-Sanz et al., 1990; Yue et al., 2004; Zuckerman et al., 1993) and also in MSCs when differentiated completely into adipocytes (Sekiya et al., 2004). Administration of adipocytes directly into the brain cannot be performed, therefore we tested related conditions in an attempt to induce ApoE expression without lipid droplet accumulation that occurs during adipogenic differentiation. In contrast with previous literature where adipocytes were employed (Yue et al., 2004), The PPARγ agonists gave very limited success

(Figure 2a) demonstrating that the compounds function in a cell type-dependent manner. Another series of studies demonstrated efficacy with the hydrocortisone analog, dexamethasone on murine macrophages and rat hepatocytes (Lin, 1988; Martin-Sanz et al., 1990; Zuckerman et al., 1993). We therefore tested dexamethasone at the equivalent concentration employed for adipogenic differentiation and we achieved high levels of ApoE expression without complete differentiation into adipocytes. Indomethacin and Dex also induced ApoE secretion, but we also observed high levels of unwanted adipogenesis (data not shown). We acquired the genotype of two of the eight donors and found them to be Apo ε3/3 and Apo ε2/3. These donors had comparable ApoE expression levels when compared with the other uncharacterized MSC preparations. This confirmed that MSCs with preferable Apo ε3/3 genotype would be compatible with the Dex induction strategy.

Permanent induction of ApoE would be beneficial, dismissing the need for constant drug administration. However, withdrawal of both Dex and AIM caused a reduction of ApoE output over 2 weeks. Although it is unclear whether this is due to outgrowth of a non-expressing component of MSCs or due to attenuation of expression, the extent of proliferation required to completely ablate expression is not expected in these confluent cultures. Of interest, is the reduced expression of ApoE in the AIM treated cultures, which, by day 21 have mostly differentiated into lipid-filled adipocytes. It appears that ApoE is not a prerequisite for maintenance of the terminal adipocyte phenotype. We did not observe a qualitative reduction in lipid-filled cells suggesting that dedifferentiation had not occurred, but this phenomenon cannot be completely discounted.

We found that doses as low as 0.125 μM were sufficient to maintain maximal expression of ApoE, and doses as low as 0.01 μM could sustain half maximal levels of ApoE expression. These levels are comparable with published therapeutic plasma levels of dexamethasone, which are in the region of 0.001–0.05 μM for immunomodulation (Czock et al., 2005). These results suggest that relatively safe plasma levels that can be attained clinically would be sufficient for ApoE induction by implanted MSCs.

Nevertheless, chronic Dex administration is not without serious side effects (Zoorob and Cender, 1998) such as immunological inhibition, diabetes/hyperglycemia, osteoporotic symptoms, gastric irritation, weight loss or gain, glaucoma, muscle pain/weakness, and exacerbation of psychosis. The side effects increase with duration and dose. Since expression of ApoE was maintained for at least 7 days by hMSCs after withdrawal of stimulus, it is possible that less frequent administration of Dex (every 2 days, for instance) may maintain ApoE levels while reducing the probability of harmful effects. Furthermore, corticosteroids with faster clearance and shorter effect durations, such as prednisone or hydrocortisone may improve the risk/benefit ratio (Zoorob and Cender, 1998).

In terms of efficacy, we found that maximal ApoE expression per cell was in the region of 0.0033 ng per cell in 24 hr when treated with Dex. Since the plasma concentration is about 50 mg l^{-1} (Mahley, 1988), and the average blood volume in an adult human is 5.5 l, it would take an implant containing 250 million cells about 7 days to attain 1% of normal systemic ApoE levels, a dose that is protective against atherosclerotic plaque formation (Hasty et al., 1999). However, systemically infused MSCs have the capacity to migrate to sites of injury and inflammation, suggesting that the local dose of ApoE might be much higher at the lesions (Gregory et al., 2005; Prockop, 1997; Prockop et al., 2003). Direct injection of a lower dose of MSCs into the brain may provide long term relief of AD while stimulating the local population of neural stem cells to repair existing damage (Munoz et al., 2005). In healthy humans, the blood brain barrier (BBB) is somewhat resistant to Dex penetration due to multi-drug resistance receptor action (Meijer et al., 1998) and this is a potential problem for treatment of AD. There are, however, alternative corticosteroids, such as prednisolone, which are predicted to have similar effects and have been reported to have increased permeability into the cerebrospinal fluid (Bannwarth et al., 1997; Birmingham et al., 1984; Joëls et al., 1997; Zoorob and Cender, 1998). Furthermore, there is extensive evidence that the BBB is compromised in individuals with AD suggesting that Dex may have access to implanted MSCs in severe cases (Desai et al., 2007; Donahue and Johanson, 2008; Pluta, 2006).

It can be argued that MSCs may not require pharmaceutical ApoE induction at all since there have been reports that they express various neuronal markers *in vitro* (Deng et al., 2006) and *in vivo* (Deng et al., 2006; Kopen et al., 1999; Zhao et al., 2002) and thus may spontaneously differentiate into astrocytes in the brain. Indeed, murine MSCs were shown to express nestin, β-III tubulin, neurofilament marker and GFAP (an astrocyte marker) *in vitro* (Deng et al., 2006), and GFAP, β-III tubulin, and neurofilament *in vivo* after transplantation into mice (Deng et al., 2006; Kopen et al., 1999). Human MSCs were also shown to express GFAP (Zhao et al., 2002) *in vivo*. However, it is noteworthy that in every instance where MSCs were implanted into the murine brain, only a small proportion expressed the astrocyte marker, GFAP. Therefore, although some hMSCs may differentiate into ApoE-secreting astrcocytes, it remains important to pre-treat the hMSCs with Dex to ensure that the majority of the cells secrete ApoE immediately upon implantation.

Since functional ApoE has been expressed in *E. coli* (Vogel et al., 1985) and in insect cells (Gretch et al., 1991), it is likely that the MSC-derived ApoE is also functional. Nevertheless, we confirmed that the protein could associate with cholesterol esters and could also bind to VLDLs (Figures 7 and 8). The MSC-derived ApoE also accelerated uptake of lipid by hepatocytes (Figure 8). Since the physiological role of ApoE is dependent binding of lipid and the LDL-receptor, these data suggest that the ApoE would satisfy its role *in vivo*. Of particular note, is the observation that MSCs produce high levels of ApoE in the absence of serum (Figure 7a). This raises the possibility of generating ApoE preparations for therapeutic use without the necessity for MSC administration. Since MSC conditioned media inherently contains neuroprotective cytokines (Munoz et al., 2005), dialysed conditioned media containing ApoE may represent an efficacious neuroprotective cocktail for clinical use.

RESULTS

Culture and Characterization of Human MSCs

We employed MSCs from a total of eight donors for the study. Human MSCs were recovered from the mononuclear fraction of whole bone marrow and cultured as described in the Materials and Methods. The adherent component of the cultures, containing hMSCs is relatively pure, but frequently contains traces of contaminating osteoblasts, fibroblasts, and senescent cells. To assay for enrichment of multipotent hMSCs, we performed differentiation assays to osteoblasts, adipocytes, and chondrocytes. The hMSCs readily differentiated into all three lineages when subjected to the appropriate conditions (Figure 1). The MSCs formed mineralized osteoblasts as detected by the calcium binding dye, alizarin red S; they formed adipocytes with oil red O stainable lipid droplets; and formed proteoglycan-filled cartilage pellets that stained purple with toluidine blue when subjected to pellet culture in the presence of bone morphogenic protein 2 and tumor necrosis factor β.

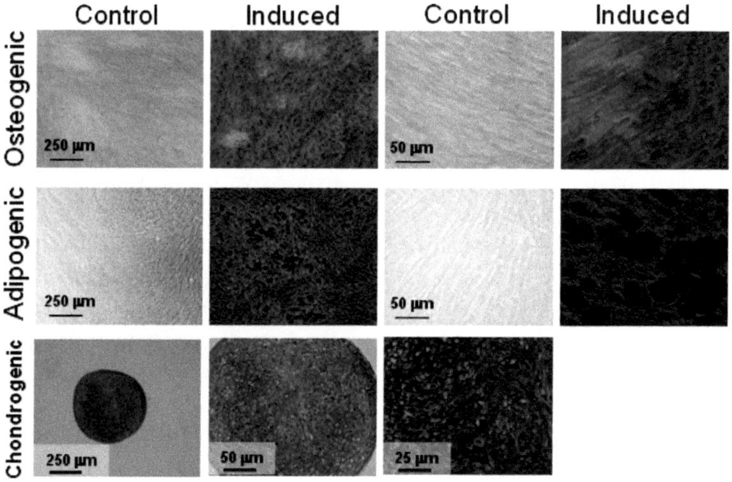

Figure 1. Differentiation of human MSCs. Characterization of MSCs by differentiation assays. One donor is presented. Row 1, high (right) and low power (left) micrographs of osteogenic MSCs stained with Alizarin Red S for calcium. Row 2, high (right) and low power (left) micrographs of adipogenic MSCs stained with oil red O for lipid. Row 3, high (right) and low power (center and left) micrographs of toluidine blue (purple) stained sections of MSC pellets induced to form chondrocytes and cartilage. All donors were assayed for adipogenesis and osteogenesis with the exception of chondrogenesis, where two donors were assayed.

Induction of ApoE Production

Unmanipulated hMSCs did not secrete detectable levels of ApoE when the conditioned culture media was assayed by ELISA as shown in the controls in Figures 2, 4, 5, and 6. Since previous studies have reported successful induction of ApoE secretion from other cell types, we decided to screen some candidates for ApoE inducing activity. A total of nine conditions were tested; 0.5 μM dexamethasone (Dex), neural stem cell conditioned media (NSC-CM), AIM, osteogenic media (ost), 30 μM ciglitazone (cig 30), 3 μM ciglitazone (cig 3), 100 μM troglitazone (trog 100), 10 μM troglitazone (trog 10). Confluent MSC monolayers from two donors were cultured in the experimental conditions for 21 days. At 2 day increments, conditioned medium was recovered for ApoE ELISA. Of the conditions tested, five induced ApoE expression after 10 days of treatment; these were Dex, NSC-CM, AIM, ost, and cig 30 (Figure 2a). The

Cig 30 transiently induced ApoE secretion by day 10 of culture but these levels were absent at subsequent time points. The Ost maintained ApoE expression to day 21, the end point of the experiment, but the levels remained very low. Since mMSCs were shown to secrete ApoE in brains of mice (Peister et al., 2006), we tested conditioned media from murine neural stem cells. Transient expression of ApoE was induced after 10 days of culture, but these levels were undetectable at later time points. Since the ELISA detects only human ApoE, the levels were derived from the hMSCs rather than trace levels in the conditioned media itself. In contrast, Dex and AIM induced high and robust expression of ApoE, which persisted until the end of the experiment at 21 days.

a.

	Days of treatment, values are ApoE secreted (ng day^{-1}) n=3			
	7	10	14	21
Vehicle	0	0	0	0
Dex	0	12.43±1.94	42.40±6.51	43.64±7.99
NSC-CM	0	10.40±3.35	0	0
AIM	0	14.50±10.36	28.77±8.70	27.04±2.58
Ost	0	6.61±3.70	5.60±2.00	12.92±3.29
Cig 30	0	15.16±3.44	0	0
Cig 3	0	0	0	0
Trog 100	0	0	0	0
Trog 10	0	0	0	0

Vehicle, dimethyl sulphoxide; Dex, dexamethasone; NSC-CM, murine neural stem cell conditioned medium; AIM, adipo-inductive medium; Ost, osteogenic medium; Cyg, cyglitazone at 3 and 30 μM; Troglitazone at 10 and 100 μM.

c.

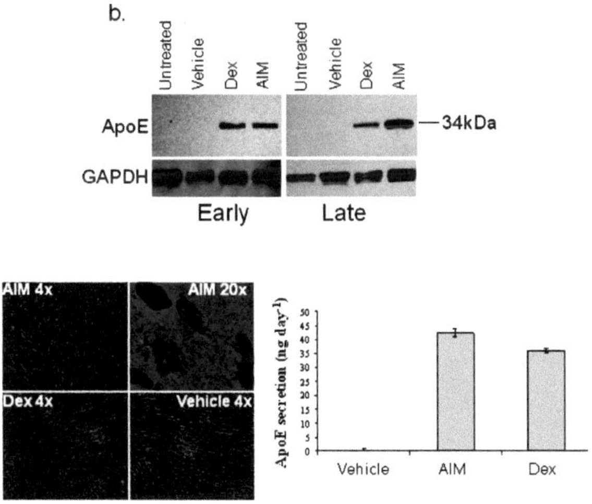

Figure 2. (a) Assays of ApoE production. Some conditions known to induce ApoE production in other cells and their effect upon MSCs. The NSC conditioned media AIM and osteogenic conditions are also included. Experiment was repeated with two donors and data from one of the donors is presented, n = 3, average ± standard deviation is shown. (b) Detection of ApoE in MSCs by western blotting. Western blot demonstrating ApoE (34 kD) production (upper) in early (passage 2, left column) and late (passage 8, right column) passage MSCs. Lanes were normalized to GAPDH expression (lower). Experiment was repeated five donors. (c) Dex-mediated expression of ApoE in MSCs is not accompanied by adipocyte differentiation. The ApoE expression by MSCs was induced by exposure to Dex or AIM. After 21 days, the monolayers were stained with oil red O to visualize lipid droplets (left). Lipid droplets were evident in AIM treated, but not Dex treated MSCs. However, ApoE expression was high in both cases when media was assayed by ELISA (right).

a.

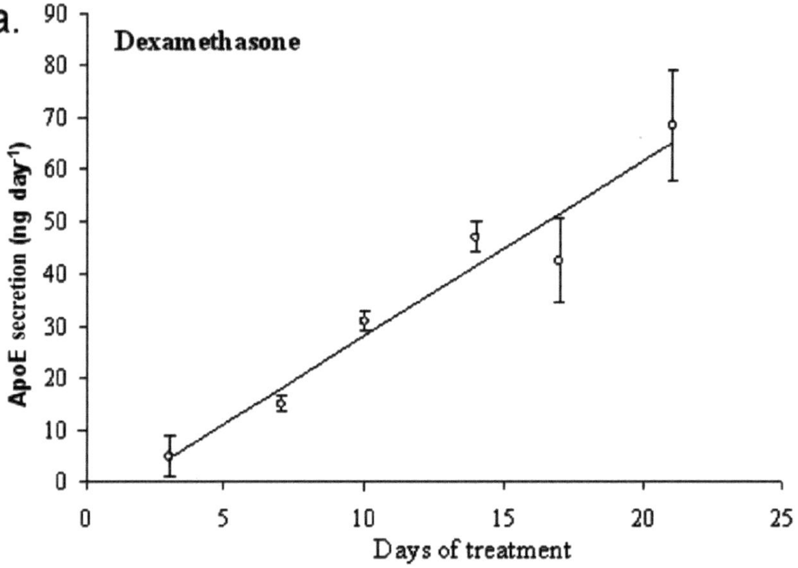

b.

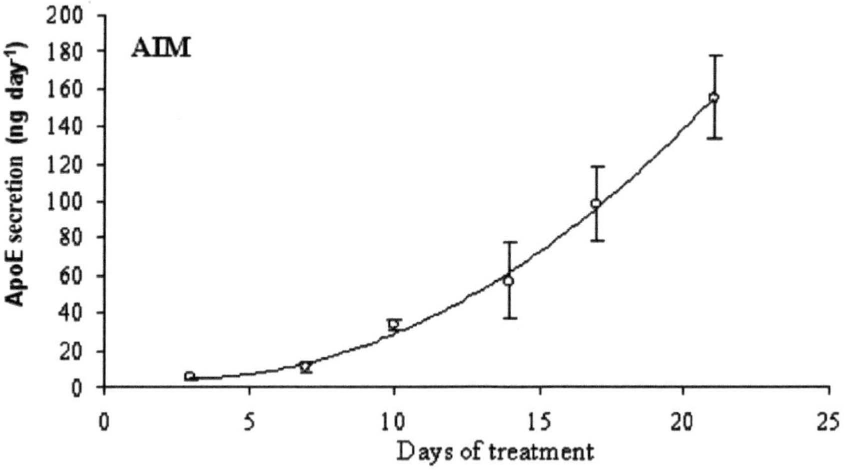

Figure 3. ApoE production kinetics. ApoE production during 21 days of treatment with 0.5 μM dexamethasone (panel a) or adipoinductive media (panel b). Experiment was repeated for eight donors, data from one donor is presented, n = 3, error bars are standard deviations.

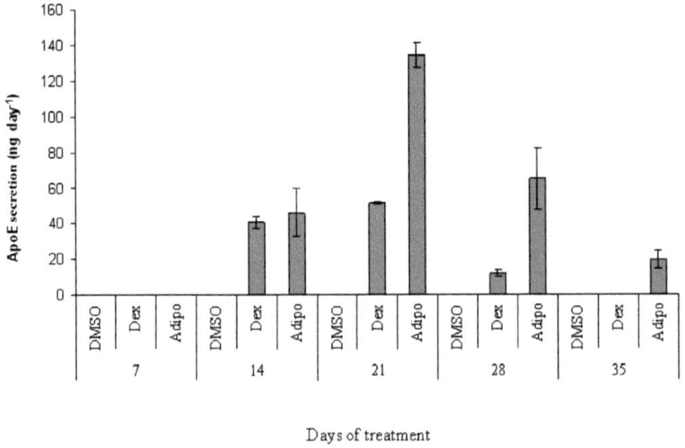

Figure 4. ApoE production following withdrawal of inductive media. The MSCs were treated with the inductive media (0.5 µM dexamethasone (Dex) or AIM (Adipo)) through for 21 days, then with CCM for a further 2 weeks. ApoE levels drop abruptly after day 21. Experiment was repeated three donors, data from one donor is presented, n = 3, error bars are standard deviations.

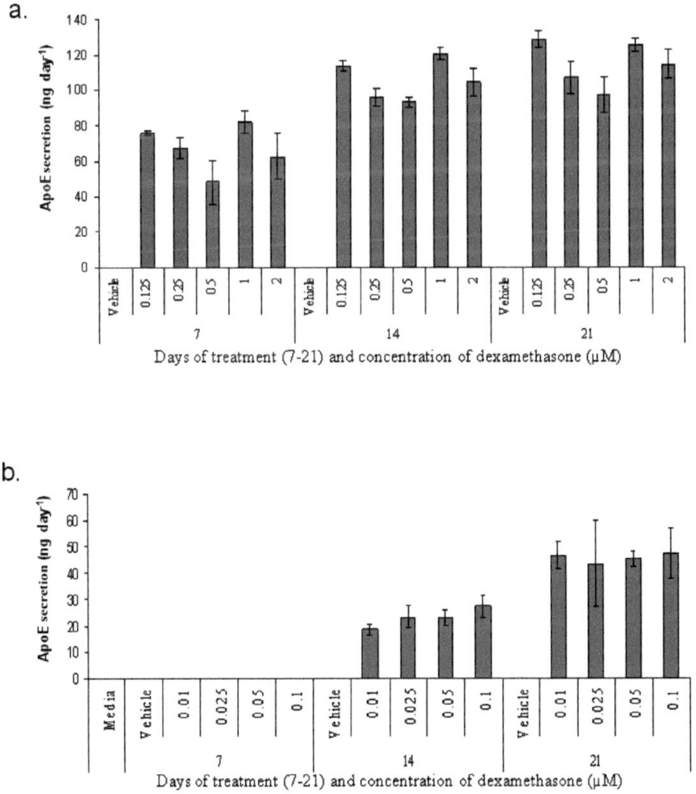

Figure 5. Dose responses. Dexamethasone dose response (high dose, panel a, and low dose, panel b). Experiments were repeated with two donors, data from one of the donors is presented, n = 3, error bars are standard deviations.

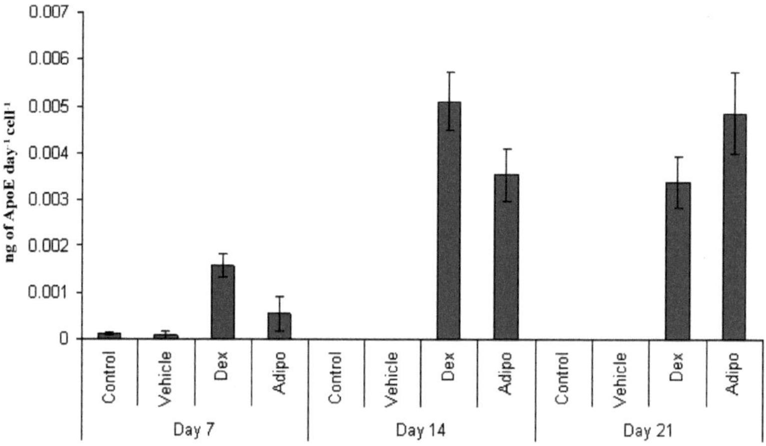

Figure 6. ApoE production per cell. Rate of ApoE production normalized to cell number. Cells were treated with inductive media (0.5 μM dexamethasone (Dex) or AIM (Adipo)) for 7–21 days. Experiment was performed on one donor, n = 3, error bars are standard deviations.

To confirm ELISA data, ApoE was also detected in protein extracts from MSCs treated with Dex, AIM, and control media, containing an appropriate level of vehicle DMSO, by western blotting. A single band (34 kDa) corresponding to ApoE was present only in the Dex and AIM treated MSCs (Figure 2b). The position of this band was later confirmed by comparison to immunoblotted recombinant human ApoE (data not shown). To confirm that Dex was solely responsible for the induction of ApoE secretion, we tested whether the two additional components of AIM induced ApoE expression. Isobutyl-methyl xanthine, a phosphodiesterase inhibitor, and indomethacin, a ligand of the adipogenesis master-regulator peroxisome proliferator-activated receptor, both failed to induce ApoE expression alone or in combination, nor did they induce terminal adipogenesis (data not shown). Furthermore, Dex did not appear to induce ApoE as a by-product of terminal adipogenesis, since lipid droplets could not be detected in long term treated cultures (Figure 2c). Thereafter, Dex and AIM were the selected conditions for subsequent experiments.

Kinetics and Maintenance of ApoE Production

To examine the kinetics, longevity, and donor-dependency of the inducible ApoE secretion, a series of time course experiments were performed with hMSCs from eight donors. In the first series of experiments, we examined the rate of response to Dex and AIM in terms of attaining maximal ApoE secretion. Confluent monolayers of hMSCs were established from passage 2 (approximately 15 doublings per cell) cultures. Cells were treated with Dex or AIM and for controls, the cells were treated with either vehicle (DMSO) or not at all. At 2–3 day intervals, media were recovered and ApoE levels were measured by ELISA (Figure 3). For all MSC preparations tested the control cultures did not secrete ApoE over the entire experimental period (data not shown). For the AIM and Dex conditions, maximal ApoE expression was attained after 21 days and was sustained for up to 35 days. After long term culture (about 35 days), the ApoE yield dropped due to apoptosis of the MSCs that frequently occurs after sustained culture at confluency. The ApoE yields were comparable between all of the MSC preparations at about 70–100 ng day-1 for the Dex (Figure 3a) and 100–140 ng day-1 for the AIM conditions (Figure 3b). There were no correlations between the rate of response to stimulus and donor age or sex. When stimulated by Dex only, there was a linear increase in the rate of ApoE secretion from hMSCs. However, there was an exponential increase in the rate of ApoE secretion when treated with AIM and this was accompanied by differentiation into adipocytes. Since adipocytes are a source of ApoE *in vivo*, this probably accounts for the higher overall ApoE output, and the accelerated rate of secretion.

The next study was designed to address the longevity of ApoE secretion after withdrawal of stimulus. Confluent passage two MSC cultures were incubated in Dex and AIM media for 21 days to attain maximal expression of ApoE. The cells were then cultured in the absence of stimulus for an additional 2 weeks (Figure 4). After 2 weeks, ApoE expression dropped to about 8% of the maximum for AIM treated cells and the Dex treated cells expressed barely detectable levels. This suggested that for sustained ApoE expression, induction is required at least weekly.

In consideration of the prospect of clinical application, we examined the dose dependency of ApoE induction on MSCs. Although AIM media was most effective in inducing ApoE secretion by MSCs, the compounds have not been safely co-administered *in vivo*. On the other hand, dexamethasone is a standard therapeutic and would be acceptable for administration to humans at low doses. We performed dose response curves ranging from 0.125 μM to 2 μM and 0.01 μM to 0.1 μM found that the dose of Dex could be reduced from 0.5 μM to 0.125 μM with insignificant reduction in ApoE secretion (Figure 5a). The lower dose response series demonstrated that approximately half maximal ApoE expression could be attained (Figure 5b).

ApoE Production and Cell Number

To provide insights on cell viability and proliferative potential during induction, we examined ApoE secretion on a per cell basis. The MSCs were allowed to reach 70% confluency before beginning treatment with AIM or Dex. Media and cells were collected at day 7, 14, and 21. At each time point, the amount of ApoE secreted per day was normalized to the number of cells in the monolayer. Overall cell recovery was slightly reduced when compared to the untreated controls suggesting that DMSO primarily affected MSC proliferation (data not shown). However, the presence of Dex and AIM did not affect long term viability, since the cultures slowly expanded over the 21 day experimental period. In the case of AIM, normalized ApoE levels reflected the unmodified measurements (Figure 3b) with a continuous increase in ApoE levels over time suggesting that as the cells divide in culture, they retain their ApoE secretion potential. In the case of the Dex conditions, normalized ApoE levels dropped slightly, suggesting expansion of some cells with limited or no potential for ApoE secretion (Figure 6).

We then tested the ability of the ApoE to bind to VLDLs. To reduce background, ApoE expression was induced for 2 days by Dex treatment in serum free media. The

MSC viability was not significantly affected during the brief exposure to serum free conditions and ApoE expression occurred at levels comparable to expression in serum containing media (Figure 7b). The conditioned media was then incubated with biotinylated VLDLs and then subjected to a series of biotin-mediated depletions using streptavidin coated microtiter plates (Figure 7a). Upon ELISA of the depleted media, ApoE levels were significantly reduced when compared to controls that were treated identically, but lacked VLDL (Figure 7b). This suggests that the MSC-derived ApoE meets at least one of its *in vivo* functions. The ApoE also binds to the LDL receptor and facilitates internalization by hepatocytes, macrophages and astrocytes. To examine the potential of MSC-derived ApoE to accelerate lipid uptake, we generated synthetic micelles containing fluorescently labeled cholesterol ester and free cholesterol. When such lipid micelles were added to serum free media conditioned by the ApoE (Figure 8a), it bound to them and could be enriched from the media by centrifugation (Figure 8b). When compared to untreated controls, the ApoE conditioned media catalyzed the formation of larger micelle aggregates, many of which could be identified by the naked eye (data not shown). Furthermore, ApoE conditioned media accelerated the uptake of the fluorescent lipid aggregates by huh-7 hepatocytes (Figure 8c).

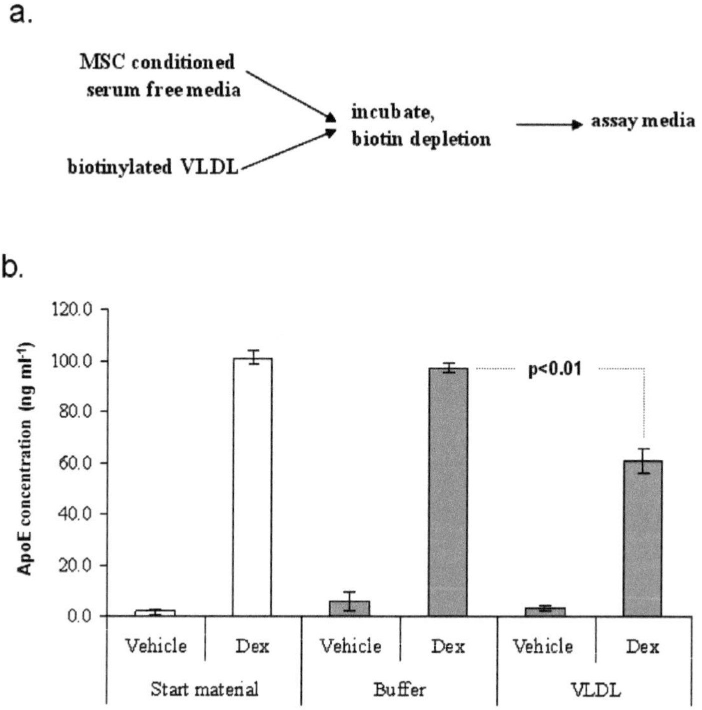

Figure 7. Binding of ApoE to VLDL. ApoE was secreted into serum free media by MSCs. The conditioned media was then added to biotinylated VLDLs (panel a). After biotin depletion, the remaining ApoE in the conditioned medium was measured by ELISA (panel b). When compared with buffer alone, biotinylated VLDLs depleted the ApoE from the conditioned medium. Data from one of two donors is presented, n = 3, error bars are standard deviations.

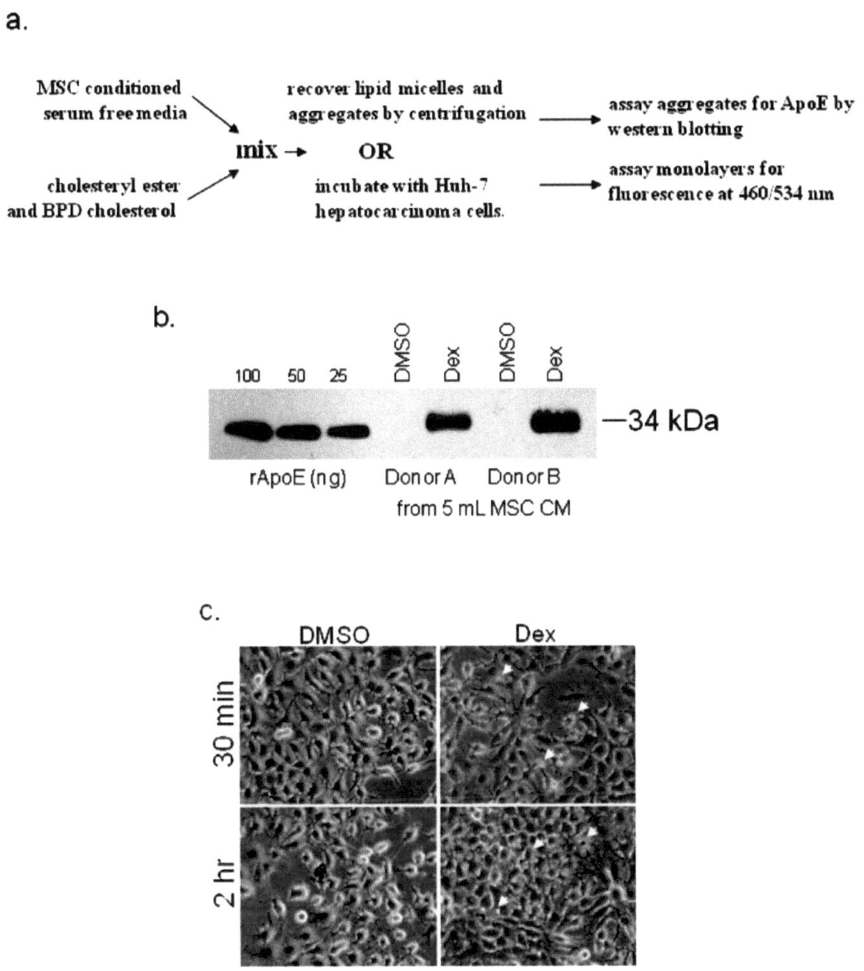

Figure 8. Binding of ApoE to synthetic micelles and uptake by hepatocyte cells. The ApoE was secreted into serum free media by MSCs. Fluorescent cholesterol-ester and cholesterol was then added to the media (panel a). Upon recovery of the micelles by centrifugation, ApoE could be detected when analyzed by western blotting (panel b). When ApoE conditioned media was mixed with lipids and incubated with huh-7 hepatocarcinoma cells, it accelerated uptake when compared with control media. Phase contrast/fluorescent merge indicating hepatocytes taking up fluorescent cholesterol (green) from the medium (panel c).

CONCLUSION

In this study we have shown that expression of potentially therapeutic levels of functional ApoE by hMSCs can be induced with dexamethasone. These data demonstrate that co-administration of hMSCs genotyped for homozygous expression of ApoE ε3 and chronic cortisol treatment may represent a novel therapy for severe instances of ApoE related diseases.

KEYWORDS

- **Adipo-inductive media**
- **Apolipoprotein E**
- **Complete culture medium**
- **Multipotent mesenchymal stromal cells**
- **Phosphate buffered saline**

AUTHORS' CONTRIBUTIONS

Suzanne Zeitouni conceptualized experimental strategy, carried out experiments, interpreted data, and co-wrote manuscript. Brian S. Ford carried out experiments and interpreted data. Sean M. Harris carried out experiments. Mandolin J. Whitney prepared some of the MSCs, carried out experiments. Carl A. Gregory conceptualized experimental strategy, interpreted data, and co-wrote manuscript. Darwin J. Prockop conceptualized experimental strategy, interpreted data, and co-wrote manuscript. All authors read and approved the final manuscript.

ACKNOWLEDGMENTS

We would like to thank Dina Gaupp, Center for Gene Therapy, Tulane Health Sciences Center for histology. We thank Dr. Jeffrey Spees, Department of Medicine, Cardiovascular Research Institute, University of Vermont for NSCs. We thank Srikanta Dash, Tulane Health Sciences Center for the Huh-7 cells. The work was supported in part by grants from the Amon Carter Foundation, the NIH (P40 RR17447) and the Louisiana Gene Therapy Research Consortium.

Chapter 17

Cationic Nanoparticles for Delivery of Amphotericin B

Dbora B. Vieira and Ana M. Carmona-Ribeiro

INTRODUCTION

Particulate systems are well known to be able to deliver drugs with high efficiency and fewer adverse side effects, possibly by endocytosis of the drug carriers. On the other hand, cationic compounds and assemblies exhibit a general antimicrobial action. In this work, cationic nanoparticles built from drug, cationic lipid and polyelectrolytes are shown to be excellent and active carriers of amphotericin B (AmB) against *Candida albicans*.

Assemblies of AmB and cationic lipid at extreme drug to lipid molar ratios were wrapped by polyelectrolytes forming cationic nanoparticles of high colloid stability and fungicidal activity against *Candida albicans*. Experimental strategy involved dynamic light scattering for particle sizing, zeta-potential analysis, colloid stability, determination of AmB aggregation state by optical spectra and determination of activity against *Candida albicans in vitro* from colony-forming unit (CFU) countings.

Novel and effective cationic particles delivered AmB to *C. albicans in vitro* with optimal efficiency seldom achieved from drug, cationic lipid, or cationic polyelectrolyte in separate. The multiple assembly of antibiotic, cationic lipid, and cationic polyelctrolyte, consecutively nanostructured in each particle produced a strategical and effective attack against the fungus cells.

In the recent years, much work has been devoted to characterize nanoparticles and their biological effects and applications. These include bottom–up and molecular self-assembly, biological effects of naked nanoparticles and nano-safety, drug encapsulation and nanotherapeutics, and novel nanoparticles for use in microscopy, imaging, and diagnostics (Soloviev, 2007). Particulate drug delivery systems such as polymeric microspheres (Liu et al., 2000). nanoparticles (de Verdiere et al., 1997; Moghimi and Hunter, 2000). liposomes (Booser et al., 2002; Romsicki and Sharom, 1997), and solid lipid nanoparticles (SLNs) (Wong et al., 2004), offer great promise to achieve the goal of improving drug accumulation inside cancer cells without causing side effects. Particulate systems are well known to be able to deliver drugs with higher efficiency with fewer adverse side effects (Booser et al., 2002; Lamprecht et al., 2005). A possible mechanism is increase of cellular drug uptake by endocytosis of the drug carriers (Lee et al., 1992; Nori et al., 2003; Soma et al., 1999). The emergence of the newer forms of SLN such as polymer-lipid hybrid nanoparticles, nanostructured lipid carriers, and long-circulating SLN may further expand the role of this versatile drug carrier aiming at chemotherapy with cancer drugs (Wong et al., 2007). Recently, new nanoparticulate delivery systems for AmB have been developed by means of the polyelectrolyte complexation technique (Tiyaboonchai and Limpeanchob, 2007; Tiyaboonchai et al., 2001). Two oppositely charged polymers were used to form nanoparticles through electrostatic interaction as usual for the layer-by-layer approach (LbL). This approach creates homogeneous ultrathin films on solid supports based on the electrostatic attraction between opposite charges (Lvov et al., 1993). Consecutively alternating adsorption of anionic and cationic polyelectrolytes or amphiphiles from their aqueous solution leads to the formation of multilayer assemblies (Decher and Hong, 1991).

On the other hand, some double-chained synthetic lipids such as dioctadecyldimethylammonium bromide (DODAB) or sodium dihexadecylphosphate (DHP) self-assemble in aqueous solution yielding closed bilayers (vesicles) or disrupted vesicles (bilayer fragments, BF, or disks) depending on the procedure used for dispersing the lipid (Carmona-Ribeiro, 2003). The DODAB, in particular, bears a quaternary ammonium moiety as cationic polar head, which imparts to this cationic lipid outstanding anti-infective properties (Carmona-Ribeiro et al., 2006). Both AmB and miconazole self-assemble and solubilize at hydrophobic sites of DODAB or DHP BFs in water solution exhibiting *in vivo* therapeutic activity (Lincopan et al., 2003, 2005; Pacheco and Carmona-Ribeiro, 2003; Vieira and Carmona-Ribeiro, 2001). Over the last decade, our group has been describing the anti-infective properties of cationic bilayers composed of the synthetic lipid DODAB (Campanha et al., 2011, 1999; Carmona-Ribeiro, 2003; Carmona-Ribeiro et al., 2006; Lincopan et al., 2003, 2005; Martins et al., 1997; Sicchierolli et al., 1995; Tapias et al., 1994). Adsorption of DODAB cationic bilayers onto bacterial cells changes the sign of the cell surface potential from negative to positive with a clear relationship between positive charge on bacterial cells and cell death (Campanha et al., 1999). Regarding the mechanism of DODAB action, neither bacterial cell lysis nor DODAB vesicle disruption takes place Martins et al., 1997). Recently, it was shown that the critical phenomenon determining antifungal effect of cationic surfactants and lipids is not cell lysis but rather the reversal of cell surface charge from negative to positive (Vieira and Carmona-Ribeiro, 2006). In this work, we combine the SLN and the LbL approaches to develop novel and effective cationic particles to deliver AmB to *C. albicans*. Cationic microbicides self-assemble in a single supramolecular structure. The first attack against the fungus comes from an outer cationic polyelectrolyte layer. Thereafter the inert carboxymethylcellulose (CMC) layer is unwrapped so that monomeric AmB solubilized at the edges of DODAB BFs and the BF themselves can contact the fungus cell. Maybe this design represents a very effective cocktail against multidrug resistance. Complete loss of fungus viability could not be achieved before at the same separate doses of each component.

MATERIALS AND METHODS

Drug, Lipid, Polyelectrolytes, and Microorganism

The DODAB, 99.9% pure was obtained from Sigma Co. (St. Louis, MO, USA). Carboxymethyl cellulose sodium salt (CMC) with a nominal mean degree of substitution (DS) of 0.60–0.95, poly(diallyldimethylammonium chloride) (PDDA) with Mv 100,000–200,000 and polylysines (PL) were obtained from Sigma (Steinheim, Germany) and used without further purification. The AmB (batch 008000336) was purchased from Bristol-Myers Squibb (Brazil) and was initially prepared as a 1 g/l stock solution in DMSO/methanol 1:1. *Candida albicans* ATCC 90028 was purchased from American Type Culture Collection (ATCC) and reactivated in Sabouraud liquid broth 4% before plating for incubation at 37°C/24 hr. In order to prepare fungal cell suspension for antifungal activity assays, three to four colonies were picked from the plate and washed twice either in isotonic glucose phosphate buffer (IGP; 1 mM potassium phosphate buffer, pH 7.0, supplemented with 287 mM glucose as an osmoprotectant) (Helmerhorst et al., 1999; Wei and Bobek, 2004) or in Milli-Q water by centrifugation (3000 rpm/10 min), pelleting, and resuspension. The final fungal cell suspension was prepared by adjusting the inoculum to 2×10^7 cfu/ml and then diluting by a factor of 1:10 either in IGP or in Milli-Q water yielding 2×10^6 cfu/ml.

Preparation of Lipid Dispersion and Analytical Determination of Lipid Concentration

The DODAB was dispersed in water or IGP buffer, using a titanium macrotip probe (Carmona-Ribeiro, 1992). The macrotip probe was powered by ultrasound at a nominal output of 90 W (10 min, 70°C) to disperse 32 mg of DODAB powder in 25 ml water solution. The dispersion was centrifuged (60 min, 10,000 g, 4°C) in order to eliminate residual titanium ejected from the macrotip. This procedure dispersed the amphiphile powder in aqueous solution using a high-energy input, which not only produced bilayer vesicles but also disrupted these vesicles, thereby generating open BF (Carmona-Ribeiro, 1992; Carmona-Ribeiro and Chaimovich, 1983). Analytical concentration of DODAB was determined by halide microtitration (Schales and Schales, 1941). and adjusted to 2 mM.

Determination of Zeta-Average Diameter and Zeta-Potential for Dispersions

Stock solutions of AmB were prepared at 1 mg/ml in 1:1 DMSO/methanol. Stock solutions of PDDA, CMC, and PL were prepared at 20 mg/ml and diluted in the final dispersion to yield the desired final concentration. The stock solution of AmB (1 mg/ml) was added to DODAB BF dispersions to yield low and high drug to lipid molar proportions (P). At low P, dispersions contained final concentrations of drug, DODAB, CMC and PDDA equal to 0.005 mM (5 micrograms/ml), 1 mM (631 micrograms/ml), 0.01–2.00 mg/ml and 0.01–10.00 mg/ml, respectively. Firstly, DODAB BF and drug were allowed to interact for 10 min. Thereafter, CMC was added and allowed to interact for 20 min before adding PDDA, which was also allowed to interact for 20 min, before determining zeta-average diameter and zeta-potentials. At high P, a similar procedure was done this time at final concentrations of drug, DODAB, CMC, and PDDA equal to 0.050 mM (50 micrograms/ml), 0.1 mM (63.1 micrograms/ml), 0.01–2.00 mg/ml, and 0.01–10.00 mg/ml, respectively. At high P, drug particles were obtained at 0.050 mM AmB in IGP buffer yielding particles with 75 nm zeta-average diameter and –27 mV zeta-potential (Lincopan and Carmona-Ribeiro, 2006). These drug particles were firstly covered by DODAB BF and then wrapped by the polyelectrolytes over the quoted range of concentrations. Sizes and zeta-potentials were determined by means of a ZetaPlus Zeta-Potential Analyser (Brookhaven Instruments Corporation, Holtsville,

NY, USA) equipped with a 570 nm laser and dynamic light scattering at 90° for particle sizing (Grabowski and Morrison, 1983). The zeta-average diameters referred to in this work from now on should be understood as the mean hydrodynamic diameters D_z. Zeta-potentials (ζ) were determined from the electrophoretic mobility μ and Smoluchowski's equation, $\zeta = \mu\eta/\varepsilon$, where η and ε are medium viscosity and dielectric constant, respectively. All D_z and ζ were obtained at 25°C, 1 hr after mixing.

Optical Spectra and Aggregation State of AmB in the Formulations

The UV-visible optical spectra (280–450 nm) for characterization of AmB aggregation state were obtained in the double-beam mode by means of a Hitachi U-2000 Spectrophotometer against a blank of DODAB BF or DODAB BF/CMC (without drug), to separate light scattered by the dispersions from light absorption by the drug. All spectra were obtained at room temperature (25°C) at about 20 min after mixing DODAB BF and AmB at low or high drug to lipid P or after adding CMC to DODAB BF/drug assemblies.

Determination of Cell Viability for *C. albicans* ATCC 90028 as a Function of Polyelectrolytes Concentration at Low and High Drug to Lipid Molar Proportion (P)

At low or high P, DODAB/drug assemblies were wrapped by two layers of oppositely charged polyelectrolytes so that CFU were counted as a function of CMC and/or PDDA concentrations at 1 hr of interaction time between *C. albicans* (1×10^6 cfu/ml) and formulations. Plating on agar plates for CFU counts was performed by taking 0.1 ml of a 1,000-fold dilution in Milli-Q water of the mixtures. After spreading, plates were incubated for 2 days at 37°C. The CFU counts were made using a colony counter. At low P, final DMSO/methanol concentration is 0.5% whereas at high P it is 5%. No effect of the solvent mixture at 0.5% on cells viability was previously detected (Campanha et al., 2011). For further studies *in vivo* and at high P, it will be advisable to perform a dialysis step for the cationic nanoparticles aiming at complete elimination of the toxic solvent mixture.

DISCUSSION AND RESULTS

Colloid Stability and Antifungal Activity of Cationic Bilayer Fragments/Amphotericin B/Carboxymethyl Cellulose/Poly(Diallyldimethylammonium) Chloride at Low Drug-to-lipid Molar Proportion

Chemical structures of AmB, CMC, PDDA, and the cationic lipid DODAB are on Table 1. DODAB self-assembly in water dispersion yields BF by ultrasonic input with a macrotip probe.

The existence of BFs from synthetic lipids such as DHP, or DODAB or chloride obtained by sonication with tip has been supported by the following evidences: (i) osmotic non-responsiveness of the dispersion indicative of absence of inner vesicle compartment (Carmona-Ribeiro and Chaimovich, 1983). (ii) the TEM micrographs with electronic staining (Carmona-Ribeiro et al., 1991). (iii) cryo-TEM micrographs (Hammarstroem et al., 1995). (iv) fluid and solid state coexistence and complex formation with oppositely charged surfactant (Cocquyt et al., 2004). (v) solubilization of hydrophobic drugs at the borders of DODAB BFs, which does not occur for DODAB closed bilayer vesicles (Carmona-Ribeiro, 2006; Lincopan et al., 2003; Pacheco and Carmona-Ribeiro, 2003; Vieira and Carmona-Ribeiro, 2001; Vieira et al., 2006). They differ from the closed vesicles by providing hydrophobic borders at their edges that are absent in closed bilayer systems such as vesicles or liposomes. Under conditions of low ionic strength, due to electrostatic repulsion, the charged BFs remain colloidally stable in aqueous dispersions (Carmona-Ribeiro, 2006; Lincopan et al., 2003; Pacheco and Carmona-Ribeiro, 2003; Vieira and Carmona-Ribeiro, 2001; Vieira et al., 2006).

Table 1. Sizing and zeta-potential of drug, cationic lipid and anionic polyelectrolyte in separate or as assemblies.

Dispersion	[DODAB] (mM)	[AmB] (mM)	[CMC] (mg/mL)	$D \pm \delta$ (nm)	$\zeta \pm \delta$ (mV)
AmB in water	---	0.005	---	433 ± 5	-26 ± 3
DODAB BF	1	---	---	79 ± 2	41 ± 2
DODAB BF/AmB	1	0.005	---	79 ± 1	42 ± 2
DODAB BF/AnB/CMC	1	0.005	0.01	88 ± 1	40 ± 1
	1	0.005	0.1	145 ± 1	32 ± 2
	1	0.005	1	90 ± 2	-50 ± 2
AmB in water	---	0.050	---	360 ± 4	-26 ± 3
AmB in IGP	---	0.050	---	75 ± 2	-27 ± 1
DODAB BF in IGP	0.1	---	---	75 ± 1	40 ± 1
AmB/DODAB BF	0.1	0.050	---	195 ± 3	9 ± 1
AmB/DODAB BF/CMC	0.1	0.050	0.001	199 ± 1	16 ± 1
	0.1	0.050	0.01	1280 ± 80	4 ± 1
	0.1	0.050	0.1	230 ± 2	-34 ± 1

In fact, DODAB BF have been used to solubilize AmB (Vieira and Carmona-Ribeiro, 2001) at room temperature as schematically shown in Figure 1. This solubilization takes place at low drug-to-lipid molar proportions (low P) and presents certain limitations: (1) hydrophobic edges of BFs have a limited capacity of solubilizing the hydrophobic drug; (2) the bilayer core in the rigid gel state is too rigid to allow solubilization of AmB at room temperature being a poor solubilizer for this difficult, hydrophobic drug (Lincopan and Carmona-Ribeiro, 2006; Pacheco and Carmona-Ribeiro, 2003; Vieira and Carmona-Ribeiro, 2001; Vieira et al., 2006). On the other hand, at high P, AmB aggregates in water solution can be considered as drug particles. These can be surrounded by a thin cationic DODAB bilayer as previously described (Lincopan and Carmona-Ribeiro, 2006). (Figure 1).

Chemical structure or assemblies	Name and abbreviation
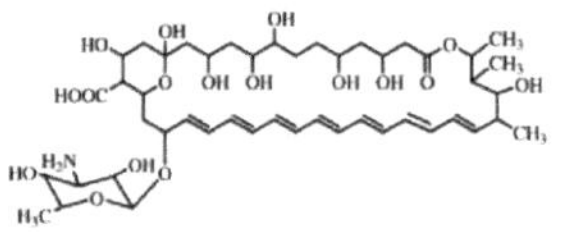	Amphotericin B (AmB)
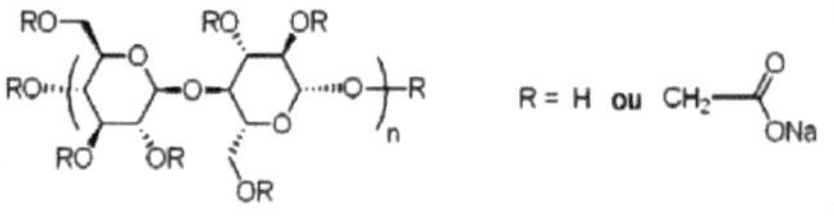	Carboxymethyl cellulose (CMC)
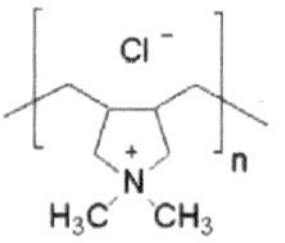	Poly(diallyldimethylammonium chloride) (PDDA)
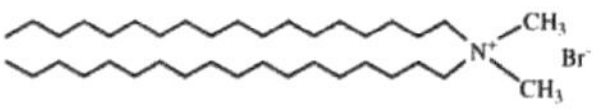	Dioctadecyldimethylammonium bromide (DODAB)
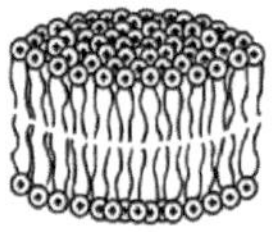	Cationic DODAB bilayer fragments (BF)
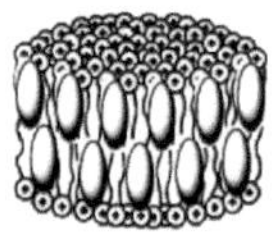	At low drug to lipid molar proportion (P), solubilization of drug molecules at the rim of DODAB BF.
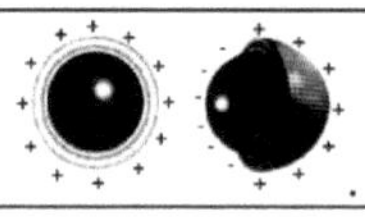	At high P, bilayer-covered drug particle

Figure 1. Chemical structure or schematic assemblies of compounds used to formulate amphotericin B. Each molecule of amphotericin B that was solubilized at the edges of DODAB bilayer fragments was represented by an ellipsoid whereas aggregated drug forming a particle was represented by solid spheres.

The physical properties of different dispersions such as size and zeta-potential are given in Table 1 both at low and high P. The drug in water exhibits substancial aggregation (Dz = 360–433 nm), as expected from its hydrophobic character. The drug particle presents a negative zeta-potential of –26 mV explained by dissociation of its carboxylate moiety at the pH of water (Lincopan and Carmona-Ribeiro, 2006). Upon changing the medium to IGP buffer, as previously reported, a decrease in size for AmB aggregates was observed (Dz = 75 nm) (Table 1), due to the chaotropic (dispersing) effect of dihydrogenphosphate anion on AmB aggregates (Lincopan and Carmona-Ribeiro, 2006). Both types of AmB aggregates interacted with DODAB BF yielding either loaded BF fragments at low P or DODAB covered drug particles at high P. The characteristics of these cationic assemblies before and after their interaction with oppositely charged CMC over a range of concentrations (0.001–1.0 mg/ml) are in Table 1. At low P, charge reversal took place above 1 mg/ml CMC whereas at high P, it occurred above 0.1 mg/ml CMC (Table 1).

At low P, the effect of CMC concentration on DODAB BF/CMC (unloaded control) or DODAB BF/AmB/CMC properties is in Figure 2. At low P and 1 mg/ml CMC, DODAB BF/AmB/CMC anionic complexes present 90 nm mean diameter and –50 mV of zeta-potential. The low size and large surface potential mean high colloid stability, so that this was the condition chosen for coverage with cationic polyelectrolytes. In the presence of CMC, there are two regions of colloid stability for cationic or anionic assemblies characterized by small sizes: regions I and III, and one region of instability: region II, characterized by aggregation and large sizes (Figure 1). Charged particles covered by oppositely charged polyelectrolytes exhibited similar profiles for the colloid stability as a function of polyelectrolyte concentration (Araújo et al., 2005; Correia et al., 2004).

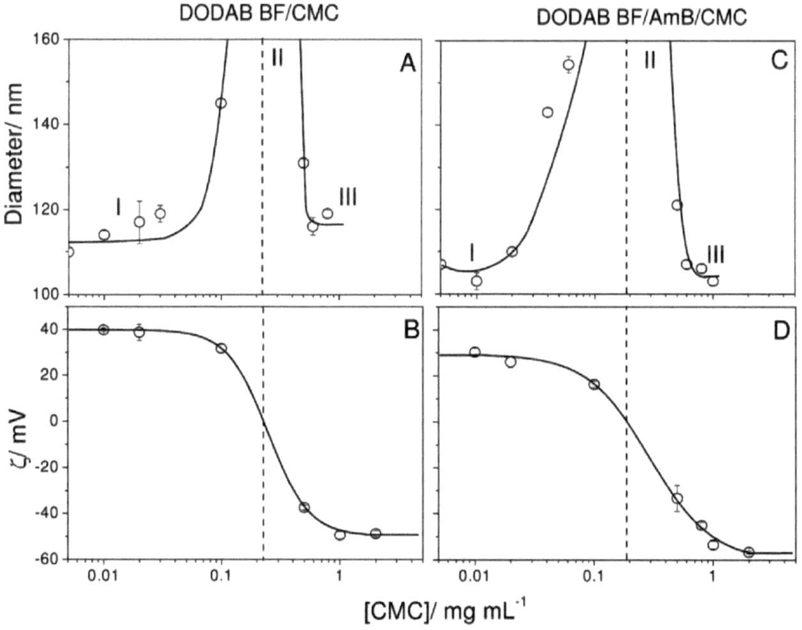

Figure 2. Amphotericin B solubilized in cationic bilayer fragments adsorbs a layer of carboxymethyl cellulose. Effect of CMC concentration on zeta-average diameter (A, C) and zeta-potential (B, D) of unloaded DODAB BF (A, B) or DODAB BF/AmB (C, D) at low drug-to-lipid molar proportion. Final DODAB and/or AmB concentrations are 1 and 0.005 mM, respectively. The three different moieties of the curves were named I, II, and III corresponding to positive, zero, and negative zeta-potentials, respectively.

The aggregation state of AmB at low P was evaluated from optical spectra (Figure 3). The drug in DMSO:methanol 1:1 yields a spectrum of completely solubilized, non-aggregated drug since this organic solvent mixture is the one of choice for AmB solubilization (Figure 3A). The drug in water exhibits the typical spectrum of aggregated AmB (Figure 3B). As depicted from AmB spectrum in DODAB BF (Figure 3C) or DODAB BF/AmB/CMC (Figure 3D), the drug is found in its monomeric state and completely solubilized. In fact, solubilization of AmB in DODAB BF, at low P, was previously described (Vieira and Carmona-Ribeiro, 2001). This formulation employing DODAB BF at low P was very effective *in vivo* (Lincopan et al., 2003) and exhibited low nephrotoxicity (Lincopan et al., 2005).

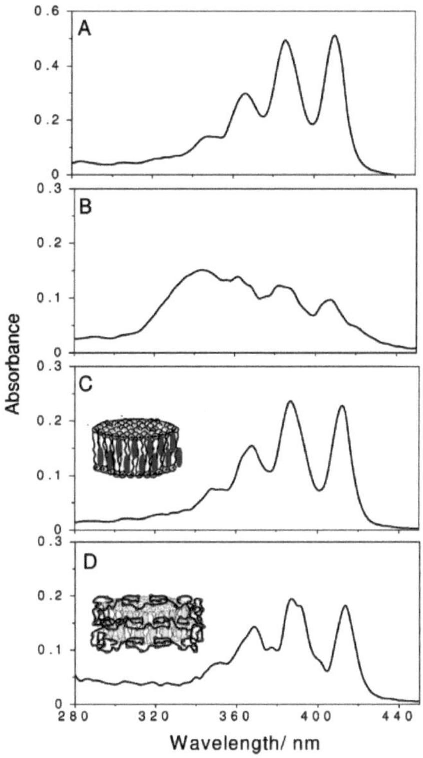

Figure 3. Adsorption of carboxy methylcellulose onto amphotericin B-cationic lipid assemblies preserves monomeric state of the drug at the edges of cationic bilayer fragments. Optical spectra of AmB in: 1:1 DMSO: methanol (best organic solvent mixture) (A); water (B); DODAB BF (C); or DODAB BF/AmB/CMC complexes (D). Final DODAB, AmB and/or CMC concentration are 1 mM, 0.005 mM and 1 mg.ml^{-1}, respectively.

At low P, the effect of (PDDA) on sizes and zeta-potentials of DODAB BF/AmB/CMC assemblies at 1 mM DODAB, 0.005 mM AmB, and 1 mg/ml CMC is on Figure 4. The region of PDDA concentrations for size minimization and high colloid stability was very narrow and around 1 mg/ml PDDA. Below and above this concentration, about 300 nm and negative zeta-potentials, or 500–700 nm of zeta-average diameter and positive zeta-potentials were obtained, respectively (Figure 4). Size minimization at Dz = 171 nm and zeta-potential = 24 mV for the DODAB BF/AmB/CMC/PDDA assembly was not related to optimal fungicidal activity as depicted from the 79% of *C. albicans* viability (Table 2). Possibly, the total positive charge on the assembly was not sufficient to substantially reduce fungus viability. For final coverage with PL of increasing molecular weight at 1 mg/ml PL, there was an increase in the final zeta-potential modulus and a larger loss of viability (Table 2). The DODAB BF/AmB/CMC/PDDA formulation at low P was 100% effective against the fungus only at 5 mg/ml PDDA (Figure 5D).

Table 2. Sizing, zeta-potential and antifungal activity of drug, cationic lipid, and polyelectrolyte(s) assemblies.

Cationic Lipid, Drug and Polyelectrolyte Assemblies	[DODAB] (mM)	[AmB] (mM)	[CMC] (mg/mL)
DODAB BF (0.6)/AmB (0.005)/CMC (1)/PDDA(1)	171 ± 1	24 ± 2	79 ± 5
DODAB BF (0.6)/AmB (0.005)/CMC (I)/$PL_{5000-10000}$(I)	92 ± 4	40 ± 1	71 ± 4
DODAB BF (0.6)/AmB (0.005)/CMC (I)/$PL_{30000-70000}$ (1)	138 ± 5	50 ± 3	21 ± 9
DODAB BF (0.6)/AmB (0.005)/CMC (I)/$PL_{70000-150000}$ (1)	148 ± 5	60 ± 3	13 ± 5
AmB (0.05)/DODAB BF (0.06)/CMC (0.1)/PDDA (1)	280 ± 2	35 ± 1	27 ± 2
AmB (0.05)/DODAB BF (0.06)/CMC (0.1)/$PL_{5000-10000}$ (1)	238 ± 1	25 ± 7	37 ± 1
AmB (0.05)/DODAB BF (0.06)/CMC (0.1)/$PL_{30000-70000}$ (1)	326 ± 5	36 ± 3	23 ± 6
AmB (0.05)/DODAB BF (0.06)/CMC (0.1)/$PL_{70000-150000}$ (1)	417 ± 3	47 ± 5	11 ± 3

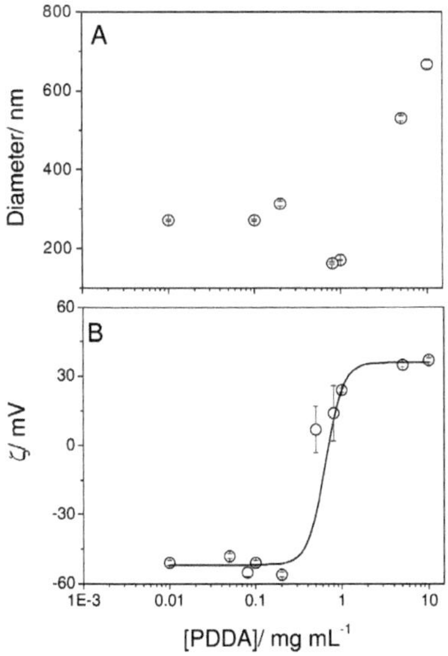

Figure 4. Adsorption of poly(diallyldimethylammonium) chloride onto carboxy methyl cellulose layer of amphotericin B- cationic bilayer fragment. Effect of PDDA concentration on z-average diameter (A) and zeta-potential (B) for DODAB BF/AmB/CMC/PDDA assemblies. Final DODAB, AmB and CMC concentrations were 1 mM, 0.005 mM and 1 mg.ml^{-1}, respectively. Interaction time between DODAB BF/AmB and CMC is 20 min. Thereafter, the interaction between DODAB BF/AmB/CMC and PDDA lasted 30 min.

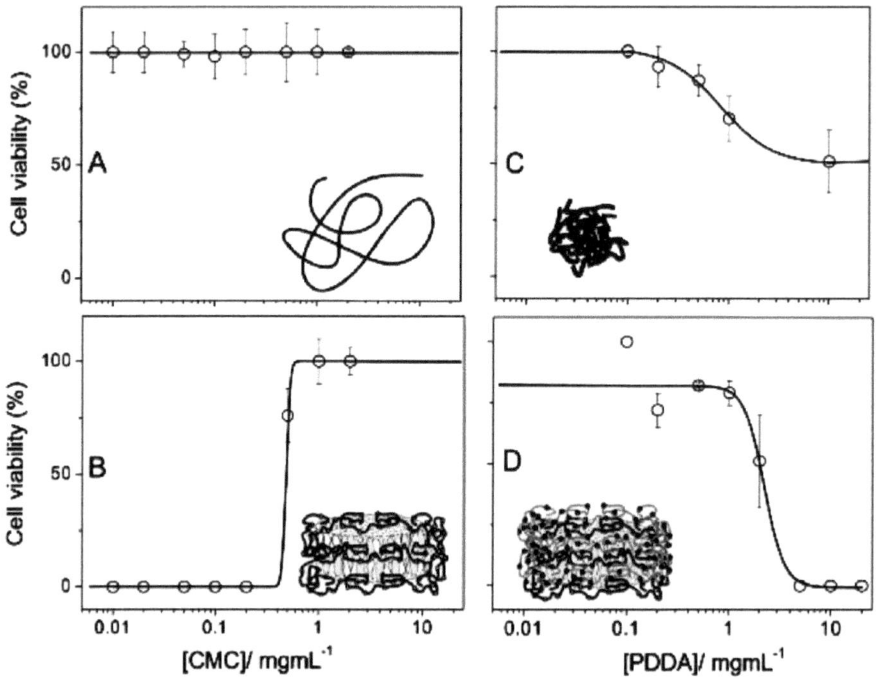

Figure 5. Fungicidal activity of different assemblies at low P against fungus. Cell viability (%) of *Candida albicans* (1 x 10^6 cfu/ml) as a function of polyelectrolytes concentration. Cells and CMC (A); DODAB/AmB/CMC (B); CMC/PDDA (C); and DODAB/AmB/CMC/PDDA (D) interacted for 1 hr before dilution and plating on agar of 0.1 ml of the diluted mixture (1:1,000 dilution).

The importance of large positive zeta-potentials for high efficiency of drug assemblies with DODAB BF and polyelectrolytes can be clearly seen from Figure 5. Negatively charged assemblies like those in Figures 5A, B yielded 100% of cell viability. Positively charged assemblies obtained upon increasing (PDDA) reduced cell viability to 50% (CMC/PDDA) (Figure 5C) or to 0% (DODAB BF/AmB/CMC/PDDA above 5 mg/ml PDDA) (Figure 5D). The schematic drawing in Figure 5D illustrates the layered assembly of microbicides in a single supramolecular assembly. The first attack comes from the outer cationic polyelectrolyte layer. Upon unwrapping this first layer and the second inert CMC layer, monomeric AmB contacts the fungus cell followed by the also effective DODAB action. Maybe this design represents a very effective assembly against multidrug resistance. Complete loss of fungus viability can seldom be achieved at the same separate doses of each component (Campanha et al., 2011).

Colloid Stability and Antifungal Activity of AmB/DODAB BF/CMC/PDDA at High P

The complexation between DODAB BF and CMC was previously studied in detail by our group (Correia et al., 2004). DODAB BF at 0.1 mM DODAB and CMC (0.001–2 mg/ml) are, in fact, electrostatically driven to complexation from the electrostatic attraction (Figures 6A, B).

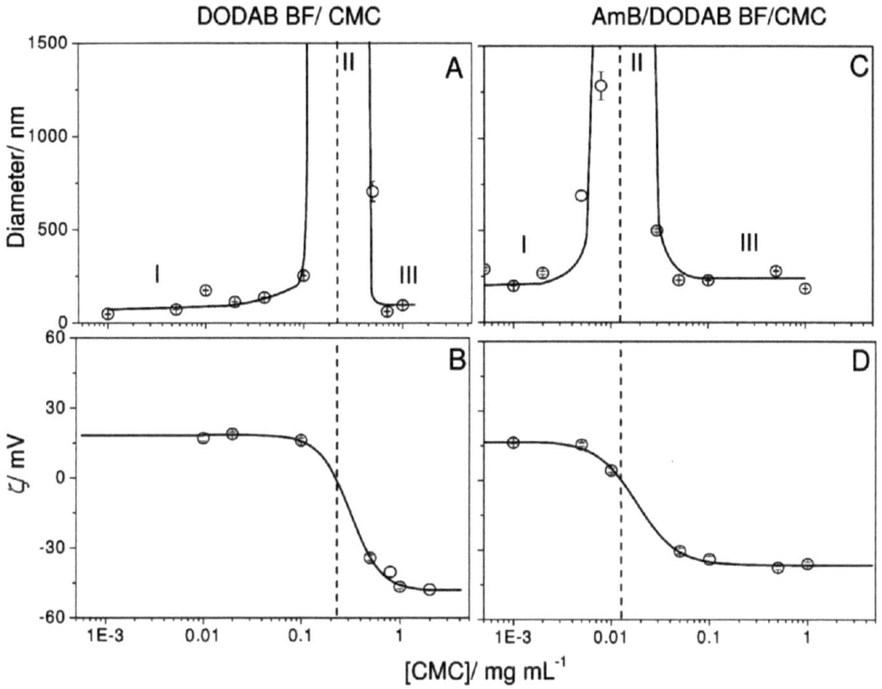

Figure 6. Amphotericin B aggregates covered by a layer of cationic lipid adsorb a layer of carboxymethyl cellulose. Effect of CMC concentration on zeta-average diameter (A, C) and zeta-potential (B, D) of DODAB BF (A, B) or AmB/DODAB BF (C, D) at high P. Final DODAB and/or AmB concentrations were 0.1 and 0.05 mM, respectively. The three different moieties of the curves were named I, II, and III corresponding to positive, zero and negative zeta-potentials, respectively. Interactions DODAB BF/CMC or AmB/DODAB BF/CMC took place over 20 min before measurements. One should notice that, at high P, (DODAB) concentration is 20 times smaller than at low P (Figure 1) surrounding drug aggregates as a thin layer of cationic lipid (Carmona-Ribeiro, 2006).

At high P, 0.1 mM DODAB BF is sufficient to cover all AmB particles present in dispersion at 0.05 mM AmB with a thin, possibly bilayered, 6–8 nm DODAB cationic shell as previously described (Lincopan and Carmona-Ribeiro, 2006). This cationic interface is expected to interact with the oppositely charged CMC polyelectrolyte. At 0.1 mg/ml CMC, AmB/DODAB BF/CMC anionic complexes present high colloid stability, 230 nm mean diameter and –34 mV of zeta-potential (Figures 6C, D). This condition was chosen for further coverage with cationic polylectrolytes.

Regarding the aggregation state of AmB, as expected, at 0.05 mM AmB, the majority of drug molecules were found in the aggregated state. Spectra in IGP buffer (Figure 7A), after drug particle coverage with 0.1 mM DODAB BF (Figure 7B) or with 0.1 mM DODAB BF plus 0.1 mg/ml CMC (Figure 7C) revealed the typical profile of aggregated drug. The spectrum in Figure 7C indicates a certain amount of monomeric drug not present in the other spectra (Figures 7A, B). Possibly, CMC sterically stabilized DODAB BF preserving hydrophobic sites of DODAB BF to be occupied by the monomeric drug. In absence of CMC, DODAB BF might fuse diminishing drug solubilization at their rim.

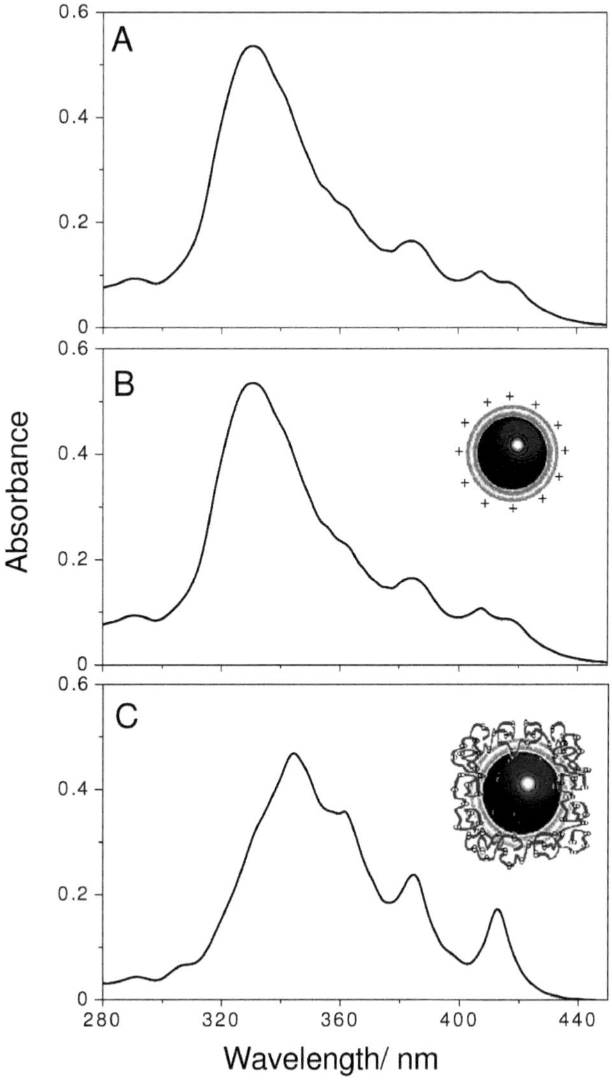

Figure 7. Amphotericin B is found as in the aggregated state (drug particles) covered by a thin layer of cationic lipid further surrounded by a layer of carboxymethyl cellulose at high P. Optical spectra of AmB in isotonic glucose buffer (A); AmB/DODAB BF (B); or AmB/DODAB/CMC complexes (C). Final DODAB, AmB and/or CMC concentration were 0.1 mM, 0.05 mM e 0.1 $mg.ml^{-1}$, respectively. These conditions yield complexes at high P.

At the chosen condition for the AmB/DODAB BF/CMC assembly, the effect of increasing (PDDA) was an initial colloid stabilization (decrease in size) around 1 mg/ml PDDA followed by further destabilization (increase in size) above this concentration (Figure 8A), possibly due to bridging flocculation (Vieira et al., 2003). Zeta-potential displayed the usual sigmoidal dependence on (PDDA) (Figure 8B).

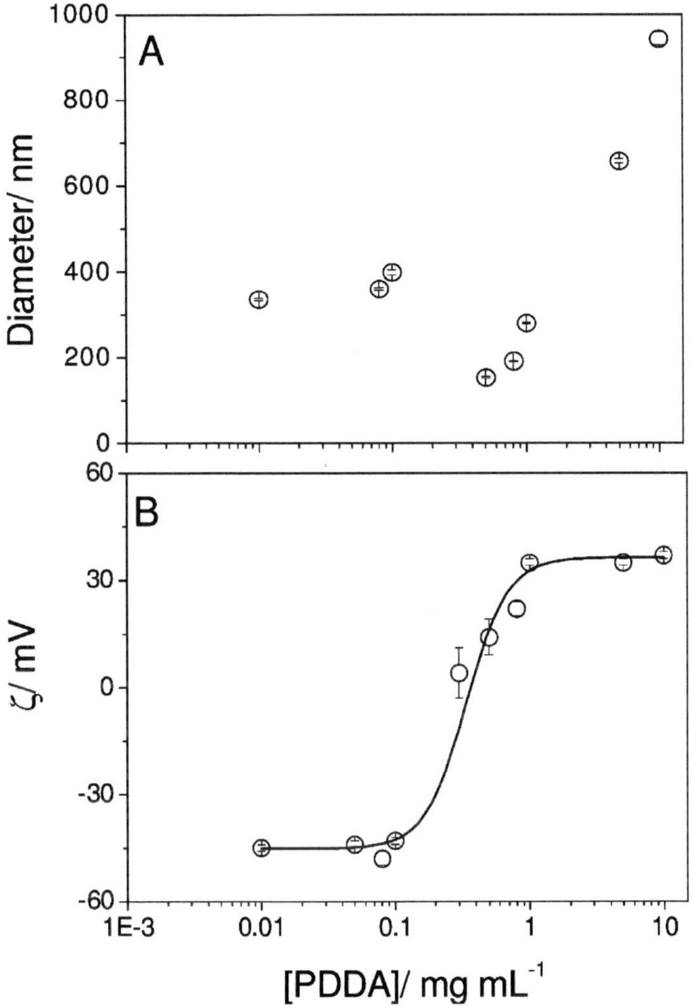

Figure 8. Amphotericin B particles covered by a thin layer of cationic lipid, at high P, and surrounded by a layer of carboxymethyl cellulose further adsorb a layer of cationic polyelectrolyte. Effect of PDDA concentration on zeta-average diameter (A) and zeta-potential (B) for AmB/DODAB BF/CMC/PDDA complexes. Final DODAB, AmB and CMC concentrations were 0.1 mM, 0.05 mM, and 0.1 $g.l^{-1}$, respectively. Interactions DODAB BF/AmB and CMC took place over 20 min and AmB/DODAB BF/CMC and PDDA, over 30 min.

The importance of positively charged assemblies at high P for fungicidal activity is emphasized in Figure 9. *Candida albicans* remains 100% viable in the presence of negatively charged CMC only (Figure 9A), 70% viable in the presence of negatively charged AmB/DODAB BF/CMC at high P (Figure 9B), 50–60% viable in the presence of CMC/PDDA at (PDDA) > 1 mg/ml and 0% viable in the presence of AmB/DODAB BF/CMC/PDDA at PDDA ≥ 2 mg/ml (Figure 9D).

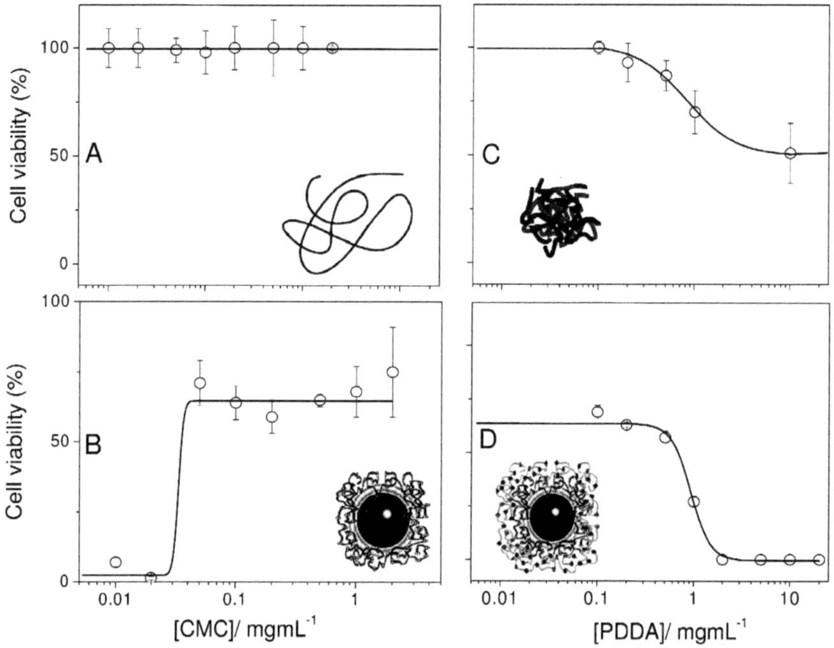

Figure 9. Fungicidal activity of different assemblies at high P against fungus. Cell viability (%) of *Candida albicans* (1 x 10^6 cfu/ml) as a function of CMC (A, B) or PDDA (C, D) concentration in the presence of different assemblies: CMC only (A); AmB/DODAB/CMC (B); CMC/PDDA (C); and AmB/DODAB/CMC/PDDA (D). The assemblies interacted with cells for 1 hr before dilution (1:1000) and plating on agar of 0.1 ml of the diluted mixture.

Alternatively, PDDA was replaced by PL (Table 2). At high P, the effect of increasing PL molecular weight was an increase in size, an increase in zeta-potential and a decrease of % of cell viability (Table 2). Table 1 summarized the different properties of assemblies at low and high P. One should notice that coverage of a drug particle with a thin DODAB layer led to a positive zeta-potential of only 9 mV. The CMC was slightly attracted to the covered particle producing a looser assembly than the one obtained with CMC coverage of DODAB BF, where electrostatic attraction is due to a higher zeta-potential on the BFs, typically 41 mV. The particles are loosely or tightly packed depending on the electrostatic attraction between oppositely charged components (cationic layer and CMC) depicted from zeta-potentials. This certainly made a large difference for occasion of drug delivery to the fungus cell. Having a loose or a more tightly packed assembly originated considerable differences in the profile of cell viability as a function of zeta-potential (Figure 10). For the less tightly packed drug particles at high P, drug delivery was more efficient leading to drug release and cell death at lower zeta-potentials (Figure 10). The reason for this high efficiency at low zeta-potential is associated both with the high P, meaning high drug dose, and with the loosely packed nanoparticle assembly.

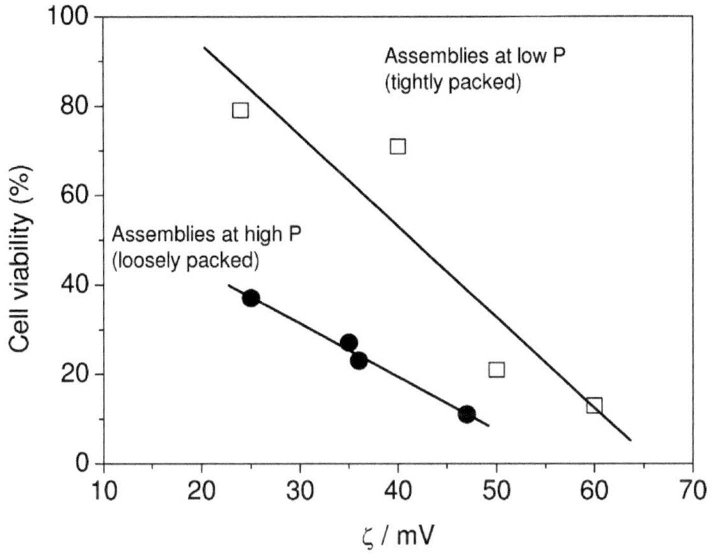

Figure 10. Correlation between *Candida albicans* viability (%) and zeta-potential (mV) for AmB formulation at low (□) and high P (●). At high P, formulations are more loosely packed and efficiently deliver the aggregated drug to the fungus at low zeta-potentials. On the other hand, at low P, formulations are more tightly packed and efficiently deliver the monomeric drug (solubilized at the edges of the bilayer fragments) to the fungus at high zeta-potentials. Both formulations lead to 0% of fungus viability, a situation that cannot be achieved for cationic components of the particles in separate.

Fungizon (AmB in deoxycholate) and DODAB BF/AmB (formulation at low P) were previously evaluated in mice with systemic candidiasis (Lincopan et al., 2003). Both formulations yielded equivalent therapeutic results. However, DODAB BF/AmB was better from the point of view of reduced nephrotoxicity (Lincopan et al., 2005). Furthermore, cationic surfactants and polymers have an effect on integrity of red blood cells (Vieira and Carmona-Ribeiro, 2006). Therefore, similar studies should be performed for the formulations described in this chapter.

CONCLUSION

Optimal colloid stability and maximal fungicidal activity of monomeric or aggregated AmB in cationic lipid was achieved for cationic formulations at low or high drug to lipid molar proportions. At 0.005 mM drug, 1 mM DODAB, 1 mg/ml CMC and $\geq$ 5 mg/ml PDDA, monomeric AmB was found in DODAB BF enveloped by the two oppositely charged polyelectrolytes yielding 0% *C. albicans* viability. At 0.05 mM drug, 0.1 mM DODAB, 0.1 mg/ml CMC and PDDA $\geq$ 2 mg/ml, AmB/DODAB BF/CMC/PDDA assembly contained AmB in the aggregated state forming drug particles sequentially covered by DODAB BF, CMC, and PDDA yielding also 0% fungus viability. The less tightly packed assembly turned out to be the one at high P, and high drug concentration which easily delivered the drug to cells at the lower zeta-potentials. The more tightly packed assembly was the one at low P, delivering drug to cells at higher zeta-potentials and lower drug concentration. *In vitro* both types of AmB formulations yielded complete fungicidal effect against *Candida albicans* (1×10^6 cfu/ml) representing good candidates to further tests *in vivo*.

KEYWORDS

- **Bilayer fragments**
- **Carboxymethylcellulose**
- **Dioctadecyldimethylammonium bromide**
- **Poly diallyldimethylammonium chloride**
- **Polylysines**
- **Solid lipid nanoparticles**

AUTHORS' CONTRIBUTIONS

Dbora B. Vieira did all of the experiments and data analysis in the laboratory, Ana M. Carmona-Ribeiro coordinated experiments, provided important advice for the experiments and financial support. Both authors read and approved the final manuscript.

ACKNOWLEDGMENTS

This work was supported by the Conselho Nacional de Desenvolvimento Científico e Tecnológico (CNPq) and by the Fundação de Âmparo à Pesquisa do Estado de São Paulo.

COMPETING INTERESTS

The authors declare that they have no competing interests.

Permissions

Chapter 1: Nanotechnology-based Drug Delivery Systems was originally published as "Nanotechnology-based Drug Delivery Systems" in *BioMed Central Ltd* 12:1, 2007. Reprinted with permission under the Creative Commons Attribution License or equivalent.

Chapter 2: Novel Multi-component Nanopharmaceuticals for Anti-HIV Effects was originally published as "Novel multi-component nanopharmaceuticals derived from poly (ethylene) glycol, retro-inverso-Tat-nonapeptideand saquinavir demonstrate combined anti-HIV effects" in *BioMed Central Ltd* 4:24, 2006. Reprinted with permission under the Creative Commons Attribution License or equivalent.

Chapter 3: Hydroxycamptothecin-loaded Nanoparticles to Enhance Drug Delivery was originally published as "Hydroxycamptothecin-loaded nanoparticles enhance target drug delivery and anticancer effect" in *BioMed Central Ltd* 5:4, 2008. Reprinted with permission under the Creative Commons Attribution License or equivalent.

Chapter 4: Targeted Drug-carrying Phage Nanomedicines was originally published as "Killing cancer cells by targeted drug-carrying phage nanomedicines" in *BioMed Central Ltd* 4:3, 2008. Reprinted with permission under the Creative Commons Attribution License or equivalent.

Chapter 5: Artemisinin-derived Antimalarial Dry Suspensions for Pediatric Usewas originally published as "Post-marketing assessment of content and efficacy of preservatives in artemisinin-derived antimalarial dry suspensions for paediatric use" in *BioMed Central Ltd* 1:26, 2007. Reprinted with permission under the Creative Commons Attribution License or equivalent.

Chapter 6: Inhibition of Cell Growth and Invasion by Epidermal Growth Factor-targeted Phagemid Particles was originally published as "Inhibition of cell growth and invasion by epidermal growth factor-targeted phagemid particles carrying siRNA against focal adhesion kinase in the presence of hydroxycamptothecin" in *BioMed Central Ltd* 9:18, 2008. Reprinted with permission under the Creative Commons Attribution License or equivalent.

Chapter 7: PET-PLA/Drug Nanoparticles Synthesis for Controlled Drug Release was originally published as "PET-PLA/Drug Nanoparticles Synthesis for Controlled Drug Release" in *Hindawi Publishing Corporation* 4:4, 2008. Reprinted with permission under the Creative Commons Attribution License or equivalent.

Chapter 8: Nanotechnology Approaches to Crossing the Blood-Brain Barrier and Drug Delivery to the CNS was originally published as "Nanotechnology approaches to crossing the blood-brain barrier and drug delivery to the CNS" in *BioMed Central Ltd* 12:10, 2008. Reprinted with permission under the Creative Commons Attribution License or equivalent.

Chapter 9: Quantum Dot Imaging for Embryonic Stem Cells was originally published as "Quantum dot imaging for embryonic stem cells" in *BioMed Central Ltd* 10:9, 2007. Reprinted with permission under the Creative Commons Attribution License or equivalent

Chapter 10: Nanoporous Platforms for Cellular Sensing and Delivery was originally published as "Nanoporous Platforms for Cellular Sensing and Delivery" in *sensors* ISSN 1424-8220© 2002 by MDPI3:20, 2002. Reprinted with permission under the Creative Commons Attribution License or equivalent.

Chapter 11: Skin Permeation Mechanism and Bioavailability Enhancement of Celecoxibwas originally published as "Skin permeation mechanism and bioavailability enhancement of celecoxib from transdermally applied nanoemulsion" in *BioMed Central Ltd* 7:9, 2008. Reprinted with permission under the Creative Commons Attribution License or equivalent.

Chapter 12: Raft-dependent Endocytosis of Autocrine Motility Factor/Phosphoglucose Isomerase was originally published as “”Raft-Dependent Endocytosis of Autocrine Motility Factor/Phosphoglucose Isomerase: A Potential Drug Delivery Route for Tumor Cells in *PloS ONE* 10:31, 2008. Reprinted with permission under the Creative Commons Attribution License or equivalent.

Chapter 13: Adenovirus Dodecahedron, as a Drug Delivery Vector was originally published as “Adenovirus Dodecahedron, as a Drug Delivery Vector” in *PloS ONE* 5:15, 2009. Reprinted with permission under the Creative Commons Attribution License or equivalent.

Chapter 14: Exon Skipping Oligonucleotides and Concomitant Dystrophin Expression in Skeletal Muscle of mdx Mice was originally published as “Nanopolymers improve delivery of exon skipping oligonucleotides and concomitant dystrophin expression in skeletal muscle of mdx mice” in *BioMed Central Ltd* 4:2, 2008. Reprinted with permission under the Creative Commons Attribution License or equivalent.

Chapter 15: *In Vitro* Drug Release Behavior was originally published as “*In vitro* drug release behavior from a novel thermosensitive composite hydrogel based on Pluronic f127 and poly (ethylene glycol)-poly (ε-caprolactone)-poly (ethylene glycol) copolymer” in *BioMed Central Ltd* 2:11, 2009. Reprinted with permission under the Creative Commons Attribution License or equivalent.

Chapter 16: Pharmaceutical Induction of ApoE Secretion was originally published as “Pharmaceutical induction of ApoE secretion by multipotentmesenchymal stromal cells (MSCs)” in *BioMed Central Ltd* 9:29, 2008. Reprinted with permission under the Creative Commons Attribution License or equivalent.

Chapter 17: Cationic Nanoparticles for Delivery of Amphotericin Bwas originally published as “Cationic nanoparticles for delivery of amphotericin B: preparation, characterization and activity *in vitro*” in *BioMed Central Ltd* 7:7, 2008. Reprinted with permission under the Creative Commons Attribution License or equivalent.

References

1

Anderson, M. E. and Siahaan, T. J. (2003). Targeting ICAM-1/LFA-1 interaction for controlling autoimmune diseases: Designing peptide and small molecule inhibitors. *Peptides* **24**, 487–501.

Andrews, R. K. and Berndt, M. C. (2004). Platelet physiology and thrombosis. *Thromb. Res.* **114**, 447–453.

Arap, W., Pasqualini, R. R., and Ruoslahti, E. (1998). Cancer treatment by targeted drug delivery to tumor vasculature in a mouse model. *Science* **279**, 377–380.

Balland, O., Pinto-Alphandary, H., Viron, A., Puvion, E., Andremont, A., and Couvreur, P. (1996). Intracellular distribution of ampiciUin in murine macrophages infected with *Salmonella typhimurium* and treated with (3H)ampicillin-loaded nanoparticles. *J. Antimicrob. Chemotherapy* **37**, 105–115.

Bhadra, D., Bhadra, S., Jain, S., and Jain, N. K. (2003). A PEGylated dendritic nanoparticulate carrier of fluorouracil. *Int. J. Pharm.* **257**(1–2), 111–124.

Brannon-Peppase, L. and Blanchette, J. Q. (2004). Nanoparticle and targeted systems for cancer therapy. *Adv. Drug. Deliv. Rev.* **56**(11), 1649–1659.

Chen, A. A., Derfus, A. M., Khetani, S. R., and Bhatia, S. N. (2005). Quantum dots to monitor RNAi delivery and improve gene silencing. *Nucleic Acids Res.* **33**(22), e190.

Chen, X., Plasencia, C., Hou, Y., and Neamati, N. (2005). Synthesis and biological evaluation of dimeric RGD peptide-paclitaxel conjugate as a model for integrin-targeted drug delivery. *J. Med. Chem.* **48**, 1098–1106.

Christofori, G. (2003). Changing neighbours, changing behaviour: Cell adhesion molecule-mediated signalling during tumour progression. *EMBO J.* **22**, 2318–2323.

Costantino, L., Gandolfi, F., Tosi, G., Rivasi, F., Vandelli, M. A., and Forni, F. (2005). Peptide-derivatized biodegradable nanoparticles able to cross the blood-brain barrier. *J. Control Release* **108**(1), 84–96.

Dunehoo, A. L., Anderson, M., Majumdar, S., Kobayashi, N., Berkland, C., and Siahaan, T. J. (2006). Cell adhesion molecules for targeted drug delivery. *J. pharmaceutical Sci.* **95**, 1856–1872.

Fenniri, H., Deng, B. L., Ribbe, A. E., Hallenga, K., Jacob, J., and Thiyagarajan, P. (2002). Entropically driven self-assembly of multichannel rosette nanotubes. *Proc. Nat. Acad. Sci.* **99**, 6487–6492.

Fenniri, H., Mathivanan, P., Vidale, K. L., Sherman, D. M., Hallenga, K., Wood, K. V., and Stowell, J. G. (2001). Helical rosette nanotubes: Design, self-assembly, and characterization. *J. Am. Chem. Soc.* **123**, 3854–3855.

Fonseca, C., Simoes, S., and Gaspar, R. (2002). Paclitaxel-loaded PLGA nanoparticles: Preparation, physicochemical characterization and *in vitro* anti-tumoral activity. *J. Control Release* **83**(2), 273–286.

Gaspar, R., Préat, V., Opperdoes, F. R., and Roland, M. (1992). Macrophage activation by polymeric nanoparticles of polyalkylcyanoacrylates: activity against intracellular *Leishmania donovani* associated with hydrogen peroxide production. *Pharmaceu. Res.* **9**(6), 782–787.

Grady, W. M. (2005). Epigenetic events in the colorectum and in colon cancer. *Biochem. Soc. Trans.* **33**, 684–688.

Groneberg, D. A., Rabe, K. F., and Fischer, A. (2006). Novel concepts of neuropeptide-based therapy: Vasoactive intestinal polypeptide and its receptors. *Eu. J. Pharmacol.* **533**, 182–194.

Gupta, A. S., Huang, G., Lestini, B. J., Sagnella, S., Kottke-Marchant, K., and Marchant, R. E. (2005). RGD modified liposomes targeted to activated platelets as a potential vascular drug delivery system. *Thromb. Haemost.* **93**, 106–114.

Gupta, S. and Viyas, S. P (2007). Development and characterization of amphotericin B bearing emulsomes for passive and active macrophage targeting. *J. Drug Target* **15**(3), 206–217.

Haass, N. K., Smalley, K. S., Li, L., and Herlyn, M. (2005). Adhesion, migration and communication in melanocytes and melanoma. *Pigment Cell Res.* **18**, 150–159.

Howard, K. A., Rahbek, U. L., Liu, X., Damgaard, C. K., Glud, S. Z., Andersen, M. Ø., Hovgaard, M. B., Schmitz, A., Nyengaard, J. R., Besenbacher, F., and Kjems, J. (2006). RNA interference *in vitro* and *in vivo* using a novel chitosan/siRNA nanoparticle system. *Mol. Ther.* **14**(4), 476–484.

Hynes, R. O. (2002). A reevaluation of integrins as regulators of angiogenesis. *Nat. Med.* **8**, 918–921.

Hynes, R. O. and Zhao, Q. (2000). The evolution of cell adhesion. *J. Cell Biol.* **24**, F89–F96.

Kipp, J. E. (2004). The role of solid nanoparticle technology in the parenteral delivery of poorly water-soluble drugs. *Int. J. Pharm.* **284**(1–2), 109–122.

Koziara, J. M., Lockman, P. R., Allen, D. D., and Mumper, R. J. (2004). Paclitaxel nanoparticles for the potential treatment of brain tumors. *J. Control Release* **99**(2), 259–269.

Koziara, J. M., Whisman, T. R., Tseng, M. T., and Mumper, R. J. (2006). *In-vivo* efficacy of novel paclitaxel nanoparticles in paclitaxel-resistant human colorectal tumors. *J. Control Release* **112**(3), 312–319.

Kreuter, J., Shamenkov, D., Petrov, V., Ramge, P., Cychutek, K., Koch-Brandt, C., and Alyautdin, R. (2002). Apolipoprotein-mediated transport of nanoparticle-bound drugs across the blood-brain barrier. *J. Drug Target* **10**(4), 317–325.

Li L, Wartchow, C. A., Danthi, S. N., Shen, Z., Dechene, N., Pease, J., Choi, H. S., Doede, T., Chu, P., Ning, S., Lee, D. Y., Bednarski, M. D., and Knox, S. J. (2004). A novel antiangiogenesis therapy using an integrin antagonist or anti-Flk-1 antibody coated 90Y-labeled nanoparticles. *Int. J. Radiat. Oncol. Biol. Phy.* **58**(4), 1215–1227.

Michaelis, K., Hoffmann, M. M., Dreis, S., Herbert, E., Alyautdin, R. N., Michaelis, M., Kreuter, J., and Langer, K. (2006). Covalent linkage of apolipoprotein E to albumin nanoparticles strongly enhances drug transport into the brain. *J. Pharmacol. Exp. Ther.* **317**(3), 1246–1253.

Ould-Ouali, L., Noppe, M., Langlois, X., Willems, B., Te Riele, P., Timmerman. P., Brewster, M. E., Arien, A., and Preat, V. (2005). Self-assembling PEG-p(CL-co-TMC) copolymers for oral delivery of poorly water-soluble drugs: a case study with risperidone. *J. Control Release* **102**(3), 657–668.

Pancioli, A. M. and Brott, T. G. (2004). Therapeutic potential of platelet glycoprotein IIb/IIIa receptor antagonists in acute ischaemic stroke: Scientific rationale and available evidence. *CNS Drugs* **18**, 981–988.

Panyam, J. and Labhasetwar, V. (2004). Sustained cytoplasmic delivery of drugs with intracellular receptors using biodegradable nanoparticles. *Mol. Pharm.* **1**(1), 77–84.

Park, J. H., Kwon, S., Nam, J. O., Park, R. W., Chung, H., Seo, S. B., Kim, I. S., Kwon, I. C., and Jeong, S. Y. (2004). Self-assembled nanoparticles based on glycol chitosan bearing 5beta-cholanic acid for RGD peptide delivery. *J. Control Release* **95**(3), 579–588.

Pison, U., Welte, T., Giersing, M., and Groneberg, D. A. (2006). Nanomedicine for respiratory diseases. *Eu. J. Pharmacol.* **533**, 341–350.

Schatzlein, A. G. (2006). Delivering cancer stem cell therapies—a role for nanomedicines? *Eur. J. Cancer*, **42**(9), 1309–1315.

Schiffelers, R. M., Koning, G. A., ten Hagen, T. L., Fens, M. H., Schraa, A. J., Janssen, A. P., Kok, R. J., Molema, G., and Strom, G. (2003). Anti-tumor efficacy of tumor vasculature-targeted liposomal doxorubicin. *J. Control Rel* **91**, 115–122.

Shimaoka, M. and Springer, T. A. (2004). Therapeutic antagonists and the conformational regulation of the β2 integrins. *Curr. Top. Med. Chem.* **4**, 1485–1495.

Shinde, R. R., Bachmann, M. H., Wang, Q., Kasper, R., and Contag, C. H. (2007). *PEG-PLA/PLGA Nanoparticles for In-Vivo RNAi Delivery.* NSTI Nano tech., California.

Steiniger, S. C., Kreuter, J., Khalansky, A. S., Skidan, I. N., Bobruskin, A. I., Smirnova, Z. S., Severin, S. E., Uhl, R., Kock, M., Geiger, K. D., and Gelperina, S. E. (2004). Chemotherapy of glioblastoma in rats using doxorubicin-loaded nanoparticles. *Int. J. Cancer* **109**(5), 759–767.

Stylios, G. K., Giannoudis, P. V., and Wan, T. (2005). Applications of nanotechnologies in medical practice. *Injury* **36**, S6–13.

Sumner, J. P. and Kopelman, R. (2005). Alexa Fluor 488 as an iron sensing molecule and its application in PEBBLE nanosensors. *Analyst* **130**(4), 528–533.

Tan, W. B., Jiang, S., and Zhang, Y. (2007). Quantum-dot based nanoparticles for targeted silencing of *HER2/neu* gene via RNA interference. *Biomaterials* **28**(8), 1565–1571.

Yokoyama, M. (2005). Drug targeting with nano-sized carrier systems. *J. Artif. Organs* **8**(2), 7784.

Yoo, H. S., Lee, K. H., Oh, J. E., and Park, T. G. (2000). *In vitro* and *in vivo* anti-tumor activities of nanoparticles based on doxorubicin-PLGA conjugates. *J. Control Release* **68**(3), 419–431.

Yusuf-Makagiansar, H., Anderson, M. E., Yakovleva, T. V., Murray, J. S., and Siahaan, T. J. (2002). Inhibition of LFA-1/ICAM-1 and VLA-4/VCAM-1 as a therapeutic approach to inflammation and autoimmune diseases. *Med. Res. Rev.* **22**, 146–167.

Zhang, D., Tan, T., Gao, L., Zhao, W., and Wang, P. (2007). Preparation of azithromycin nanosuspensions by high pressure homogenization and its physicochemical characteristics studies. *Drug Dev. Ind. Pharm.* **33**(5), 569–575.

Zhang, N. and Berkland, C. (2006). Synthesis of PLGA Nanoparticles with conjugated CLABL as targeted vascular delivery vehicles. *Science Talks.* Higuchi Biosciences Center, University of Kansas, Lawrence..

Zhang, Y., Sun, C., Kohler, N., and Zhang, M. (2004). Self-assembled coatings on individual monodisperse magnetite nanoparticles for efficient intracellular uptake. *Biomedical Microdevices* **6**, 33–40.

Zhuang, S. and Schnellmann, R. G. (2006). A death-promoting role for extracellular signal-regulated kinase. *J. Pharmacol. Exp. Ther.* **319**, 991–997.

2

Aungst, B. J. (1999). P-glycoprotein, secretory transport, and other barriers to the oral delivery of anti-HIV drugs. *Adv. Drug. Deliv. Rev.* **39**, 105–116.

Baba, M., Nishimura, O., Kanzaki, N., Okamoto, M., Sawada, H., Iizawa, Y., Shiraishi, M., Aramaki, Y., Okonogi, K., Ogawa, Y., et al. (1999). A small-molecule, nonpeptide CCR5 antagonist with highly potent and selective anti-HIV-1 activity. *Proc. Natl. Acad. Sci. USA* **96**, 5698–5703.

Bangsberg, D. R., Hecht, F. M., Charlebois, E. D., Zolopa, A. R., Holodniy, M., Sheiner, L., Bamberger, J. D., Chesney, M. A., and Moss, A. (2000). Adherence to protease inhibitors, HIV-1 viral load, and development of drug resistance in an indigent population. *AIDS* **14**, 357–366.

Brenchley, J. M., Schacker, T. W., Ruff, L. E., Price, D. A., Taylor, J. H., Beilman, G. J., Nguyen, P. L., Khoruts, A., Larson, M., Haase, A. T., and Douek, D. C. (2004). CD4+ T cell depletion during all stages of HIV disease occurs predominantly in the gastrointestinal tract. *J. Exp. Med.* **200**, 749–759.

Caliceti, P. and Veronese, F. M. (2003). Pharmacokinetic and biodistribution properties of poly(ethylene glycol)-protein conjugates. *Adv. Drug. Deliv. Rev.* **55**, 1261–1277.

Castagna, A., Biswas, P., Beretta, A., and Lazzarin, A. (2005). The appealing story of HIV entry inhibitors: From discovery of biological mechanisms to drug development. *Drugs* **65**, 879–904.

Chen, L. L., Frankel, A. D., Harder, J. L., Fawell, S., Barsoum, J., and Pepinsky, B. (1995). Increased cellular uptake of the human immunodeficiency virus-1 Tat protein after modification with biotin. *Anal. Biochem.* **227**, 168–175.

Chorev, M. and Goodman, M. (1995). Recent developments in retro peptides and proteins–an ongoing topochemical exploration. *Trend. Biotechnol.* **13**, 438–445.

Choudhury, I., Wang, J., Rabson, A. B., Stein, S., Pooyan, S., Stein, S., and Leibowitz, M. J. (1998). Inhibition of HIV-1 replication by a Tat RNA-binding domain peptide analog. *J. Acquir.*

Immune. Defic. Syndr. Hum. Retrovirol. **17**, 104–111.

Choudhury, I., Wang, J., Stein, S., Rabson, A., and Leibowitz, M. J. (1999). Translational effects of peptide antagonists of Tat protein of human immunodeficiency virus type 1. *J. Gen. Virol.* **80**(Pt 3), 777–782.

Cole, S. P., Bhardwaj, G., Gerlach, J. H., Mackie, J. E., Grant, C. E., Almquist, K. C., Stewart, A. J., Kurz, E. U., Duncan, A. M., and Deeley, R. G. (1992). Overexpression of a transporter gene in a multidrug-resistant human lung cancer cell line. *Science* **258**, 1650–1654.

Conover, C. D., Pendri, A., Lee, C., Gilbert, C. W., Shum, K. L., and Greenwald, R. B. (1997). Camptothecin delivery systems: The antitumor activity of a camptothecin-20-0-polyethylene glycol ester transport form. *Anticancer. Res.* **17**, 3361–3368.

Davis, S., Abuchowski, A., Park, Y. K., and Davis, F. F. (1981). Alteration of the circulating life and antigenic properties of bovine adenosine deaminase in mice by attachment of polyethylene glycol. *Clin. Exp. Immunol.* **46**, 649–652.

Debouck, C. (1992). The HIV-1 protease as a therapeutic target for AIDS. *AIDS Res. Hum. Retrovir.* **8**, 153–164.

Doranz, B. J., Grovit-Ferbas, K., Sharron, M. P., Mao, S. H., Goetz, M. B., Daar, E. S., Doms, R. W., and O'Brien, W. A. (1997). A small-molecule inhibitor directed against the chemokine receptor CXCR4 prevents its use as an HIV-1 coreceptor. *J. Exp. Med.* **186**, 1395–1400.

Flexner, C. (1998). HIV-protease inhibitors. *N. Engl. J. Med.* **338**, 1281–1292.

Foroutan, S. M. and Watson, D. G. (1999). The *in vitro* evaluation of polyethylene glycol esters of hydrocortisone 21-succinate as ocular prodrugs. *Int. J. Pharm.* **182**, 79–92.

Frankel, A. D. and Pabo, C. O. (1988). Cellular uptake of the tat protein from human immunodeficiency virus. *Cell* **55**, 1189–1193.

Fromme, B., Eftekhari, P., Van Regenmortel, M., Hoebeke, J., Katz, A., and Millar, R. (2003). A novel retro-inverso gonadotropin-releasing hormone (GnRH) immunogen elicits antibodies that neutralize the activity of native GnRH. *Endocrinology* **144**, 3262–3269.

Ghezzi, S., Noonan, D. M., Aluigi, M. G., Vallanti, G., Cota, M., Benelli, R., Morini, M., Reeves, J. D., Vicenzi, E., Poli, G., and Albini, A. (2000). Inhibition of CXCR4-dependent HIV-1 infection by extracellular HIV-1 Tat. *Biochem. Biophys. Res. Commun.* **270**, 992–996.

Goldie, J. H. and Coldman, A. J. (1984). The genetic origin of drug resistance in neoplasms: implications for systemic therapy. *Cancer Res.* **44**, 3643–3653.

Gunaseelan, S., Debrah, O., Wan, L., Leibowitz, M. J., Rabson, A. B., Stein, S., and Sinko, P. J. (2004). Synthesis of poly(ethylene glycol)-based saquinavir prodrug conjugates and assessment of release and anti-HIV-1 bioactivity using a novel protease inhibition assay. *Bioconjug. Chem.* **15**, 1322–1333.

Hamy, F., Brondani, V., Florsheimer, A., Stark, W., Blommers, M. J., and Klimkait, T. (1998). A new class of HIV-1 Tat antagonist acting through Tat-TAR inhibition. *Biochemistry* **37**, 5086–5095.

Harris, J. M. and Chess, R. B. (2003). Effect of pegylation on pharmaceuticals. *Nat. Rev. Drug Discov.* **2**, 214–221.

Hauber, J., Malim, M. H., and Cullen, B. R. (1989). Mutational analysis of the conserved basic domain of human immunodeficiency virus Tat protein. *J. Virol.* **63**, 1181–1187.

Jeang, K. T., Xiao, H., and Rich, E. A. (1999). Multifaceted activities of the HIV-1 transactivator of transcription, Tat. *J. Biol. Chem.* **274**, 28837–28840.

Jones, K., Bray, P. G., Khoo, S. H., Davey, R. A., Meaden, E. R., Ward, S. A., and Back, D. J. (2001). P-Glycoprotein and transporter MRP1 reduce HIV protease inhibitor uptake in CD4 cells: Potential for accelerated viral drug resistance? *AIDS* **15**, 1353–1358.

Kaushik, N., Basu, A., Palumbo, P, Myers, R. L., and Pandey, V. N. (2002). Anti-TAR polyamide nucleotide analog conjugated with a membrane-permeating peptide inhibits human immunodeficiency virus type 1 production. *J. Virol.* **76**, 3881–3891.

Kilby, J. M., Hopkins, S., Venetta, T. M., DiMassimo, B., Cloud, G. A., Lee, J. Y., Alldredge, L., Hunter, E., Lambert, D., Bolognesi, D., et al.

(1998). Potent suppression of HIV-1 replication in humans by T-20, a peptide inhibitor of gp41-mediated virus entry. *Nat. Med.* **4**, 1302–1307.

Larder, B. A. (1995). Viral resistance and the selection of antiretroviral combinations. *J. Acquir. Immune. Defic. Syndr. Hum. Retrovirol.* **10**(Suppl 1), S28–33.

Lazzarin, A., Clotet, B., Cooper, D., Reynes, J., Arasteh, K., Nelson, M., Katlama, C., Stellbrink, H. J., Delfraissy, J. F., Lange, J., et al. (2003). Efficacy of enfuvirtide in patients infected with drug-resistant HIV-1 in Europe and Australia. *N. Engl. J. Med.* **348**, 2186–2195.

Lee, H. J. and Pardridge, W. M. (2001). Pharmacokinetics and delivery of tat and tat-protein conjugates to tissues *in vivo*. *Bioconjug. Chem.* **12**, 995–999.

Lohr, M., Kibler, K. V., Zachary, I., Jeang, K. T., and Selwood, D. L. (2003). Small HIV-1-Tat peptides inhibit HIV replication in cultured T-cells. *Biochem. Biophys. Res. Commun.* **300**, 609–613.

Madore, S. J. and Cullen, B. R. (1993). Genetic analysis of the cofactor requirement for human immunodeficiency virus type 1 Tat function. *J. Virol.* **67**, 3703–3711.

Nieuwkerk, P. T., Sprangers, M. A., Burger, D. M., Hoetelmans, R. M., Hugen, P. W., Danner, S. A., van Der Ende, M. E., Schneider, M. M., Schrey, G., Meenhorst, P. L., et al. (2001). Limited patient adherence to highly active antiretroviral therapy for HIV-1 infection in an observational cohort study. *Arch. Intern. Med.* **161**, 1962–1968.

Nori, A., Jensen, K. D., Tijerina, M., Kopeckova, P., and Kopecek, J. (2003). Tat-conjugated synthetic macromolecules facilitate cytoplasmic drug delivery to human ovarian carcinoma cells. *Bioconjug. Chem.* **14**, 44–50.

O'Brien, W. A., Sumner-Smith, M., Mao, S. H., Sadeghi, S., Zhao, J. Q., and Chen, I. S. (1996). Anti-human immunodeficiency virus type 1 activity of an oligocationic compound mediated via gp120 V3 interactions. *J. Virol.* **70**, 2825–2831.

Opravil, M., Hirschel, B., Lazzarin, A., Furrer, H., Chave, J. P., Yerly, S., Bisset, L. R., Fischer, M., Vernazza, P., Bernasconi, E., et al. (2002). A randomized trial of simplified maintenance therapy with abacavir, lamivudine, and zidovudine in human immunodeficiency virus infection. *J. Infect. Dis.* **185**, 1251–1260.

Paterson, D. L., Swindells, S., Mohr, J., Brester, M., Vergis, E. N., Squier, C., Wagener. M. M., and Singh, N. (2000). Adherence to protease inhibitor therapy and outcomes in patients with HIV infection. *Ann. Intern. Med.* **133**, 21–30.

Roberts, N. A., Martin, J. A., Kinchington, D., Broadhurst, A. V., Craig, J. C., Duncan, I. B., Galpin, S. A., Handa, B. K., Kay, J., Krohn, A., et al. (1990). Rational design of peptide-based HIV proteinase inhibitors. *Science* **248**, 358–361.

Ruben, S., Perkins, A., Purcell, R., Joung, K., Sia, R., Burghoff, R., Haseltine, W. A., and Rosen. C. A. (1989). Structural and functional characterization of human immunodeficiency virus tat protein. *J. Virol.* **63**, 1–8.

Sawchuk, R. J. and Yang, Z. (1999). Investigation of distribution, transport and uptake of anti-HIV drugs to the central nervous system. *Adv. Drug Deliv. Rev.* **39**, 5–31.

Schrager, L. K. and D'Souza, M. P. (1998). Cellular and anatomical reservoirs of HIV-1 in patients receiving potent antiretroviral combination therapy. *JAMA* **280**, 67–71.

Sinko, P. J., Kunta, J. R., Usansky, H. H., Perry, B. A. (2004). Differentiation of gut and hepatic first pass metabolism and secretion of saquinavir in ported rabbits. *J. Pharmacol. Exp. Ther.* **310**, 359–366.

Turpin, J. A., Song, Y., Inman, J. K., Huang, M., Wallqvist, A., Maynard, A., Covell, D. G., Rice, W. G., and Appella, E. (1999). Synthesis and biological properties of novel pyridinioalkanoyl thiolesters (PATE) as anti-HIV-1 agents that target the viral nucleocapsid protein zinc fingers. *J. Med. Chem.* **42**, 67–86.

Wang, J. (1997). *Development of an HIV-1 Tat Antagonist Based on TAR RNA as the Strategic Target*. Graduate Program in Chemistry, Rutgers University.

Wender, P. A., Mitchell, D. J., Pattabiraman, K., Pelkey, E. T., Steinman, L., and Rothbard, J. B. (2000). The design, synthesis, and evaluation of molecules that enable or enhance cellular uptake: Peptoid molecular transporters. *Proc. Natl. Acad. Sci. USA* **97**, 13003–13008.

Wild, C. T., Shugars, D. C., Greenwell, T. K., McDanal, C. B., and Matthews, T. J. (1994). Peptides corresponding to a predictive alpha-helical domain of human immunodeficiency virus type 1 gp41 are potent inhibitors of virus infection. *Proc. Natl. Acad. Sci. USA* **91**, 9770–9774.

Williams, G. C., Liu, A., Knipp, G., and Sinko, P. J. (2002). Direct evidence that saquinavir is transported by multidrug resistance-associated protein (MRP1) and canalicular multispecific organic anion transporter (MRP2). *AntimicrobAgents Chemother* **46**, 3456–3462.

Xiao, H., Neuveut, C., Tiffany, H. L., Benkirane, M., Rich, E. A., Murphy, P. M., and Jeang, K. T. (2000). Selective CXCR4 antagonism by Tat: Implications for *in vivo* expansion of coreceptor use by HIV-1. *Proc. Natl. Acad. Sci. USA* **97**, 11466–11471.

Zhang, X., Wan, L., Pooyan, S., Su, Y., Gardner, C. R., Leibowitz, M. J., Stein, S., and Sinko, P. J. (2004). Quantitative assessment of the cell penetrating properties of RI-Tat-9: Evidence for a cell type-specific barrier at the plasma membrane of epithelial cells. *Mol. Pharm.* **1**, 145–155.

3

Ding, X. Q., Wang, A. X., Kong, Q. Y., Chen, H. Z., and Chen, Y. (2002). Anticancer effect of hydroxycampothecin on oral squamous carcinoma cell line. *Ai. Zheng.* **21**(4), 3–88.

Dong, A. J., Deng, L. D., Sun, D. X., Zhang, Y. T., Jin, J. Z., and Yuan, Y. J. (2004). Studies on paclitaxel-loaded nanoparticles of amphiphilic block copolymer. *Yao. Xue. Xue. Bao.* **39**(2), 149–152.

Jeong, Y. I., Kang, M. K., Sun, H. S., Kang, S. S., Kim, H. W., Moon, K. S., Lee, K. J., Kim, S. H., and Jung, S. (2004). All-*trans*-retinoic acid release from core-shell type nanoparticles of poly(epsilon-caprolactone)/poly(ethylene glycol) diblock copolymer. *Int. J. Pharm.* **273**(1–2), 95–107.

Jeong, Y. I., Nah, J. W., Lee, H. C., Kim, S. H., and Cho, C. S. (1999). Adriamycin release from flower-type polymeric micelle based on star-block copolymer composed of poly(gamma-benzyl L-glutamate) as the hydrophobic part and poly(ethylene oxide) as the hydrophilic part. *Int. J. Pharm.* **188**(1), 49–58.

Kim, T. E., Park, S. Y., Hsu, C. H., Dutschman, G. E., and Cheng, Y. C. (2004). Synergistic antitumor activity of troxacitabine and camptothecin in selected human cancer cell lines. *Mol. Pharmacol.* **66**(2), 285–292.

Li, S., Jiang, W. Q., Wang, A. X., Guan, Z. Z., and Pan, S. R. (2004). Studies on 5-FU/PEG-PBLG nano-micelles: Preparation, characteristics, and drug releasing *in vivo*. *Ai. Zheng.* **23**(4), 381–385.

Li, Y. F. and Zhang, R. (1996). Reversed-phase high-performance liquid chromatography method for the simultaneous quantitation of the lactone and carboxylate forms of the novel natural product anticancer agent 10-hydroxycamptothecin in biological fluids and tissues. *J. Chromatogr. B. Biomed. Appl.* **686**(2), 257–265.

Machida, Y., Onishi, H., Kurita, A., Hata, H., and Morikawa, A. (2000). Pharmacokinetics of prolonged-release CPT-11-loaded microspheres in rats. *J. Control. Release.* **66**(2–3), 159–175.

Mainardes, R. M. and Silva, L. P. (2004). Drug delivery systems: Past, present, and future. *Curr. Drug Targets* **5**(5), 449–455.

Onishi, H. and Machida, Y. (2003). Antitumor properties of irinotecan-containing nanoparticles prepared using poly(DL-lactic acid) and poly(ethylene glycol)-block-poly(propylene glycol)-block-poly(ethylene glycol). *Biol. Pharm. Bull.* **26**(1), 116–119.

Ping, Y. H., Lee, H. C., Lee, J. Y., Wu, P. H., Ho, L. K., Chi, C. W., Lu, M. F., and Wang, J. J. (2006). Anticancer effects of low-dose 10-hydroxycamptothecin in human colon cancer. *Oncol. Rep.* **15**(5), 1273–1279.

Sanchez, A., Tobio, M., Gonzalez, L., Fabra, A., and Alonso, M. J. (2003). Biodegradable micro- and nanoparticles as long-term delivery vehicles for interferon-alpha. *Eur. J. Pharm. Sci.* **18**(3–4), 221–229.

Wang, A. X., Li, S., Ding, X. Q., Chen, Y., and Chen, D. (2005). Antitumor effects of ring-closed and ring-opened hydroxycamptothecin on oral squamous carcinoma cell line Tca8113. *Ai. Zheng.* **24**(8), 970–974.

Wang, M. D., Shin, D. M., Simons, J. W., and Nie, S. (2007). Nanotechnology for targeted cancer therapy. *Expert Rev. Anticancer Ther.* 7(6), 833–837.

Williams, J., Lansdown, R., Sweitzer, R., Romanowski, M., LaBell, R., Ramaswami, R., and Unger, E. (2003). Nanoparticle drug delivery system for intravenous delivery of topoisomerase inhibitors. *J. Control Release* **91**(1–2), 167–172.

Zentner, G. M., Rathi, R., Shih, C., McRea, J. C., Seo, M. H., Oh, H., Rhee, B. G., Mestecky, J., Moldoveanu, Z., Morgan, M., and Weitman, S. (2001). Biodegradable block copolymers for delivery of proteins and water-insoluble drugs. *J. Control Release* **72**(1–3), 203–215.

Zhang, R., Li, Y., Cai, Q., Liu, T., Sun, H., and Chambless, B. (1998). Preclinical pharmacology of the natural product anticancer agent 10-hydroxycamptothecin, an inhibitor of topoisomerase I. *Cancer Chemother Pharmacol.* **41**(4), 257–267.

Zhang, X., Pan, S. R., Hu, H. M., Wu, G. F., Feng, M., Zhang, W., and Luo, X. (2007). Poly(ethylene glycol)-block-polyethylenimine copolymers as carriers for gene delivery: Effects of PEG molecular weight and PEGylation degree. *J. Biomed. Mater. Res. A.*

Zhang, Z. R. and Lu, W. (1997). Study on liver targeting and sustained release hydroxycamptothecin polybutylcyanoacrylate nanoparticles. *Yao. Xue. Xue. Bao.* **32**(3), 222–227.

Zhou, J. J., Liu, J., and Xu, B. (2001). Relationship between lactone ring forms of HCPT and their antitumor activities. *Acta Pharmacol. Sin.* **22**(9), 827–830.

4

Albright, C. F., Graciani, N., Han, W., Yue, E., Stein, R., Lai, Z., Diamond, M., Dowling, R., Grimminger, L., Zhang, S. Y., Behrens, D., Musselman, A., Bruckner, R., Zhang, M., Jiang, X., Hu, D., Higley, A., Dimeo, S., Rafalski, M., Mandlekar, S., Car, B., Yeleswaram, S., Stern, A., Copeland, R. A., Combs, A., Seitz, S. P., Trainor, G. L., Taub, R., Huang, P., and Oliff, A. (2005). Matrix metalloproteinase-activated doxorubicin prodrugs inhibit HT1080 xenograft growth better than doxorubicin with less toxicity. *Mol. Cancer Ther.* 4(5), 751–760.

Andersson, L., Davies, J., Duncan, R., Ferruti, P., Ford. J., Kneller, S., Mendichi, R., Pasut, G., Schiavon, O., Summerford, C., Tirk, A., Veronese, F. M., Vincenzi, V., and Wu, G. (2005). Poly(ethylene glycol)-poly(ester-carbonate) block copolymers carrying PEG-peptidyl-doxorubicin pendant side chains: synthesis and evaluation as anticancer conjugates. *Biomacromolecules* 6(2), 914–926.

Austin, C. D., Wen, X., Gazzard, L., Nelson, C., Scheller, R. H., and Scales, S. J. (2005). Oxidizing potential of endosomes and lysosomes limits intracellular cleavage of disulfide-based antibody-drug conjugates. *Proc. Natl. Acad. Sci. USA* 102(50), 17987–17992.

Becerril, B., Poul, M. A., and Marks, J. D. (1999). Toward selection of internalizing antibodies from phage libraries. *Biochem. Biophys. Res. Commun.* 255(2), 386–393.

Brannon-Peppas, L. and Blanchette, J. O. (2004). Nanoparticle and targeted systems for cancer therapy. *Adv. Drug Deliv. Rev.* 56(11), 1649–1659.

Carter, P. and Merchant, A. M. (1997). Engineering antibodies for imaging and therapy. *Curr. Opin. Biotechnol.* 8(4), 449–454.

Chari, R. V. (1998). Targeted delivery of chemotherapeutics: tumor-activated prodrug therapy. *Adv. Drug Deliv. Rev.* 31(1-2), 89–104.

Doronina, S. O., Mendelsohn, B. A., Bovee, T. D., Cerveny, C. G., Alley, S. C., Meyer, D.L., Oflazoglu, E., Toki, B. E., Sanderson, R. J., Zabinski, R. F., Wahl, A. F., and Senter, P. D. (2006). Enhanced activity of monomethylauristatin F through monoclonal antibody delivery: Effects of linker technology on efficacy and toxicity. *Bioconjug. Chem.* 17(1), 114–124.

Dubowchik, G. M. and Firestone, R. A. (1998). Cathepsin B-sensitive dipeptide prodrugs. 1. A model study of structural requirements for efficient release of doxorubicin. *Bioorg. Med. Chem. Lett.* 8(23), 3341–3346.

Duncan, R. (2006). Polymer conjugates as anticancer nanomedicines. *Nat. Rev. Cancer* 6(9), 688–701.

Dziubla, T. D., Shuvaev, V. V., Hong, N. K., Hawkins, B. J., Madesh, M., Takano, H., Simone, E., Nakada, M. T., Fisher, A., Albelda, S. M., and Muzykantov, V. R. (2008). Endothelial targeting of semi-permeable polymer nanocarriers for enzyme therapies. *Biomaterials* 29(2), 215–227.

Endo, N., Umemoto, N., Kato, Y., Takeda, Y., and Hara, T. (1987). A novel covalent modification of antibodies at their amino groups with retention of antigen-binding activity. *J. Immunol. Methods* 104(1–2), 253–258.

Enshell-Seijffers, D., Smelyanski, L., and Gershoni, J. M. (2001). The rational design of a "type 88" genetically stable peptide display vector in the filamentous bacteriophage fd. *Nucleic Acids Res.* 29(10), E50

Erickson, H. K., Park, P. U., Widdison, W. C., Kovtun, Y. V., Garrett, L. M., Hoffman, K., Lutz, R. J., Goldmacher, V. S., and Blattler, W. A. (2006). Antibody-maytansinoid conjugates are activated in targeted cancer cells by lysosomal degradation and linker-dependent intracellular processing. *Cancer Res.* 66(8), 4426–4433.

Ferrari, M. (2005). Cancer nanotechnology: opportunities and challenges. *Nat. Rev. Cancer* 5(3), 161–171.

Gallois, L., Fiallo, M., and Garnier-Suillerot, A. (1998). Comparison of the interaction of doxorubicin, daunorubicin, idarubicin and idarubicinol with large unilamellar vesicles. Circular dichroism study. *Biochim. Biophys. Acta.* 1370(1), 31–40.

Gao, G., Mao, S., Ronca, F., Zhuang, S., Quaranta, V., Wirsching, P., and Janda, K. D. (2003). De novo identification of tumor-specific internalizing human antibody–receptor pairs by phage-display methods. *J. Immunol. Methods* 274, 185–197.

Hajitou, A., Rangel, R., Trepel, M., Soghomonyan, S., Gelovani, J. G., Alauddin, M. M., Pasqualini, R., and Arap, W. (2007). Design and construction of targeted AAVP vectors for mammalian cell transduction. *Nat. Protoc.* 2(3), 523–531.

Hajitou, A., Trepel, M., Lilley, C. E., Soghomonyan, S., Alauddin, M. M., Marini, F. C. 3rd, Restel, B. H., Ozawa, M. G., Moya, C. A., Rangel, R., Sun, Y., Zaoui, K., Schmidt, M., von Kalle, C., Weitzman, M. D., Gelovani, J. G., Pasqualini, R., and Arap, W. (2006). A hybrid vector for ligand-directed tumor targeting and molecular imaging. *Cell* 125(2), 385–398.

Iyer, A. K., Khaled, G., Fang, J., and Maeda, H. (2006). Exploiting the enhanced permeability and retention effect for tumor targeting. *Drug Discov. Today* 11(17-18), 812–818.

Kassner, P. D., Burg, M. A., Baird, A., and Larocca, D. (1999). Genetic selection of phage engineered for receptor-mediated gene transfer to mammalian cells. *Biochem. Biophys. Res. Commun.* 264(3), 921–928.

King, H. D., Dubowchik, G. M., Mastalerz, H., Willner, D., Hofstead, S. J., Firestone, R. A., Lasch, S. J., and Trail, P. A. (2002). Monoclonal antibody conjugates of doxorubicin prepared with branched peptide linkers: Inhibition of aggregation by methoxytriethyleneglycol chains. *J. Med. Chem.* 45(19), 4336–4343.

King, H. D., Yurgaitis, D., Willner, D., Firestone, R. A., Yang, M. B., Lasch, S. J., Hellstrom, K. E., and Trail, P. A. (1999). Monoclonal antibody conjugates of doxorubicin prepared with branched linkers: A novel method for increasing the potency of doxorubicin immunoconjugates. *Bioconjug. Chem.* 10(2), 279–288.

Kobayashi, H., Shirakawa, K., Kawamoto, S., Saga, T., Sato, N., Hiraga, A., Watanabe, I., Heike, Y., Togashi, K., Konishi, J., Brechbiel, M. W., and Wakasugi, H. (2002). Rapid accumulation and internalization of radiolabeled herceptin in an inflammatory breast cancer xenograft with vasculogenic mimicry predicted by the contrast-enhanced dynamic MRI with the macromolecular contrast agent G6-(1B4M-Gd)(256). *Cancer Res.* 62(3), 860–866.

Kovtun, Y. V. and Goldmacher, V. S. (2007). Cell killing by antibody-drug conjugates. *Cancer Lett.* 255(2), 232–240.

Kreitman, R. J. (1999). Immunotoxins in cancer therapy. *Curr. Opin. Immunol.* 11, 570–578.

Larocca, D. and Baird, A. (2001). Receptor-mediated gene transfer by phage-display vectors: Applications in functional genomics and gene therapy. *Drug Discov. Today* 6(15), 793–801.

Larocca, D., Jensen-Pergakes, K., Burg, M. A., and Baird, A. (2001). Receptor-targeted gene delivery using multivalent phagemid particles. *Mol. Ther.* 3(4), 476–484.

Liu, B., Conrad, F, Roth, A., Drummond, D. C., Simko, J. P., and Marks, J. D. (2007). Recombinant full-length human IgG1s targeting hormone-refractory prostate cancer. *J. Mol. Med.* 85(10), 1113–1123.

Luo, Y. and Prestwich, G. D. (2002). Cancer-targeted polymeric drugs. *Curr. Cancer. Drug. Targets* 2(3), 209–226.

MacDiarmid, J. A., Mugridge, N. B., Weiss, J. C., Phillips, L., Burn, A. L., Paulin, R. P., Haasdyk, J, E., Dickson, K. A., Brahmbhatt, V. N., Pattison, S. T., James, A. C., Al Bakri, G., Straw, R. C., Stillman, B., Graham, R. M., and Brahmbhatt, H. (2007). Bacterially derived 400 nm particles for encapsulation and cancer cell targeting of chemotherapeutics. *Cancer Cell* 11(5), 431–445.

Maeda, H., Wu, J., Sawa, T., Matsumura, Y., and Hori, K. (2000). Tumor vascular permeability and the EPR effect in macromolecular therapeutics: A review. *J. Control Release* 65(1–2), 271–284.

Mazor, Y., Barnea, I., Keydar, I., and Benhar, I. (2007). Antibody internalization studied using a novel IgG binding toxin fusion. *J. Immunol. Methods* 321(1–2), 41–59.

Medina, O.P., Zhu, Y., and Kairemo, K. (2004). Targeted liposomal drug delivery in cancer. *Curr. Pharm. Des.* 10(24), 2981–2989.

Merril, C. R., Biswas, B., Carlton, R., Jensen, N. C., Creed, G. J., Zullo, S., and Adhya, S. (1996). Long-circulating bacteriophage as antibacterial agents. *Proc. Natl. Acad. Sci. USA* 93(8), 3188–3192.

Muro, S., Dziubla, T., Qiu, W., Leferovich, J., Cui, X., Berk, E., and Muzykantov, V. R. (2006). Endothelial targeting of high-affinity multivalent polymer nanocarriers directed to intercellular adhesion molecule 1. *J. Pharmacol. Exp. Ther.* 317(3), 1161–1169.

Nam, K. T., Kim, D. W., Yoo, P. J., Chiang, C. Y., Meethong, N, Hammond, P. T., Chiang, Y. M., and Belcher, A. M. (2006). Virus-enabled synthesis and assembly of nanowires for lithium ion battery electrodes. *Science* 312(5775), 885–888.

Nielsen, U. B. and Marks, J. D. (2000). Internalizing antibodies and targeted cancer therapy: Direct selection from phage display libraries. *Pharm. Sci. Technolo. Today* 3(8), 282–291.

Petty, N. K., Evans, T. J., Fineran, P. C., and Salmond, G. P. (2007). Biotechnological exploitation of bacteriophage research. *Trends Biotechnol.* 25(1), 7–15.

Poul, M. A., Becerril, B., Nielsen, U. B., Morisson, P., and Marks, J. D. (2000). Selection of tumor-specific internalizing human antibodies from phage libraries. *J. Mol. Biol.* 301(5), 1149–1161.

Poul, M. A. and Marks, J. D. (1999). Targeted gene delivery to mammalian cells by filamentous bacteriophage. *J. Mol. Biol.* 288(2), 203–211.

Sarikaya, M., Tamerler, C., Jen, A. K., Schulten, K., and Baneyx, F. (2003). Molecular biomimetics: Nanotechnology through biology. *Nat. Mater.* 2(9), 577–585.

Schrama, D., Reisfeld, R. A., and Becker, J. C. (2006). Antibody targeted drugs as cancer therapeutics. *Nat, Rev, Drug, Discov*, 5(2), 147–159.

Sidhu, S. S. (2001). Engineering M13 for phage display. *Biomol. Eng.* 18(2), 57–63.

Smith Lab Phage Display Vectors. (http://www.biosci.missouri.edu/smithgp/PhageDisplayWebsite/vectors.doc).

Souza, G. R., Christianson, D. R., Staquicini, F. I., Ozawa, M. G., Snyder, E. Y., Sidman, R. L., Miller, J. H., Arap, W., and Pasqualini, R. (2006). Networks of gold nanoparticles and bacteriophage as biological sensors and cell-targeting agents. *Proc. Natl. Acad. Sci. USA* 103(5), 1215–1220.

Staros, J. V., Wright, R. W., and Swingle, D. M. (1986). Enhancement by N-hydroxysulfosuccinimide of water-soluble carbodiimide-mediated coupling reactions. *Anal. Biochem.* 156(1), 220–222.

Stephenson, S. M., Low, P. S., and Lee, R. J. (2004). Folate receptor-mediated targeting of liposomal drugs to cancer cells. *Methods Enzymol.* 387, 33–50.

Sweeney, R. Y., Park, E. Y., Iverson, B. L., and Georgiou, G. (2006). Assembly of multimeric phage nanostructures through leucine zipper interactions. *Biotechnol. Bioeng.* 95(3), 539–545.

Torchilin, V. P. (2006). Multifunctional nanocarriers. *Adv. Drug Deliv. Rev.* 58(14), 1532–1555.

Ulbrich, K. and Subr, V. (2004). Polymeric anticancer drugs with pH-controlled activation. *Adv. Drug. Delivery Rev.* 56, 1023–1050.

Urbanelli, L., Ronchini, C., Fontana, L., Menard, S., Orlandi, R., and Monaci, P. (2001). Targeted gene transduction of mammalian cells expressing the HER2/neu receptor by filamentous phage. *J. Mol. Biol.* 313, 965–976.

von Minckwitz, G., Harder, S., Hovelmann, S., Jager, E., Al-Batran, S. E., Loibl, S., Atmaca, A., Cimpoiasu, C., Neumann, A., Abera, A., Knuth, A., Kaufmann, M., Jager, D., Maurer, A. B., and Wels, W. S. (2005). Phase I clinical study of the recombinant antibody toxin scFv(FRP5)-ETA specific for the ErbB2/HER2 receptor in patients with advanced solid malignomas. *Breast Cancer Res.* 7(5), R617–626.

Wels, W., Harwerth, I. M., Mueller, M., Groner, B., and Hynes, N. E. (1992). Selective inhibition of tumor cell growth by a recombinant single-chain antibody-toxin specific for the erbB-2 receptor. *Cancer Res.* 52(22), 6310–6317.

Wu, A. M. and Senter, P. D. (2005). Arming antibodies: prospects and challenges for immunoconjugates. *Nat. Biotechnol.* 23(9), 1137–1146.

Wu, G., Barth, R. F., Yang, W., Kawabata, S., Zhang, L., and Green-Church, K. (2006). Targeted delivery of methotrexate to epidermal growth factor receptor-positive brain tumors by means of cetuximab (IMC-C225) dendrimer bioconjugates. *Mol. Cancer Ther.* 5(1), 52–59.

Yacoby, I., Bar, H., and Benhar, I. (2007). Targeted drug-carrying bacteriophages as antibacterial nanomedicines. *Antimicrob. Agents Chemother.* 51(6), 2156–2163.

Yacoby, I., Shamis, M., Bar, H., Shabat, D., and Benhar, I. (2006). Targeting antibacterial agents by using drug-carrying filamentous bacteriophages. *Antimicrob. Agents Chemother.* 50(6), 2087–2097.

Yip, W. L., Weyergang, A., Berg, K., Tonnesen, H. H., and Selbo, P. K. (2007). Targeted delivery and enhanced cytotoxicity of cetuximab-saporin by photochemical internalization in EGFR-positive cancer cells. *Mol. Pharm.* 4(2), 241–251.

Zou, J., Dickerson, M. T., Owen, N. K., Landon, L. A., and Deutscher, S. L. (2004). Biodistribution of filamentous phage peptide libraries in mice. *Mol. Biol. Rep.* 31(2), 121–129.

5

Anger, C. B., Rupp, D., and Lo, P. (1996). Preservation of dispersed systems. In *Pharmaceutical Dosage forms*. Vol. 2 and 2nd edition. H. A. Lieberman, M. M. Rieger, and G. S. Banker (Eds.). Marcel Dekker, New York, pp 377–435.

Atemnkeng, M. A., De Cock, K., and Plaizier-Vercammen, J. (2007). Quality control of active ingredients in artemisinin-derivative antimalarials within Kenya and DR Congo. *Trop. Med. Int. Health* **12**, 68–74.

European Pharmacopoeia IV (2003). *European Directorate for the Quality of Medicines for the Council of Europe*, Strasbourg.

Haines, A. and Smith, R. (1997). Working together to reduce poverty's damage. *BMJ* **314**, 5–29.

International Committee on Harmonization (1992). *Specifications and Control Tests on the Finished Product*, Directive 75/318/EEC.

Klocker, N., Kramer, A., Verse, T., Sikora, C., Rudolph, P., and Daeschlein, G. (2004). Antimicrobial safety of a preservative-free nasal multidose drug administration system. *Eur. J. Pharmaceut. Biopharmaceut.* **57**, 489–493.

Koundourellis, J. E., Malliou, E. T., and Broussalli, A. (2000). High performance liquid chromatographic determination of ambroxol in the presence of different preservatives in pharmaceutical formulations. *J. Pharm. Biomed. Anal.* **23**, 469–475.

Lon, C. T., Tsuyuoka, R., Phanouvoug, S., Nivanna, N., Socheat, D., Sokhan, C., Blum, N., Christophel, E. M., and Smine, A. (2006), Counterfeit and substandard antimalarial drugs in Cambodia. *Trans. R. Soc. Trop. Med. Hyg.* **100**, 1019–1024.

Martin, A., Swarbrick, J., and Cammarata, A. (1983). Physical pharmacy. In *Physical Chemical Principles in the Pharmaceutical Sciences*. 3rd edition. Lea and Febiger Press, Philadelphia.

Martindale (1999). *The Complete Drug Reference*. 32nd edition. Pharmaceutical Press, Massachusetts.

Newton, P. N., Dondorp, A., Green, M., Mayxay, M., and White, N. J. (2003). Counterfeit artesunate antimalarials in southeast Asia. *Lancet* **362**, 1–69.

Ofner III, C. M., Schnaare, R. L., and Schwartz, J. B. (1996). Reconstitutible oral suspensions. In *Pharmaceutical Dosage Forms*. Vol. 2 and 2nd edition. H. A. Lieberman, M. M. Rieger, and G. S. (Eds.). Banker. Marcel Dekker, New York, pp, 243–259.

Rowe, R., Sheskey, P., and Weller, P. (Eds.) (2005). *Handbook of Pharmaceutical Excipients*. 5th edition. Pharmaceutical Press, London.

Soni, M. G., Burdock, G. A., Taylor, S. L., and Greenberg, N. A. (2001). Safety assessment of propylparaben: A review of published literature. *Food Chem. Toxicol.* **39**, 513–532.

The Japanese standards of cosmetic ingredients-with commentary (1984). In *The Society of Japanese Pharmacopoeia*. 2nd edition. Yakug-inippousha, Tokyo.

Van der Meersch, H. (2005). Review of the use of artemisinin and its derivatives in the treatment of malaria (article in French). *J. Pharm. Belg.* **60**, 23–29.

Wilson, L. A., Kuehne, J. W., Hall, S. W., and Ahearn, D. G. (1971). Microbial contamination in ocular cosmetics. *Am. J. Ophthalmol.* **71**, 1298–1302.

6

Burg, M. A., Jensen-Pergakes, K., Gonzalez, A. M., Ravey, P., Baird, A., and Larocca, D. (2002). Enhanced phagemid particle gene transfer in camptothecin-treated carcinoma cells. *Cancer Res.* **62**, 977–981.

Cai, X. M., Tao, B. B., Wang, L. Y., Liang, Y. L., Jin, J. W., Yang, Y., Hu, Y. L., and Zha, X. L. (2005). Protein phosphatase activity of PTEN inhibited the invasion of glioma cells with epidermal growth factor receptor mutation type III expression. *Int. J. Cancer*. **117**, 905–912.

Carelli, S., Zadra, G., Vaira, V., Falleni, M., Bottiglieri, L., Nosotti, M., Giulio, A. M., Gorio, A., and Bosari, S. (2006). Up-regulation of focal adhesion kinase in non-small cell lung cancer. *Lung Cancer* **53**, 263–271.

Chen, J., Gamou, S., Takayanagi, A., Ohtake, Y., Ohtsubo, M., and Shimizu, N. (1998). Receptor-mediated gene delivery using the Fab fragments of anti-epidermal growth factor receptor antibodies: Improved immunogene approach. *Cancer Gene Ther*. **5**, 357–364.

Giovine, M. D., Salone, B., Martina, Y., Amati, V., Zambruno, G., Cundari, E., Failla, C. M., and Saggio, I. (2001). Binding properties, cell delivery and gene transfer of adenoviral penton base displaying bacteriophage. *Virology* **282**, 102–112.

Han, E. K., Mcgonigal, T., Wang, J., Giranda, V. L., and Luo, Y. (2004). Functional analysis of focal adhesion kinase (FAK) reduction by small inhibitory RNAs. *Anticancer Res*. **24**, 3899–3905.

Jiang, H., Cai, X., Shi, B., Zhang, J., Li, Z., and Gu, J. (2008). Development of efficient RNA interference system using EGF-displaying phagemid particles. *Acta. Pharm. Sinica*. **29**, 437–442.

Kassner, P. D., Burg, M. A., Baird, A., and Larocca, D. (1999). Genetic selection of phage engineered for receptor-mediated gene transfer to mammalian cells. *Biochem. Biophys. Res. Commun*. **264**, 921–928.

Kornberg, L. J. (1998). Focal adhesion kinase and its potential involvement in tumor invasion and metastasis. *Head Neck* **20**, 745–752.

Larocca, D., Kassner, P. D., Witte, A., Ladner, R. C., Pierce, G. F., and Baird, A. (1999). Gene transfer to mammalian cells using genetically targeted filamentous bacteriophage. *FASEB J.* **13**, 727–734.

Larocca, D., Witte, A., Johnson, W., Pierce, G. F., and Baird, A. (1998). Targeting bacteriophage to mammalian cell surface receptors for gene delivery. *Hum. Gene Ther*. **9**, 2393–2399.

Li, Z. H., Jiang, H., Zhang, J., Shi, B. Z., and Gu, J. R. (2006). Cell targeted phagemid particles preparation using *E. coli* bearing ligand-pIII encoding helper phage genome. *Bio. Techniques* **41**, 706–707.

Li, Z. H., Zhang, J., Zhao, R. J., Xu, Y. H., and Gu, J. R. (2005). Preparation of peptide-targeted phagemid particles using a protein III-modified helper phage. *Biotechniques* **39**, 493–497.

Liang, Y., Shi, B., Zhang, J., Jiang, H., Xu, Y., Li, Z., and Gu, J. (2006). Better gene expression by (–)gene than by (+)gene in phage gene delivery systems. *Biotechnol. Prog*. **22**, 626–630.

Mitra, S. K., Lim, S. T., Chi, A., and Schlaepfer, D. D. (2006). Intrinsic focal adhesion kinase activity controls orthotopic breast carcinoma metastasis via the regulation of urokinase plasminogen activator expression in a syngeneic tumor model. *Oncogene* **25**, 4429–4440.

Oktay, M. H., Oktay, K., Hamele, D., Buyuk, A., and Koss, L. G. (2003). Focal adhesion kinase as a marker of malignant phenotype in breast and cervical carcinomas. *Hum. Pathol.* **34**, 240–245.

Poul, M. A., and Marks, J. D. (1999). Targeted gene delivery to mammalian cells by filamentous bacteriophage. *J. Mol. Biol.* **288**, 203–211.

Qing, K., Wang, X. S., Kube, D. M., Ponnazhagan, S., Bajpai, A., and Srivastava, A. (1997). Role of tyrosine phosphorylation of a cellular protein in adeno-associated virus 2-mediated transgene expression. *Proc. Natl. Acad. Sci. USA* **94**, 10879–10884.

Rondot, S., Koch, J., Breitling, F., and Dübe, S. (2001). A helper phage to improve single-chain antibody presentation in pahge display. *Nat. Biotechnol.* **19**, 75–78.

Sood, A. K., Coffin, J. E., and Schneider, G. B. (2005). Biological significance of focal adhesion kinase in ovarian cancer: role in migration and invasion. *Am. J. Pathol.* **165**, 1087–1095.

Zhou, G. F., Ye, F., Cao, L. H., and Zha, X. L. (2000). Over expression of integrin alpha 5 beta 1 in human hepatocellular carcinoma cell line suppresses cell proliferation *in vitro* and tumorigenicity in nude mice. *Mol. Cell Biochem.* **207**, 49–55.

7

Beck, L. R., Cowsar, D. R., Lewis, D. H., et al., (1979). A new long-acting injectable microcapsule system for the administration of progesterone. *Fert. Ster.* **31**(5), 545–551.

Bruijn, E. A., Oosterom, A. T., and Tjaden, U. S. (1989). Site specific delivery of 5Fu with 5-deoxy-5-florouridine. *Regional Cancer Treatment* **2**, 61–76.

Eldrige, J. H., Staas, J. K., Meulbroek, J. A., McGhee, J. R., Tice, T. R., and Gilley, R. M. (1991). Biodegradable microspheres as a vaccine delivery system. *Molec. Immunol.* **28**(3), 287–294.

Kennay, J. F. (1978). Reaction products of specific antimony compounds with a carboxylate of zinc calcium or manganese and an alcohol or glycol, US patent 4122107.

Lai, M. -K., Chang, C. -Y., Lien, Y. -W., and Tsiang, R. C.-C., (2006). Application of gold nanoparticles to microencapsulation of thioridazine. *J. Contr. Rel.* **111**(3), 352–361.

O'Hagan, D. T., McGee, J. P., Holmgren, J., et al., (1993). Biodegradable microparticles for oral immunization. *Vaccine* **11**(2), 149–154.

Olewnik, E., Czerwiński, W., Nowaczyk, J., et al., (2007). Synthesis and structural study of copolymers of L-lactic acid and bis(2-hydroxyethyl terephthalate). *Eur. Poly. J.* **43**(3), 1009–1019.

Pignatello R., Amico, D., Chiechio, S., Spadaro, C., Puglisi, G., and Giunchedi, P., (2001). Preparation and analgesic activity of eudragit RS100® microparticles containing diflunisal. *Drug Delivery* **8**(1), 35–45.

Salhi, S., Tessier, M., Blais, J.-C., Gharbi, R. El., and Fradet, A., (2004). Synthesis of aliphatic-aromatic copolyesters by a high temperature bulk reaction between poly(ethylene terephthalate) and cyclodi(ethylene succinate). *Macromol. Chem. Phys.* **205**(18), 2391–2397.

Selvaraj, V. and Alagar, M., (2007). Analytical detection and biological assay of antileukemic drug 5-fluorouracil using gold nanoparticles as probe. *Intern. J. Pharmac.* **337**(1–2), 275–281.

Selvaraj, V., Alagar, M., and Hamerton, I., (2006). Analytical detection and biological assay of antileukemic drug using gold nanoparticles. *Electrochimica Acta* **52**(3), 1152–1160.

Uchida, T., Martin, S., Foster, T. P., Wardley, R. C., and Grimm, S. (1994). Dose and load studies for subcutaneous and oral delivery of poly(lactide-co-glycolide) microspheres containing ovalbumin. *Pharmaceu. Res.* **11**(7), 1009–1015.

van Nostrum, C. F., Veldhuis, T. F. J., Bos, G. W., and Hennik, W. E., (2004). Hydrolytic degradation of oligo(lactic acid): a kinetic and mechanistic study. *Polymer* **45**(20), 6779–6787.

Yuan, X., Mak, A. F. T., and Yao, K., (2002). Comparative observation of accelerated degradation of poly(L-lactic acid) fibres in phosphate buffered saline and a dilute alkaline solution. *Poly. Degrad. and Stabil.* **75**(1), 45–53.

Yuan, X., Mak, A. F. T., and Yao, K., (2003). Surface degradation of poly(L-lactic acid) fibres in a concentrated alkaline solution. *Poly. Degrad. and Stabil.* **79**(1), pp. 45–52.

8

Alyautdin, R. N., Petrov, V. E., Langer, K., Berthold, A, Kharkevich, D. A., and Kreuter, J. (1997). Delivery of loperamide across the blood-brain barrier with polysorbate 80-coated polybutylcyanoacrylate nanoparticles. *Pharm. Res.* **14**, 325–328.

Alyaudtin, R. N., Reichel, A., Lobenberg, R., Ramge, P., Kreuter, J., and Begley, D. J. (2001). Interaction of poly(butylcyanoacrylate) nanoparticles with the blood-brain barrier *in vivo* and *in vitro*. *J. Drug. Target* **9**, 209–221.

Alyautdin, R. N., Tezikov, E. B., Ramge, P., Kharkevich, D. A., Begley, D. J., and Kreuter, J. (1998). Significant entry of tubocurarine into the brain of rats by adsorption to polysorbate 80-coated polybutylcyanoacrylate nanoparticles: An *in situ* brain perfusion study. *J. Microencapsul.* **15**, 67–74.

Brigger, I., Morizet, J., Aubert, G., Chacun, H., Terrier-Lacombe, M. J., Couvreur, P., and Vassal, G. (2002). Poly(ethylene glycol)-coated hexadecylcyanoacrylate nanospheres display a combined effect for brain tumor targeting. *J. Pharmacol. Exp. Ther.* **303**, 928–936.

Calvo, P., Gouritin, B., Villarroya, H., Eclancher, F., Giannavola, C., Klein, C., Andreux, J. P., and Couvreur, P. (2002). Quantification and localization of PEGylated polycyanoacrylate nanoparticles in brain and spinal cord during experimental allergic encephalomyelitis in the rat. *Eur. J. Neurosci.* **15**, 1317–1326.

Dupas, B., Berreur, M., Rohanizadeh, R., Bonnemain, B., Meflah, K., and Pradal, G. (1999). Electron microscopy study of intrahepatic ultrasmall superparamagnetic iron oxide kinetics in the rat. Relation with magnetic resonance imaging. *Biol. Cell* **91**, 195–208.

Ercolini, A. M. and Miller, S. D. (2006). Mechanisms of immunopathology in murine models of central nervous system demyelinating disease. *J. Immunol.* **176**, 3293–3298.

Feng, S. S., Mu, L., Win, K. Y., and Huang, G. (2004). Nanoparticles of biodegradable polymers for clinical administration of paclitaxel. *Curr. Med. Chem.* **11**, 413–424.

Friese, A., Seiller, E., Quack, G., Lorenz, B., and Kreuter, J. (2000). Increase of the duration of the anticonvulsive activity of a novel NMDA receptor antagonist using poly(butylcyanoacrylate) nanoparticles as a parenteral controlled release system. *Eur. J. Pharm. Biopharm.* **49**, 103–109.

Gulyaev, A. E., Gelperina, S. E., Skidan, I. N., Antropov, A. S., Kivman, G. Y., and Kreuter, J. (1999). Significant transport of doxorubicin into the brain with polysorbate 80-coated nanoparticles. *Pharm. Res.* **16**, 1564–1569.

Kanwar, J. R. (2005). Anti-inflammatory immunotherapy for multiple sclerosis/experimental autoimmune encephalomyelitis (EAE) disease. *Curr. Med. Chem.* **12**, 2947–2962.

Kreuter, J., Alyautdin, R. N., Kharkevich, D. A., and Ivanov, A. A. (1995). Passage of peptides through the blood-brain barrier with colloidal polymer particles (nanoparticles). *Brain Res.* **674**, 171–174.

Olbrich, C., Gessner, A., Kayser, O., and Muller, R. H. (2002). Lipid-drug-conjugate (LDC) nanoparticles as novel carrier system for the hydrophilic antitrypanosomal drug diminazenediaceturate. *J. Drug Target* **10**, 387–396.

Pathak, S., Cao, E., Davidson, M.C., Jin, S., and Silva, G. A. (2006). Quantum dot applications to neuroscience: New tools for probing neurons and glia. *J. Neurosci.* **26**, 1893–1895.

Peira, E., Marzola, P., Podio, V., Aime, S., Sbarbati, A., and Gasco, M. R. (2003). *In vitro* and *in vivo* study of solid lipid nanoparticles loaded with superparamagnetic iron oxide. *J. Drug Target* **11**, 19–24.

Rousselle, C., Clair, P., Smirnova, M., Kolesnikov, Y., Pasternak, G. W., Gac-Breton, S., Rees, A. R., Scherrmann, J. M., and Temsamani, J. (2003). Improved brain uptake and pharmacological activity of dalargin using a peptide-vector-mediated strategy. *J. Pharmacol. Exp. Ther.* **306**, 371–376.

Schroeder, U., Sommerfeld, P., Ulrich, S., and Sabel, B. A. (1998). Nanoparticle technology for delivery of drugs across the blood-brain barrier. *J. Pharm. Sci.* **87**, 1305–1307.

Silva, G. A. (2007). Nanotechnology approaches for drug and small molecule delivery across the blood brain barrier. *Surg. Neurol.* **67**, 113–116.

Steiniger, S. C., Kreuter, J., Khalansky, A. S., Skidan, I. N., Bobruskin, A. I., Smirnova, Z. S., Severin, S. E., Uhl, R., Kock, M., Geiger, K. D, Gelperina, S. E. (2004). Chemotherapy of glioblastoma in rats using doxorubicin-loaded nanoparticles. *Int. J. Cancer* **109**, 759–767.

Vinogradov, S. V., Batrakova, E. V., and Kabanov, A. V. (2004). Nanogels for oligonucleotide delivery to the brain. *Bioconjug. Chem.* **15**, 50–60.

Zhang, Y., Calon, F., Zhu, C., Boado, R. J., and Pardridge, W. M. (2003). Intravenous nonviral gene therapy causes normalization of striatal tyrosine hydroxylase and reversal of motor impairment in experimental parkinsonism. *Hum. Gene. Ther.* **14**, 1–12.

9

Abeyta, M. J., Clark, A. T., Rodriguez, R. T., Bodnar, M. S., Pera, R. A., and Firpo, M. T. (2004). Unique gene expression signatures of independently-derived human embryonic stem cell lines. *Hum. Mol. Genet.* **13**(6), 601–608.

Akerman, M. E., Chan, W. C., Laakkonen, P., Bhatia, S. N., and Ruoslahti, E. (2002). Nanocrystal targeting *in vivo*. *Proc. Natl. Acad. Sci. USA* **99**(20), 12617–12621.

Boheler, K. R., Czyz, J., Tweedie, D., Yang, H. T., Anisimov, S. V., and Wobus, A. M. (2002). Differentiation of pluripotent embryonic stem cells into cardiomyocytes. *Circ. Res.* **91**(3), 189–201.

Bruder, S. P., Kurth, A. A., Shea, M., Hayes, W. C., Jaiswal, N., and Kadiyala, S. (1998). Bone regeneration by implantation of purified, culture-expanded human mesenchymal stem cells. *J. Orthop. Res.* **16**(2), 155–162.

Cao, F., Drukker, M., Lin, S., Sheikh, A. Y., Xie, X., Li, Z., Connolly, A. J., Weissman, I. L., and Wu, J. C. (2007). Molecular imaging of embryonic stem cell misbehavior and suicide gene ablation. *Cloning Stem. Cells* **9**(1), 107–117.

Cao, F., Lin, S., Xie, X., Ray, P., Patel, M., Zhang, X., Drukker, M., Dylla, S. J., Connolly, A. J., Chen, X., Weissman, I. L., Gambhir, S. S., and Wu, J. C. (2006). *In vivo* visualization of embryonic stem cell survival, proliferation, and migration after cardiac delivery. *Circulation* **113**(7), 1005–1014.

Choy, G., Choyke, P., and Libutti, S. K. (2003). Current advances in molecular imaging: Noninvasive *in vivo* bioluminescent and fluorescent optical imaging in cancer research. *Mol. Imaging.* **2**(4), 303–312.

Christoffer, B. Langerholm M.W., Lauren, A. E., Ly, D. H., Liu, H., Marcel P. B., and Alan S. W. (2004). Multicolor coding of cells with cationic peptide coated quantum dots. *Nano. Letters* **4**(10), 2019–2022.

Davie, N. J., Gerasimovskaya, E. V., Hofmeister, S. E., Richman, A. P., Jones, P. L., Reeves, J. T., and Stenmark, K. R. (2006). Pulmonary artery adventitial fibroblasts cooperate with vasa vasorum endothelial cells to regulate vasa vasorum neovascularization: A process mediated by hypoxia and endothelin-1. *Am. J. Pathol.* **168**(6), 1793–1807.

Derfus, A. M., Chan, W. C. W., and Bhatia, S. N. (2004). Probing the cytotoxicity of semiconductor quantum dots. *Nano. Letters.* **4**(1), 11–18.

Dubertret, B., Skourides, P., Norris, D. J., Noireaux, V., Brivanlou, A. H., and Libchaber, A. (2002). *In vivo* imaging of quantum dots encapsulated in phospholipid micelles. *Science* **298**(5599), 1759–1762.

Evans, M. J. and Kaufman, M. H. (1981). Establishment in culture of pluripotential cells from mouse embryos. *Nature* **292**(5819), 154–156.

Fuchs, E. and Segre, J. A. (2000). Stem cells: a new lease on life. *Cell* **100**(1), 143–155.

Gao, X., Cui, Y., Levenson, R. M., Chung, L. W., and Nie, S. (2004). *In vivo* cancer targeting and imaging with semiconductor quantum dots. *Nat. Biotechnol.* **22**(8), 969–976.

Han, M., Gao, X., Su, J. Z., and Nie, S. (2001). Quantum-dot-tagged microbeads for multiplexed optical coding of biomolecules. *Nat. Biotechnol.* **19**(7), 631–635.

Hardman, R. (2006). A toxicologic review of quantum dots: Toxicity depends on physicochemical and environmental factors. *Environ. Health. Perspect.* **114**(2), 165–172.

Jaiswal, J. K., Mattoussi, H., Mauro, J. M., and Simon, S. M. (2003). Long-term multiple color imaging of live cells using quantum dot bioconjugates. *Nat. Biotechnol.* **21**(1), 47–51.

Keller, G. M. (1995). *In vitro* differentiation of embryonic stem cells. *Curr. Opin. Cell Biol.* **7**(6), 862–869.

Kim, S., Lim, Y. T., Soltesz, E. G., De Grand, A. M., Lee, J., Nakayama, A., Parker, J. A., Mihaljevic, T., Laurence, R. G., Dor, D. M., Cohn, L. H., Bawendi, M. G., and Frangioni, J. V. (2004). Near-infrared fluorescent type II quantum dots for sentinel lymph node mapping. *Nat. Biotechnol.* **22**(1), 93–97.

Larson, D. R., Zipfel, W. R., Williams, R. M., Clark, S. W., Bruchez, M. P., Wise, F. W., and Webb, W. W. (2003). Water-soluble quantum dots for multiphoton fluorescence imaging *in vivo*. *Science* **300**(5624), 1434–1436.

Lindvall, O., Kokaia, Z., and Martinez-Serrano, A. (2004). Stem cell therapy for human neurodegenerative disorders-how to make it work. *Nat. Med.* **10**(Suppl), S42–50.

Maltsev, V. A., Wobus, A. M., Rohwedel, J., Bader, M., and Hescheler, J. (1994). Cardiomyocytes differentiated *in vitro* from embryonic stem cells developmentally express cardiac-specific genes and ionic currents. *Circ. Res.* **75**(2), 233–244.

Medintz, I. L., Uyeda, H. T., Goldman, E. R., and Mattoussi, H. (2005). Quantum dot bioconjugates for imaging, labelling and sensing. *Nat. Mater.* **4**(6), 435–446.

Michalet, X., Pinaud, F. F., Bentolila, L. A., Tsay, J. M., Doose, S., Li, J. J., Sundaresan, G., Wu, A. M., Gambhir, S. S., and Weiss, S. (2005). Quantum dots for live cells, *in vivo* imaging, and diagnostics. *Science* **307**(5709), 538–544.

Murasawa, S., Kawamoto, A., Horii, M., Nakamori, S., and Asahara, T. (2005). Niche-dependent translineage commitment of endothelial progenitor cells, not cell fusion in general, into myocardial lineage cells. *Arterioscler. Thromb. Vasc. Biol.* **25**(7), 1388–1394.

Soria, B., Skoudy, A., and Martin, F. (2001). From stem cells to beta cells: New strategies in cell therapy of diabetes mellitus. *Diabetologia* **44**(4), 407–415.

Strauer, B. E. and Kornowski, R. (2003). Stem cell therapy in perspective. *Circulation* **107**(7), 929–934.

Thomson, J. A., Itskovitz-Eldor, J., Shapiro, S. S., Waknitz, M. A., Swiergiel, J. J., Marshall, V. S., and Jones, J. M. (1998). Embryonic stem cell lines derived from human blastocysts. *Science* **282**(5391), 1145–1147.

Weibo Cai, D. W. S., Kai C., Olivier, G., Qizhen, C., Shan, X. W., Sanjiv, S. G., and Xiaoyuan, C. (2006). Peptide-labeled near-infrared quantum dots for imaging tumor vasculature in living subjects. *Nano. Letters* **6**(4), 669–676.

Wu, X., Liu, H., Liu, J., Haley, K. N., Treadway, J. A., Larson, J. P., Ge, N., Peale, F., and Bruchez, M. P. (2003). Immunofluorescent labeling of cancer marker Her2 and other cellular targets with semiconductor quantum dots. *Nat. Biotechnol.* **21**(1), 41–46.

10

Akin, T. and Najafi, K. (1994). *IEEE Trans. Biomed. Eng.* **4**(4), 305–313.

Anderson, D. J., Najafi, K., Tanghe, S. J., Evans, D. A., Levy, K. L., Hetre, J. F., Xue, X., Zappia, J. J., and Wise, K. D. (1989). *IEEE Trans. Biomed. Eng.* **36**(7), 693–704.

Baxter, G. T., Bousse, L. J., Dawes, T. D., Libby, J. M., Modlin, D. N., Owick, J. C., and Parce, J. W. (1994). *Clin. Chem.* **40**(9), 1800–1804.

Desai, T. A., Chu, W. H., Tu, J. K., Beattie, G. M., Hayek, A., and Ferrari, M. (1998). *Biotechnol. Bioeng.* 118–120.

Desai, T. A., Hansford, D., and Ferrari, M. J. (1999b). *Membr. Sci.* 221–231.

Desai, T. A., Hansford, D. J., Kulinsky, L., Nashat, A. H., Rasi, G., Tu, J., Wang, Y., Zhang, M., and Ferrari, M. (1999a). *Biomed. Microd.* 11–40.

Desai, T. A., Hansford, D. J., Leoni, L., Essenpreis, M., and Ferrari, M. (2000). Nanoporous antifouling silicon membranes for implantable biosensor applications. *Biosens. Bioelec.* **15**(9-10), 453–462.

Gourley, P. L. (1996). *Nat. Med.* **2**(8), 942–944.

Henry, S., McAllister, D. V., Allen, M. G., and Prausnitz, M. R. (1998). *J. Pharm. Sci.* 922–925.

Leoni, L. and Desai. T. A. (November 2001) Nanoporous biocapsules for the encapsulation of insulinoma cells: Biotransport and biocompatibility considerations. *IEEE Trans. Biomed. Eng.* **48**(11).

Santini, J. T. Jr., Cima, M. J., and Langer, R. (1999). *Nature (London)* 335–338.

Volkmuth, W. D., Duke, T., Austin, R. H., and Cox, E. C. (1995). Trapping of branched DNA in microfabricated structures. *Proc. Natl. Acad. Sci. USA* **92**(15), 6887–6891.

11

Baboota, S., Alazaki, A., Kohli, K., Ali, J., Dixit, N., and Shakeel, F. (2007a). Development and evaluation of a microemulsion formulation for transdermal delivery of terbenafine. *PDA J. Pharm. Sci. Technol.* **61**(4), 276–285.

Baboota, S., Shakeel, F., Ahuja, A., Ali, J., and Shafiq, S. (2007b). Design development and evaluation of novel nanoemulsions formulations for transdermal potential of celecoxib. *Acta. Pharm.* **8**, 316–332.

Babua, R. J. and Pandit, J. K. (2005). Effect of penetration enhancers on the release and skin permeation of bupranolol from reservoir-type transdermal delivery systems. *Int. J. Pharm.* **288**, 325–334.

Changez, M., Varshney, M., Chander, J., and Dinda, A. K. (2006). Effect of the composition of lecithin/n-propanol/isopropyl myristate/water microemulsions on barrier properties of mice skin for transdermal permeation of tetracaine hydrochloride: *In vitro*. *Coll. Surf. B.: Biointerf.* **50**, 18–25.

Clarys, P., Alewaeters, K., Jadoul, A., Barel, A., Manadas, R. O., and Préat, V. (1998). *In vitro* percutaneous penetration through hairless rat skin: Influence of temperature, vehicle and penetration enhancers. *Eur. J. Pharm. Biopharm.* **46**, 279–283.

Cole, L. and Heard, C. (2007). Skin permeation enhancement potential of aloe vera and a proposed mechanism of action based upon size exclusion and pull effect. *Int. J. Pharm.* **333**, 10–16.

Constantinides, P. P. (1995). Lipid microemulsions for improving drug dissolution and oral absorption and biopharmaceutical aspects. *Pharm. Res.***12,** 1561–1572.

Cotte, M., Dumas, P., Besnard, M., Tchoreloff, P., and Walter. P. (2004). Synchrotron FT-IR microscopic study of chemical enhancers in transdermal drug delivery: Example of fatty acids. *J. Control. Rel.* **97**, 269–281.

Cullander, P. A. and Guy, R. H. (1991). Sites of iontophoretic current flow into the skin: Identification and characterization with the vibrating probe electrode. *J. Invest. Dermatol.* **97**, 55–64.

Cumming, K. I. and Winfield, A. J. (1994). *In vitro* evaluation of a series of sodium carboxylates as dermal penetration enhancers. *Int. J. Pharm.* **108**, 141–148.

Dreher, F., Walde, R., Walther, R., and Wehrli, E. (1997). Interaction of a lecithin microemulsion gel with human stratum corneum and its effect on transdermal transport. *J. Control. Rel.* **45**, 131–140.

Gaurel, A., Martel, A. M., and Castaner, J. (1997). Celecoxib, anti-inflammatory, cyclo-oxygenase-2 inhibitor. *Drugs Future* **22**, 711–714.

Ghosh, M. N. (2005). *Fundamentals of Experimental Pharmacology*. Hilton and company, Kolkata, p. 192.

Golden, G. M., Guzek, D. B., Harris, R. R., McKie, J. E., and Potts, R. O. (1986). Lipid thermotropic transition in human stratum corneum. *J. Invest. Dermatol.* **86**, 255–259.

Goodman, M. and Barry, B. W. (1989). Action of penetration enhancers on human stratum corneum as assessed by differential scanning calorimetry. In *Percutaneous Absorption,* 2nd edition. R. L. Bronaugh and H. I. Maibach (Eds.). Marcel Dekker, New York and Basel, pp. 567–595.

Jalalizadeh, H., Amini, M., Ziace, V., Farsam, S. A., Shafice, A. (2004). Determination of celecoxib in human plasma by high-performance liquid chromatography. *J. Pharm. Biomed. Anal.* **35**, 665–670.

Karande, P., Jain, A., and Mitragotri, S. (2004). Development of high through screening platforms for discovery of novel transdermal permeation enhancers. *Nat. Biotech.* **22**, 192–197.

Kawakami, K., Yoshikawa, T., Moroto, Y., Kanaoka, E., Takahashi, K., Nishihara, Y., and Masuda, K. (2002a), Microemulsion formulation for enhanced absorption of poorly soluble drugs I.Prescription design. *J. Control. Rel.* **81**, 65–74.

Kawakami, K., Yoshikawa, T., Moroto, Y., Kanaoka, E., Takahashi, K., Nishihara, Y., and Masuda, K. (2002b). Microemulsion formulation for enhanced absorption of poorly soluble drugs II. *In vivo* study. *J. Control. Rel.* **81**, 75–82.

Kommuru, T. R. K., Gurley, B., Khan, M. A., and Reddy, I. K. (2001). Selfemulsifying drug delivery systems (SEDDS) of coenzyme Q10: Formulation development and bioavailability assessment. *Int. J. Pharm.* **212**, 233–246.

Lawrence, M. J. and Rees, G. D. (2000). Microemulsion-based media as novel drug delivery systems. *Adv. Drug Deliv. Rev.* **45**, 89–121.

Lee, P. J., Langer, R., and Shastri, V. P. (2005). Role of n-methyl pyrrolidone in the enhancement of aqueous phase transdermal transport. *J. Pharm. Sci.* **94**, 912–917.

Monti, D., Saettone, M. F., Giannaccini, B., and Galli-Angeli, D. (1995). Enhancement of transdermal penetration of dapiprazole through hairless mouse skin. *J. Control. Rel.* **33**, 71–77.

Narishetty, S. T. K. and Panchagnula, R. (2004). Transdermal delivery of zidovudine: Effect of terpenes and their mechanism of action. *J. Control. Rel.* **95**, 367–379.

Pagano, R. and Thompson, T. E. (1968). Spherical bilayer membranes: Electrical and isotopic studies of ion permeability. *J. Mol. Biol.* **38**, 41–57.

Panchagnula, R., Bokalial, R., Sharma, P., and Khandavilli, S. (2005). Transdermal delivery of naloxone: Skin permeation, pharmacokinetic, irritancy and stability studies. *Int. J. Pharm.* **293**, 213–223.

Panchagnula, R., Salve, P. S., Thomas, N. S., Jain, A. K., and Ramarao, P. (2001). Transdermal delivery of naloxone: Effect of water, propylene glycol, ethanol and their binary combinations on permeation through rat skin. *Int. J. Pharm.* **219**, 95–105.

Shafiq, S., Shakeel, F., Talegaonkar, S., Ahmad, F. J., Khar, R. K., and Ali, M. (2007a). Design and development of oral oil in water ramipril nanoemulsion formulation: *In vitro* and *in vivo* assessment. *J. Biomed. Nanotech.* **3**, 28–44.

Shafiq, S., Shakeel, F., Talegaonkar, S., Ahmad, F. J., Khar, R. K., and Ali, M. (2007b). Development and bioavailability assessment of ramipril nanoemulsion formulation. *Eur. J. Pharm. Biopharm.* **66**, 227–242.

Shafiq, S., Shakeel, F., Talegaonkar, S., Ali, J., Baboota, S., Ahuja, A., Khar, R. K., and Ali, M. (2007c). Formulation development and optimization using nanoemulsion technique: A technical note. *AAPS Pharm. Sci. Tech.* **8**, E28.

Shakeel, F., Baboota, S., Ahuja, A., Ali, J., Aqil, M., and Shafiq, S. (2007a). Nanoemulsions as vehicles for transdermal delivery of aceclofenac. *AAPS Pharm. Sci. Tech.* **8**, E104.

Shakeel, F., Baboota, S., Ahuja, A., Shafiq, S., Faisal, S., and Ali, J. (2007b). Enhanced transdermal delivery of aceclofenac using nanoemulsion technique. *J. Pharm. Pharmacol.* **93**(Suppl 1), 31–37.

Stott, P. W., Williams, A. C., and Barry, B. W. (2001). Mechanistic study into the enhanced transdermal permeation of a model β-blocker, propranolol, by fatty acids: A melting point depression effect. *Int. J. Pharm.* **219**, 161–176.

Vaddi, H. K., Ho, P. C., and Chan, S. Y. (2002). Terpenes in propylene glycol as skin-penetration enhancers: Permeation and partition of haloperidol, fourier transform infrared spectroscopy and differential scanning calorimetry. *J. Pharm. Sci.* **91**, 1639–1651.

Xiong, G. L., Quan, D., and Maibach, H. I. (1996). Effects of penetration enhacers on *in vitro* percutaneous absorption of low molecular weight heparin through human skin. *J. Control. Rel.* **42**, 289–296.

Yamane, M. A., Williams, A. C., and Barry, B. W. (1995). Terpenes penetration enhancers in propylene glycol/water co-solvent systems: Effectiveness and mechanism of action. *J. Pharm. Pharmacol.* **47**, 978–989.

Zhao, K. and Singh, J. (1998). Mechanisms of percutaneous absorption of tamoxifen by terpenes: Eugenol, D-limonene and menthone. *J. Control. Release.* **55**(2–3), 253–264.

12

Bareford, L. M. and Swaan, P. W. (2007). Endocytic mechanisms for targeted drug delivery. *Adv. Drug Deliv. Rev.* **59**, 748–758.

Baumann, M., Kappel, A., Brand, K., Siegfeld, W., and Paterok, E. (1990). The diagnostic validity of the serum tumor marker phosphohexose isomerase (PHI) in patients with gastrointestinal, kidney, and breast cancer. *Cancer Invest.* **8**, 351–356.

Benlimame, N., Le, P. U., and Nabi, I. R. (1998). Localization of autocrine motility factor receptor to caveolae and clathrin-independent internalization of its ligand to smooth endoplasmic reticulum. *Mol. Biol. Cell* **9**, 1773–1786.

Benlimame, N., Simard, D., and Nabi, I. R. (1995) Autocrine motility factor receptor is a marker for a distinct tubular membrane organelle. *J. Cell Biol.* **129**, 459–471.

Bodansky, O. (1954). Serum phosphohexose isomerase in cancer II. As an index of tumor growth in metastatic carcinoma of the breast. *Cancer* **7**, 1200–1226.

Chaput, M., Claes, V., Portetelle, D., Cludts, I., Cravador, A., et al. (1988). The neurotrophic factor neuroleukin is 90% homologous with phosphohexose isomerase. *Nature (Lond.)* **332**, 454–457.

Chiu, C. G., St-Pierre, P., Nabi, I. R., and Wiseman, S. M. (2008). Autocrine motility factor receptor: a clinical review. *Expert review of anticancer therapy* **8**, 207–217.

Faik, P., Walker, J. I. H., Redmill, A. A. M., and Morgan, M. J. (1988). Mouse glucose-6-phosphate isomerase and neuroleukin have identical 3′ sequences. *Nature (Lond)* **332**, 455–457.

Filella, X., Molina, R., Jo, J., Mas, E., and Ballesta, A. M. (1991) Serum phosphohexose isomerase activities in patients with colorectal cancer. *Tumor Biol.* **12**, 360–367.

Funasaka, T., Haga, A., Raz, A., and Nagase, H. (2001). Tumor autocrine motility factor is an angiogenic factor that stimulates endothelial cell motility. *Biochem. Biophys. Res. Comm.* **285**, 118–128.

Funasaka, T., Haga, A., Raz, A., and Nagase, H. (2002). Autocrine motility factor secreted by tumor cells upregulates vascular endothelial growth factor receptor (Flt-1) expression in endothelial cells. *Int. J. Cancer* **101**, 217–223.

Funasaka, T., Hu, H., Hogan, V., and Raz, A. (2007). Down-regulation of phosphoglucose isomerase/autocrine motility factor expression sensitizes human fibrosarcoma cells to oxidative stress leading to cellular senescence. *J. Biol. Chem.* **282**, 36362–36369.

Funasaka, T., Yanagawa, T., Hogan, V., and Raz, A. (2005). Regulation of phosphoglucose isomerase/autocrine motility factor expression by hypoxia. *FASEB J.* **19**, 1422–1430.

Goetz, J. G., Genty, H., St. Pierre P., Dang T., Joshi B., et al. (2007) Reversible interactions between smooth domains of the endoplasmic reticulum and mitochondria are regulated by physiological cytosolic calcium levels. *J. Cell Sci.* **120**, 3553–3564.

Goetz, J. G. and Nabi, I. R. (2006). Interaction of the smooth endoplasmic reticulum and mitochondria. *Biochem. Soc. Trans.* **340**, 370–373.

Guillemard, V. and Saragovi, H. U. (2001). Taxane-antibody conjugates afford potent cytotoxicity, enhanced solubility, and tumor target selectivity. *Cancer Res.* **61**, 694–699.

Guillemard, V. and Saragovi, H. U. (2004). Novel approaches for targeted cancer therapy. *Curr. Cancer Drug Targets* **4**, 313–326.

Guirguis, R., Javadpour, N., Sharareh, S., Biswas, C., el-Amin, W., et al. (1990). A new method for evaluation of urinary autocrine motility factor and tumor cell collagenase stimulating factor as markers for urinary tract cancers. *J. Occup. Med.* **32**, 846–853.

Gurney, M. E., Apatoff, B. R., and Heinrich, S. P. (1986a). Suppression of terminal axonal sprouting at the neuromuscular junction by monoclonal antibodies against a muscle-derived antigen of 56,000 daltons. *J. Cell Biol.* **102**, 2264–2272.

Gurney, M. E., Apatoff, B. R., Spear, G. T., Baumel, M. J., Antel, J. P., et al. (1986b).

Neuroleukin: A lymphokine product of lectin-stimulated T cells. *Science* **234**, 574–581.

Haga, A., Funasaka, T., Niinaka, Y, Raz, A., and Nagase, H. (2003). Autocrine motility factor signaling induces tumor apoptotic resistance by regulations Apaf-1 and Caspase-9 apoptosome expression. *Int. J. Cancer* **107**, 707–714.

Joshi, B., Strugnell, S. S., Goetz, J. G., Kojic, L. D., Cox, M. E., et al. (2008). Phosphorylated caveolin-1 regulates Rho/ROCK-dependent focal adhesion dynamics and tumor cell migration and invasion. *Cancer Res.,* in press.

Kanbe, K., Chigara, M., and Watanabe, H. (1994). Effects of protein kinase inhibitors on the cell motility stimulated by autocrine motility factor. *Biochim. Biophys. Acta.* **1222**, 395–399.

Kirkham, M. and Parton, R. G. (2005). Clathrin-independent endocytosis: New insights into caveolae and non-caveolar lipid raft carriers. Biochimica et Biophysica Acta (BBA). *Mol. Cell Res.* **1745**, 273–286.

Kojic, L. D., Joshi, B., Lajoie, P., Le, P. U., Leung, S., et al. (2007). Raft-dependent endocytosis of autocrine motility factor is phosphatidylinositol-3-kinase-dependent in breast carcinoma cells. *J. Biol. Chem.* **282**, 29305–29313.

Kumar, N. (1981). Taxol-induced polymerization of purified tubulin. Mechanism of action. *J. Biol. Chem.* **256**, 10435–10441.

Lajoie, P. and Nabi, I. R. (2007). Regulation of raft-dependent endocytosis. *J. Cell Mol. Med.* **11**, 644–653.

Le, P. U., Guay, G., Altschuler, Y., and Nabi, I. R. (2002). Caveolin-1 is a negative regulator of caveolae-mediated endocytosis to the endoplasmic reticulum. *J. Biol. Chem.* **277**, 3371–3379.

Le, P. U. and Nabi, I. R. (2003). Distinct caveolae-mediated endocytic pathways target the Golgi apparatus and the endoplasmic reticulum. *J. Cell Sci.* **116**, 1059–1071.

Leclerc, N., Vallée, A., Nabi, I. R. (2000). Expression of the AMF/neuroleukin receptor in developing and adult rat cerebellum. *J. Neurosci. Res.* **60**, 602–612.

Liotta, L. A., Mandler, R., Murano, G., Katz, D. A., Gordon, R. K., et al. (1986). Tumor cell autocrine motility factor. *Proc. Natl. Acad. Sci. USA* **83**, 3302–3306.

Marsh, M. and Helenius, A. (2006). Virus entry: Open sesame. *Cell* **124**, 729–740.

Nabi, I. R. and Raz, A. (1987). Cell shape modulation alters glycosylation of a metastatic melanoma cell surface antigen. *Int. J. Cancer* **40**, 396–401.

Nabi, I. R. and Raz, A. (1988). Loss of metastatic responsiveness to cell shape modulation in a newly characterized B16 melanoma adhesive variant. *Cancer Res.* **48**, 1258–1264.

Nabi, I. R., Watanabe, H., and Raz, A. (1990). Identification of B16-F1 melanoma autocrine motility-like factor receptor. *Cancer Res.* **50**, 409–414.

Niinaka, Y., Paku, S., Haga, A., Watanabe, H., and Raz, A. (1998). Expression and secretion of neuroleukin/phosphohexose isomerase/maturation factor as autocrine motility factor by tumor cells. *Cancer Res.* **58**, 2667–2674.

Patel, P. S., Rawal, G. N., Rawal, R. M., Patel, G. H., Balar, D. B., et al. (1995). Comparison between serum levels of carcinoembryonic antigen, sialic acid, and phosphohexose isomeras in lung cancer. *Neoplasia* **42**, 271–274.

Predescu, S. A., Predescu, D. N., and Malik, A. B. (2007). Molecular determinants of endothelial transcytosis and their role in endothelial permeability. *Am. J. Physiol. Lung Cell. Mol. Physiol.* **293**, L823–842.

Schwartz, M. K. (1973) Enzymes in cancer. *Clin. Chem.* **19**, 10–22.

Silletti, S., Paku, S., and Raz, A. (1996). Tumor autocrine motility factor responses are mediated through cell contact and focal adhesion rearrangement in the absence of new tyrosine phosphorylation in metastatic cells. *Am. J. Pathol.* **148**, 1649–1660.

Silletti, S., Paku, S., and Raz, A. (1998a). Autocrine motility factor and the extracellular matrix. I. Coordinate regulation of melanoma cell adhesion, spreading and migration involves focal contact reorganization. *Int. J. Cancer* **76**, 120–128.

Silletti, S., Paku, S., and Raz, A. (1998b). Autocrine motility factor and the extracellular matrix. II. Degradation or remodeling of substratum components directs the motile response of tumor cells. *Int. J. Cancer* **76**, 129–135.

Sjoblom, T., Jones, S., Wood, L. D., Parsons, D. W., Lin, J., et al. (2006). The consensus coding sequences of human breast and colorectal cancers. *Science* **314**, 268–274.

Tsai, Y. C., Mendoza, A., Mariano, J. M., Zhou, M., Kostova, Z., et al. (2007). The ubiquitin ligase gp78 promotes sarcoma metastasis by targeting KAI1 for degradation. *Nat. Med.* **13**, 1504–1509.

Tsutsumi, S., Gupta, S. K., Hogan, V., Collard, J. G., and Raz, A. (2002). Activation of small GTPase Rho is required for autocrine motility factor signaling. *Cancer Res.* **62**, 4484–4490.

Tsutsumi, S., Hogan, V., Nabi, I. R., and Raz, A. (2003). Overexpression of the autocrine motility factor/phosphoglucose isomerase induces transformation and survival of NIH-3T3 fibroblasts. *Cancer Res.* **63**, 242–249.

Tsutsumi, S., Yanagawa, T., Shimura, T., Kuwano, H., and Raz, A. (2004). Autocrine motility factor signaling enhances pancreatic cancer metastasis. *Clin. Cancer Res.* **10**, 7775–7784.

Wang, H-J., Guay, G., Pogan, L., Sauve, R., and Nabi, I. R. (2000). Calcium regulates the association between mitochondria and a smooth subdomain of the endoplasmic reticulum. *J. Cell Biol.* **150**, 1489–1498.

Watanabe, H., Takehana, K., Date, M., Shinozaki, T., and Raz, A. (1996). Tumor cell autocrine motility factor is the neuroleukin/phosphohexose isomerase polypeptide. *Cancer Res.* **56**, 2960–2963.

Xu, W., Seiter, K., Feldman, E., Ahmed, T., Chiao, J. W. (1996). The differentiation and maturation mediator for human myeloid leukemia cells shares homology with neuroleukin or phosphoglucose isomerase. *Blood* **87**, 4502–4506.

Yanagawa, T., Watanabe, H., Takeuchi, T., Fujimoto, S., Kurihara, H., et al. (2004). Overexpression of autocrine motility factor in metastatic tumor cells: possible association with augmented expression of KIF3A and GDI-beta. *Lab. Invest.* **84**, 513–522.

Yang, J. L., Qu, X. J., Russell, P. J., and Goldstein, D. (2005). Interferon-alpha promotes the anti-proliferative effect of gefitinib (ZD 1839) on human colon cancer cell lines. *Oncology* **69**, 224–238.

13

Arndt, D., Zeisig, R., Bechtel, D., and Fichtner, I. (2001). Liposomal bleomycin: Increased therapeutic activity and decreased pulmonary toxicity in mice. *Drug. Deliv.* **8**, 1–7.

Balakireva, L., Schoehn, G., Thouvenin, E., and Chroboczek, J. (2003). Binding of adenovirus capsid to dipalmitoyl phosphatidylcholine provides a novel pathway for virus entry. *J. Virol.* **77**, 4858–4866.

Berg, K., Dietze, A., Kaalhus, O., and Hogset, A. (2005) Site-specific drug delivery by photochemical internalization enhances the antitumor effect of bleomycin. *Clin. Cancer. Res.* **11** 8476–8485.

Brady, J. N., Winston, V. D., and Consigli, R. A. (1977). Dissociation of polyoma virus by the chelation of calcium ions found associated with purified virions. *J. Virol.* **23**, 717–724.

Chen, J. and Stubbe, J. (2005). Bleomycins: towards better therapeutics. *Nat. Rev. Cancer.* **5**, 102–112.

Chen, P. L., Wang, M., Ou, W. C., Lii, C. K., Chen, L. S., et al. (2001). Disulfide bonds stabilize JC virus capsid-like structure by protecting calcium ions from chelation. *FEBS Lett.* **500**, 109–113.

Cobbold, S. P., Adams, E., Graca, L., Daley, S., Yates, S., et al. (2006). Immune privilege induced by regulatory T cells in transplantation tolerance. *Immunol. Rev.* **213**, 239–255.

Demarcq, C., Bunch, R. T., Creswell, D., and Eastman, A. (1994). The role of cell cycle progression in cisplatin-induced apoptosis in Chinese hamster ovary cells. *Cell Growth Differ.* **5**, 983–993.

Eliceiri, B. P. and Cheresh, D. A. (1999). The role of alphav integrins during angiogenesis: Insights into potential mechanisms of action and clinical development. *J. Clin. Invest.* **103**, 1227–1230.

Fabry, C. M., Rosa-Calatrava, M., Conway, J. F., Zubieta, C., Cusack, S., et al. (2005). A quasi-atomic model of human adenovirus type 5 capsid. *Embo. J.* **24**, 1645–1654.

Fender, P., Boussaid, A., Mezin, P., and Chroboczek, J. (2005). Synthesis, cellular localization, and quantification of penton-dodecahedron in serotype 3 adenovirus-infected cells. *Virology* **340**, 167–173.

Fender, P., Ruigrok, R. W., Gout, E., Buffet, S., and Chroboczek, J. (1997). Adenovirus dodecahedron, a new vector for human gene transfer. *Nat. Biotechnol.* **15**, 52–56.

Fender, P., Schoehn, G., Perron-Sierra, F., Tucker, G. C., and Lortat-Jacob, H. (2008). Adenovirus dodecahedron cell attachment and entry are mediated by heparan sulfate and integrins and vary along the cell cycle. *Virology* **371**, 155–164.

Gabizon, A., Price, D. C., Huberty, J., Bresalier, R. S., and Papahadjopoulos, D. (1990). Effect of liposome composition and other factors on the targeting of liposomes to experimental tumors: Biodistribution and imaging studies. *Cancer. Res.* **50**, 6371–6378.

Gallegos, C. O. and Patton, J. T. (1989). Characterization of rotavirus replication intermediates: A model for the assembly of single-shelled particles. *Virology* **172**, 616–627.

Garcel, A., Gout, E., Timmins, J., Chroboczek J, and Fender, P. (2006). Protein transduction into human cells by adenovirus dodecahedron using WW domains as universal adaptors. *J. Gene. Med.* **8**, 524–531.

Hecht, S. M. (1994). RNA degradation by bleomycin, a naturally occurring bioconjugate. *Bioconjug. Chem.* **5**, 513–526.

Hecht, S. M. (2000). Bleomycin: New perspectives on the mechanism of action. *J. Nat. Prod.* **63**, 158–168.

Horiuchi, A., Nikaido, T., Mitsushita, J., Toki, T., Konishi, I., et al. (2000) Enhancement of antitumor effect of bleomycin by low-voltage *in vivo* electroporation: A study of human uterine leiomyosarcomas in nude mice. *Int. J. Cancer.* **88**, 640–644.

Ishizu, K. I., Watanabe, H., Han, S. I., Kanesashi, S. N., Hoque, M., et al. (2001). Roles of disulfide linkage and calcium ion-mediated interactions in assembly and disassembly of virus-like particles composed of simian virus 40 VP1 capsid protein. *J. Virol.* **75**, 61–72.

Jiang, X., Wang, M., Graham, D. Y., and Estes, M. K. (1992). Expression, self-assembly, and antigenicity of the Norwalk virus capsid protein. *J. Virol.* **66**, 6527–6532.

Kinner, A., Wu, W., Staudt, C., and Iliakis, G. (2008). Gamma-H2AX in recognition and signaling of DNA double-strand breaks in the context of chromatin. *Nucleic. Acids. Res.* **36**, 5678–5694.

Larkin, J. O., Casey, G. D., Tangney, M., Cashman, J., Collins, C. G., et al. (2008). Effective tumor treatment using optimized ultrasound-mediated delivery of bleomycin. *Ultrasound. Med. Biol.* **34**, 406–413.

Lehane, D. E., Hurd, E., and Lane, M. (1975). The effects of bleomycin on immunocompetence in man. *Cancer. Res.* **35**, 2724–2728.

Lenz, P., Day, P. M., Pang, Y. Y., Frye, S. A., Jensen, P. N., et al. (2001). Papillomavirus-like particles induce acute activation of dendritic cells. *J. Immunol.* **166**, 5346–5355.

Li, T. C., Takeda, N., Kato, K., Nilsson, J., Xing, L., et al. (2003). Characterization of self-assembled virus-like particles of human polyomavirus BK generated by recombinant baculoviruses. *Virology* **311**, 115–124.

Lock, R. B., Galperina, O. V., Feldhoff, R. C., and Rhodes, L. J. (1994). Concentration-dependent differences in the mechanisms by which caffeine potentiates etoposide cytotoxicity in HeLa cells. *Cancer. Res.* **54**, 4933–4939.

Lock, R. B. and Stribinskiene, L. (1996). Dual modes of death induced by etoposide in human epithelial tumor cells allow Bcl-2 to inhibit apoptosis without affecting clonogenic survival. *Cancer. Res.* **56**, 4006–4012.

McCarthy, M. P., White, W. I., Palmer-Hill, F., Koenig, S., and Suzich, J. A. (1998). Quantitative disassembly and reassembly of human papillomavirus type 11 viruslike particles *in vitro*. *J. Virol.* **72**, 32–41.

Mir, L. M., Tounekti, O., and Orlowski, S. (1996). Bleomycin: Revival of an old drug. *Gen. Pharmacol.* **27**, 745–748.

Mosmann, T. (1983). Rapid colorimetric assay for cellular growth and survival: Application to proliferation and cytotoxicity assays. *J. Immunol. Meth.* **65**, 55–63.

Noad, R. and Roy, P. (2003). Virus-like particles as immunogens. *Tren. Microbiol.* **11**, 438–444.

Norrby, E. (1968). Comparison of soluble components of adenovirus types 3 and 11. *J. Gen. Virol.* **2**, 135–142.

Pasqualini, R., Koivunen, E., and Ruoslahti, E. (1997). Alpha v integrins as receptors for tumor targeting by circulating ligands. *Nat. Biotechnol.* **15**, 542–546.

Poddevin, B., Orlowski, S., Belehradek, J. Jr., and Mir, L. M. (1991). Very high cytotoxicity of bleomycin introduced into the cytosol of cells in culture. *Biochem. Pharmacol.* **42**(Suppl) S67–75.

Pron, G., Mahrour, N., Orlowski, S., Tounekti, O., Poddevin, B., et al. (1999). Internalisation of the bleomycin molecules responsible for bleomycin toxicity: A receptor-mediated endocytosis mechanism. *Biochem. Pharmacol.* **57**, 45–56.

Puig, P. E., Guilly, M. N., Bouchot, A., Droin, N., Cathelin, D., et al. (2008). Tumor cells can escape DNA-damaging cisplatin through DNA endoreduplication and reversible polyploidy. *Cell Biol. Int.* **32**, 1031–1043.

Rexroad, J., Evans, R. K., and Middaugh, C. R. (2006). Effect of pH and ionic strength on the physical stability of adenovirus type 5. *J. Pharm. Sci.* **95**, 237–247.

Sebti, S. M., Jani, J. P., Mistry, J. S., Gorelik, E., and Lazo. J. S. (1991). Metabolic inactivation: A mechanism of human tumor resistance to bleomycin. *Cancer. Res.* **51**, 227–232.

Sebti, S. M. and Lazo, J. S. (1988). Metabolic inactivation of bleomycin analogs by bleomycin hydrolase. *Pharmacol. Ther.* **38**, 321–329.

Sersa, G., Miklavcic, D., Cemazar, M., Rudolf, Z., Pucihar, G., et al. (2008). Electrochemotherapy in treatment of tumours. *Eur. J. Surg. Oncol.* **34**, 232–240.

Shi, L., Sanyal, G., Ni, A., Luo, Z., Doshna, S., et al. (2005). Stabilization of human papillomavirus virus-like particles by non-ionic surfactants. *J. Pharm. Sci.* **94**, 1538–1551.

Sleijfer, S. (2001). Bleomycin-induced pneumonitis. *Chest.* **120**, 617–624.

Sliwinska, M. A., Mosieniak, G., Wolanin, K., Babik, A., Piwocka, K., et al. (2008). Induction of senescence with doxorubicin leads to increased genomic instability of HCT116 cells. *Mech. Ageing. Dev.*

Song, L., Nakaar, V., Kavita, U., Price, A., Huleatt, J., et al. (2008). Efficacious recombinant influenza vaccines produced by high yield bacterial expression: a solution to global pandemic and seasonal needs. *PLoS ONE* **3**, e2257.

Sonoda, S., Tachibana, K., Uchino, E., Yamashita, T., Sakoda, K., et al. (2007). Inhibition of melanoma by ultrasound-microbubble-aided drug delivery suggests membrane permeabilization. Cancer *Biol. Ther.* **6**, 1276–1283.

Takeshita, M., Grollman, A. P., Ohtsubo, E., and Ohtsubo, H. (1978). Interaction of bleomycin with DNA. *Proc. Natl. Acad. Sci. USA* **75**, 5983–5987.

Vives, R. R., Lortat-Jacob, H., Chroboczek, J., and Fender, P. (2004). Heparan sulfate proteoglycan mediates the selective attachment and internalization of serotype 3 human adenovirus dodecahedron. *Virology* **321**, 332–340.

Wang, C., Liu, J., Pan, W., Wang, X., Gao, Q., et al. (2008). Pingyangmycin loaded bovine serum albumin microspheres for chemoembolization therapy–*in vitro* and *in vivo* studies. *Int. J. Pharm.* **351**, 219–226.

Wickham, T. J., Mathias, P., Cheresh, D. A., and Nemerow, G. R. (1993). Integrins alpha v beta 3 and alpha v beta 5 promote adenovirus internalization but not virus attachment. *Cell* **73**, 309–319.

Yanai, H., Kubota, Y., and Nakada, T. (2002). Effects of electropermeabilization after the administration of anticancer drugs on transitional cell carcinoma. *BJU Int.* **89**, 438–442.

Zubieta, C., Schoehn, G., Chroboczek, J., and Cusack, S. (2005). The structure of the human adenovirus 2 penton. *Mol. Cell.* **17**, 121–135.

14

Aartsma-Rus, A., Bremmer-Bout, M., Janson, A. A., den Dunnen, J. T., van Ommen, G. J., and van Deutekom, J. C. (2002). Targeted exon skipping as a potential gene correction therapy for Duchenne muscular dystrophy. *Neuromuscul. Disord.* **12**(Suppl 1), S71–S77.

Aartsma-Rus, A., Janson, A. A., Kaman, W. E., Bremmer-Bout, M., den Dunnen, J. T., Baas, F., van Ommen, G. J., and van Deutekom, J. C. (2003). Therapeutic antisense-induced exon skipping in cultured muscle cells from six different DMD patients. *Hum. Mol. Genet.* **12**, 907–914.

Aartsma-Rus, A., Janson, A. A., Kaman, W. E., Bremmer-Bout, M., van Ommen, G. J., den Dunnen, J. T., and van Deutekom, J. C. (2004a). Antisense-induced multiexon skipping for Duchenne muscular dystrophy makes more sense. *Am. J. Hum. Genet.* **74**, 83–92.

Aartsma-Rus, A., Janson, A. A., van Ommen, G. J., and van Deutekom, J. C. (2007). Antisense-induced exon skipping for duplications in Duchenne muscular dystrophy. *BMC Med. Genet.* **8**, 43.

Aartsma-Rus, A., Kaman, W. E., Bremmer-Bout, M., Janson, A. A., den Dunnen, J. T., van Ommen, G. J., and van Deutekom, J. C. (2004b). Comparative analysis of antisense oligonucleotide analogs for targeted DMD exon 46 skipping in muscle cells. *Gene Ther.* **11**, 1391–1398.

Aartsma-Rus, A., Kaman, W. E., Weij, R., den Dunnen, J. T., van Ommen, G. J., and van Deutekom, J. C. (2006b). Exploring the frontiers of therapeutic exon skipping for duchenne muscular dystrophy by double targeting within one or multiple exons. *Mol. Ther.* **14**, 401–407.

Aartsma-Rus, A., van Deutekom, J. C., Fokkema, I. F., van Ommen, G. J., and den Dunnen, J. T. (2006a). Entries in the Leiden Duchenne muscular dystrophy mutation database: an overview of mutation types and paradoxical cases that confirm the reading-frame rule. *Muscle Nerve* **34**, 135–144.

Aartsma-Rus, A. and van Ommen, G. J. (2007). Antisense-mediated exon skipping: A versatile tool with therapeutic and research applications. *RNA* **13**, 1609–1624.

Adams, A. M., Harding, P. L., Iversen, P. L., Coleman, C., Fletcher, S., and Wilton, S. D. (2007). Antisense oligonucleotide induced exon skipping and the dystrophin gene transcript: Cocktails and chemistries. *BMC Mol. Biol.* **8**, 5–7.

Akinc, A., Thomas, M., Klibanov, A. M., and Langer, R. (2005). Exploring polyethylenimine-mediated DNA transfection and the proton sponge hypothesis. *J. Gene Med.* **7**, 657–663.

Alter, J., Lou, F., Rabinowitz, A., Yin, H., Rosenfeld, J., Wilton, S. D., Partridge, T. A., and Lu, Q. L. (2006). Systemic delivery of morpholino oligonucleotide restores dystrophin expression bodywide and improves dystrophic pathology. *Nat. Med.* **12**, 175–177.

Bieber, T., Meissner, W., Kostin, S., Niemann, A., and Elsasser, H. P. (2002). Intracellular route and transcriptional competence of polyethylenimine-DNA complexes. *J. Control Release* **82**, 441–454.

Boussif, O., Lezoualc'h, F., Zanta, M. A., Mergny, M. D., Scherman, D., Demeneix, B., and Behr, J. P. (1995). A versatile vector for gene and oligonucleotide transfer into cells in culture and *in vivo*: Polyethylenimine. *Proc. Natl. Acad. Sci. USA* **92**, 7297–7301.

Bremmer-Bout, M., Aartsma-Rus, A., de Meijer, E. J., Kaman, W. E., Janson, A. A., Vossen, R. H., van Ommen, G. J., den Dunnen, J. T., and van Deutekom, J. C. (2004). Targeted exon skipping in transgenic hDMD mice: A model for direct preclinical screening of human-specific antisense oligonucleotides. *Mol. Ther.* **10**, 232–240.

Brus, C., Petersen, H., Aigner, A., Czubayko, F., and Kissel, T. (2004). Physicochemical and biological characterization of polyethylenimine-graft-poly(ethylene glycol) block copolymers as a delivery system for oligonucleotides and ribozymes. *Bioconjug. Chem.* **15**, 677–684.

Fischer, D., Osburg, B., Petersen, H., Kissel, T., and Bickel, U. (2004). Effect of poly(ethylene imine) molecular weight and pegylation on organ distribution and pharmacokinetics of polyplexes with oligodeoxynucleotides in mice. *Drug Metab. Dispos.* **32**, 983–992.

Fletcher, S., Honeyman, K., Fall, A. M., Harding, P. L., Johnsen, R. D., Steinhaus, J. P., Moulton, H. M., Iversen, P. L., and Wilton, S. D. (2007). Morpholino oligomer-mediated exon skipping averts the onset of dystrophic pathology in the mdx Mouse. *Mol. Ther.* **15**(9), 1587–1592.

Fletcher, S., Honeyman, K., Fall, A. M., Harding, P. L., Johnsen, R. D., and Wilton, S. D. (2005). Dystrophin expression in the mdx mouse after localised and systemic administration of a morpholino antisense oligonucleotide. *J. Gene. Med.* **8**(2), 207–216.

Foster, K., Foster, H., and Dickson, J. G. (2006). Gene therapy progress and prospects: Duchenne muscular dystrophy. *Gene Ther.* **13**, 1677–1685.

Garcia-Blanco, M. A., Baraniak, A. P., and Lasda, E. L. (2004). Alternative splicing in disease and therapy. *Nat. Biotechnol.* **22**, 535–546.

Gebski, B. L., Mann, C. J., Fletcher, S., and Wilton, S. D. (2003). Morpholino antisense oligonucleotide induced dystrophin exon 23 skipping in mdx mouse muscle. *Hum. Mol. Genet.* **12**, 1801–1811.

Glodde, M., Sirsi, S. R., and Lutz, G. J. (2006). Physiochemical properties of low and high molecular weight PEG-grafted Poly(ethylene imine) copolymers and their complexes with oligonucleotides. *Biomacromolecules* **7**(1), 347–356.

Godbey, W. T., Wu. K. K., and Mikos, A. G. (1999). Tracking the intracellular path of poly(ethylenimine)/DNA complexes for gene delivery. *Proc. Natl. Acad. Sci. USA* **96**, 5177–5181.

Hainfeld, J. F. and Powell, R. D. (2000). New frontiers in gold labeling. *J. Histochem. Cytochem.* **48**, 471–480.

Jeong, J. H., Kim, S. W., and Park, T. G. (2003). A new antisense oligonucleotide delivery system based on self-assembled ODN-PEG hybrid conjugate micelles. *J. Control Release* **93**, 183–191.

Kichler, A. (2004). Gene transfer with modified polyethylenimines. *J. Gene Med.* **6**(Suppl 1), S3–S10.

Kole, R., Williams, T., and Cohen, L. (2004). RNA modulation, repair and remodeling by splice switching oligonucleotides. *Acta. Biochim. Pol.* **51**, 373–378.

Kunath, K., von, H. A., Petersen, H., Fischer, D., Voigt, K., Kissel, T., and Bickel, U. (2004). The structure of PEG-modified poly(ethylene imines) influences biodistribution and pharmacokinetics of their complexes with NF-kappaB decoy in mice. *Pharm. Res.* **19**, 810–817.

Lu, Q. L., Bou-Gharios, G., and Partridge, T. A. (2003a). Non-viral gene delivery in skeletal muscle: a protein factory. *Gene Ther.* **10**, 131–142.

Lu, Q. L., Liang, H. D., Partridge, T., and Blomley, M. J. (2003b). Microbubble ultrasound improves the efficiency of gene transduction in skeletal muscle *in vivo* with reduced tissue damage. *Gene Ther.* **10**, 396–405.

Lu, Q. L., Mann, C. J., Lou, F., Bou-Gharios, G., Morris, G. E., Xue, S. A., Fletcher, S., Partridge, T. A., and Wilton, S. D. (2003c). Functional amounts of dystrophin produced by skipping the mutated exon in the mdx dystrophic mouse. *Nat. Med.* **9**, 1009–1014.

Lu, Q. L., Rabinowitz, A., Chen, Y. C., Yokota, T., Yin, H., Alter, J., Jadoon, A., Bou-Gharios, G., and Partridge, T. (2005). From the Cover: Systemic delivery of antisense oligoribonucleotide restores dystrophin expression in body-wide skeletal muscles. *Proc. Natl. Acad. Sci. USA* **102**, 198–203.

Lutz, G. J., Sirsi, S. R., and Williams, J. H. (2007). PEG-PEI copolymers for oligonucleotide delivery to cells and tissues. In *Methods in Molecular Biology*, Vol. 9. 433(1) edition. J. M. Ledoux (Ed.). Humana Press, pp. 141–158.

Mann, C. J., Honeyman, K., Cheng, A. J., Ly, T., Lloyd, F., Fletcher, S., Morgan, J. E., Partridge, T. A., and Wilton, S. D. (2001). Antisense-induced exon skipping and synthesis of dystrophin in the mdx mouse. *Proc. Natl. Acad. Sci. USA* **98**, 42–47.

Mann, C. J., Honeyman, K., McClorey, G., Fletcher, S., and Wilton, S. D. (2002). Improved antisense oligonucleotide induced exon skipping in the mdx mouse model of muscular dystrophy. *J. Gene Med.* **4**, 644–654.

McClorey, G., Moulton, H. M., Iversen, P. L., Fletcher, S., and Wilton, S. D. (2006). Antisense oligonucleotide-induced exon skipping restores dystrophin expression *in vitro* in a canine model of DMD. *Gene. Ther.* **13**, 1373–1381.

Moulton, H. M., Fletcher, S., Neuman, B. W., McClorey, G., Stein, D. A., Abes, S., Wilton, S. D., Buchmeier, M. J., Lebleu, B., and Iversen, P. L. (2007). Cell-penetrating peptide-morpholino conjugates alter pre-mRNA splicing of DMD (Duchenne muscular dystrophy) and inhibit murine coronavirus replication *in vivo*. *Biochem. Soc. Trans.* **35**, 826–828.

Noh, S. M., Kim, W. K., Kim, S. J., Kim, J. M., Baek, K. H., and Oh, Y. K. (2007). Enhanced cellular delivery and transfection efficiency of plasmid DNA using positively charged biocompatible colloidal gold nanoparticles. *Biochim. Biophys. Acta.* **1770**, 747–752.

Petersen, H., Fechner, P. M., Fischer, D., and Kissel, T. (2002b). Synthesis, Characterization, and biocompatibility of polyethylenimine-graft-poly(ethylene glycol) block copolymers. *Macromolecules* **35**, 6867–6874.

Petersen, H., Fechner, P. M., Martin, A. L., Kunath, K., Stolnik, S., Roberts, C. J., Fischer, D., Davies, M. C., and Kissel, T. (2002a). Polyethylenimine-graft-poly(ethylene glycol) copolymers: Influence of copolymer block structure on DNA complexation and biological activities as gene delivery system. *Bioconjug. Chem.* **13**, 845–854.

Phelps, S. F., Hauser, M. A., Cole, N. M., Rafael, J. A., Hinkle, R. T., Faulkner, J. A., and Chamberlain, J. S. (1995). Expression of full-length and truncated dystrophin mini-genes in transgenic mdx mice. *Hum. Mol. Genet.* **4**, 1251–1258.

Schiffelers, R. M., Ansari, A., Xu, J., Zhou, Q., Tang, Q., Storm, G., Molema, G., Lu, P. Y., Scaria, P. V., and Woodle, M. C. (2004). Cancer siRNA therapy by tumor selective delivery with ligand-targeted sterically stabilized nanoparticle. *Nucleic Acids Res.* **32**, e149.

Shukla, R., Bansal, V., Chaudhary, M., Basu, A., Bhonde, R. R., and Sastry, M. (2005). Biocompatibility of gold nanoparticles and their endocytotic fate inside the cellular compartment: A microscopic overview. *Langmuir* **21**, 10644–10654.

Sirsi, S. R., Williams, J., and Lutz, G. J. (2005). Poly(ethylene imine)-polyethylene glycol copolymers facilitate efficient delivery of antisense oligonucleotides to nuclei of mature muscle cells of mdx mice. *Hum. Gene Ther.* **16**(11), 1307–1317.

Sonawane, N. D., Szoka, F. C. Jr., and Verkman, A. S. (2003). Chloride accumulation and swelling in endosomes enhances DNA transfer by polyamine-DNA polyplexes. *J. Biol. Chem.* **278**, 44826–44831.

Suh, J., Wirtz, D., and Hanes, J. (2003). Efficient active transport of gene nanocarriers to the cell nucleus. *Proc. Natl. Acad. Sci. USA* **100**, 3878–3882.

Sung, S. J., Min, S. H., Cho, K. Y., Lee, S., Min, Y. J., Yeom, Y. I., and Park, J. K. (2003). Effect of polyethylene glycol on gene delivery of polyethylenimine. *Biol. Pharm. Bull.* **26**, 492–500.

Thomas, M. and Klibanov, A. M. (2002). Enhancing polyethylenimine's delivery of plasmid DNA into mammalian cells. *Proc. Natl. Acad. Sci. USA* **99**, 14640–14645.

Thomas, M. and Klibanov, A. M. (2003a). Conjugation to gold nanoparticles enhances polyethylenimine's transfer of plasmid DNA into mammalian cells. *Proc. Natl. Acad. Sci. USA* **100**, 9138–9143.

Thomas, M. and Klibanov, A. M. (2003b). Nonviral gene therapy: Polycation-mediated DNA delivery. *Appl. Microbiol. Biotechnol.* **62**, 27–34.

Vinogradov, S., Batrakova, E., Li, S., and Kabanov, A. (1999). Polyion complex micelles with protein-modified corona for receptor-mediated delivery of oligonucleotides into cells. *Bioconjug. Chem.* **10**, 851–860.

Vinogradov, S. V., Batrakova, E. V., and Kabanov, A. V. (2003). Nanogels for oligonucleotide delivery to the brain. *Bioconjug. Chem.* **15**, 50–60.

Vinogradov, S. V., Bronich, T. K., and Kabanov, A. V. (1998). Self-assembly of polyamine-poly(ethylene glycol) copolymers with phosphorothioate oligonucleotides. *Bioconjug. Chem.* **9**, 805–812.

Wells, D. J., Wells, K. E., Asante, E. A., Turner, G., Sunada, Y., Campbell, K. P., Walsh, F. S., and Dickson, G. (1995). Expression of human full-length and minidystrophin in transgenic mdx mice: Implications for gene therapy of Duchenne muscular dystrophy. *Hum. Mol. Genet.* **4**, 1245–1250.

Wells, K. E., Fletcher, S., Mann, C. J., Wilton, S. D., and Wells, D. J. (2003). Enhanced *in vivo* delivery of antisense oligonucleotides to restore dystrophin expression in adult mdx mouse muscle. *FEBS Lett.* **552**, 145–149.

Wells, K. E., Torelli, S., Lu, Q., Brown, S. C., Partridge, T., Muntoni, F., and Wells, D. J. (2003). Relocalization of neuronal nitric oxide synthase (nNOS) as a marker for complete restoration of the dystrophin associated protein complex in skeletal muscle. *Neuromuscul. Disord.* **13**, 21–31.

Williams, J. H., Sirsi, S. R., Latta, D., and Lutz, G. J. (2006). Induction of dystrophin expression by exon skipping in mdx mice following intramuscular injection of antisense oligonucleotides complexed with PEG-PEI copolymers. *Mol. Ther.* **14**(1), 88–96.

Wilton, S. D. and Fletcher, S. (2006). Modification of pre-mRNA processing: Application to dystrophin expression. *Curr. Opin. Mol. Ther.* **8**, 131–135.

Wilton, S. D., Lloyd, F., Carville, K., Fletcher, S., Honeyman, K., Agrawal, S., and Kole, R. (1999). Specific removal of the nonsense mutation from the mdx dystrophin mRNA using antisense oligonucleotides. *Neuromuscul. Disord.* **9**, 330–338.

15

Bea, S. J., Suh, J. M., Sohn, Y. S., Bae, Y. H., Kim, S. W., and Jeong, B. (2005). Thermogelling poly(caprolactone-b-ethylene glycol-b-caprolactone) aqueous solutions. *Macromolecules* **38**, 5260–5265.

Bromberg, L. E. and Ron, E.S. (1998). Temperature-responsive gels and thermogelling polymer matrices for protein and peptide delivery. *Adv. Drug Deliver. Rev.* **31**, 197–221.

Chen, L. J., Zhang, Q., Yang, G. L., Fan, L. Y., Tang, J., Garrard, I., Ignatova, S., Fisher, D., and Sutherland, I. (2007). Rapid purification and scale-up of honokiol and magnolol using high-capacity high-speed counter-current chromatography. *J. Chromatogr. A.* **1142**, 115–122.

Chen, X., Qian, Z. Y., Gou, M. L., Chao, G. T., Zhang, Y. D., Gu, Y. C., Huang, M. J., Wang, J. W., Pan, Y. F., Wei, Y. Q., Chen, J. P., and Tu, M. J. (2008).Acute oral toxicity evaluation of biodegradable and pH-sensitive hydrogel based on polycaprolactone, poly(ethylene glycol) and methylacrylic acid (MAA). *J. Biomed. Mater. Res. A.* **84**(3), 589–597.

Choi, S. W., Choi, S. Y., Jeong, B., Kim, S. W., and Lee, D. S. (1999). Thermoreversible gelation of poly(ethylene oxide) biodegradable polyester block copolymers. II. *J. Polym. Sci., Part A. Polym. Chem.* **37**, 2207–2218.

Chung, Y. M., Simmons, K. L., Gutowska, A., and Jeong, B. (2002). Sol-gel transition temperature of PLGA-g-PEG aqueous solutions. *Biomacromolecules* **3**, 511–516.

Dimitrov, I., Trzebicka, B., Muller, A. H., Dworak, A., and Tsvetamov, C. B. (2007). Thermosensitive water-soluble copolymers with doubly responsive reversibly interacting entities. *Prog. Polym. Sci.* **32**, 1275–1343.

Gariépy, E. R. and Leroux, J. C. (2004). *In situ*-forming hydrogels–review of temperature-sensitive systems. *Eur. J. Pharm. Biopharm.* **58**, 409–426.

Gilbert, J. C., Richardson, J. L., Davies, M. C., Palin, K. J., and Hadgraft J. (1987). The effect of solutes and polymers on the gelation properties of pluronic F-127 Solutions for controlled drug delivery. *J. Control Release* **5**, 113–118.

Gong, C. Y., Qian, Z. Y., Liu, C. B., Huang, M. J., Gu, Y. C., Wen, Y. J., Kan, B., Wang, K., Dai, M., Li, X. Y., Gou, M. L., Tu, M. J., and Wei, Y. Q. (2007). A thermosensitive hydrogel based on biodegradable amphiphilic poly(ethylene glycol)-polycaprolactone-poly(ethylene glycol) block copolymers. *Smart Mater. Struct.* **16**, 927–933.

Gong, C. Y., Shi, S., Dong, P. W., Gou, M. L., Li, X. Y., Wei, Y. Q., and Qian, Z. Y. (2009). A Novel thermosensitive composite hydrogel based on poly(ethylene glycol)-poly(ε-caprolactone)-poly(ethylene glycol) (PECE) copolymer and Pluronic F127. In *Amphiphilic Block Copolymers: Theory, Self-Assembly and Applications.* Frank Columbus (Ed.). Nova Science Publishers, in press.

Gong, C. Y., Shi, S., Dong, P. W., Kan, B., Gou, M. L., Wang, X. H., Chen, L. J., Zhao, X., Wei, Y. Q., and Qian, Z. Y. (2009). Synthesis, characterization, degradation, and *in vitro* Drug release behavior of thermosensitive hydrogel based on PEG-PCL-PEG block copolymers. *Int. J. Pharm.* **365**(1–2), 89–99.

Gou, M. L., Dai, M., Li, X. Y., Wang, X. H., Gong, C. Y., Xie, Y., Wang, K., Zhao, X., Qian, Z. Y., and Wei, Y. Q. (2008). Preparation and characterization of honokiol nanoparticles. *J. Mater. Sci.: Mater. Med.* **19**, 2605–2608.

Hatefi, A. and Amsden, B. (2002). Biodegradable injectable *in situ* forming drug delivery systems. *J. Control Rel.* **80**, 9–28.

Iza, M., Stoianovici, G., Viora, L., Grossiord, J. L., and Couarraze, G. (1998). Hydrogels of poly(ethylene glycol): Mechanical characterization and release of a model drug. *J. Control Rel.* **52**, 41–51.

Jemal, A., Siegel, E., Ward, E., Hao, Y., Xu J., Murray, T., and Thun, M. J. (2008). Cancer statistics. CA. *Cancer J. Clin.* **58**, 71–96.

Jeong, B., Bae, Y. H., Lee, D.S., and Kim, S.W. (1997). Biodegradable block copolymers as injectable drug-delivery systems. *Nature* **388**, 860–862.

Jeong, B., Kim, S.W., and Bae, Y. H. (2002). Thermosensitive sol-gel reversible hydrogels. *Adv. Drug Deliver. Rev.* **54**, 37–51.

Kamath, K. R. and Park, K. (1993). Biodegradable hydrogels in drug delivery. *Adv. Drug Deliv. Rev.* 11:59–84.

Kissel, T., Li, Y., and Unger, F. (2002). ABA-triblock copolymers from biodegradable polyester A-blocks and hydrophilic poly(ethylene oxide) B-blocks as a candidate for *in situ* forming hydrogel delivery systems for proteins. *Adv. Drug Deliver. Rev.* **54**, 99–134.

Lee, K. Y. and Mooney, D. J. (2001). Hydrogels for tissue engineering. *Chem. Rev.*, **101**, 1869–1879

Li, J., Li, X., Ni, X., and Leong, K. W. (2003). Synthesis and characterization of new biodegradable amphiphilic poly(ethylene oxide)-b-poly[(R)-3-hydroxybutyrate]-b-poly(ethylene oxide) triblock copolymers. *Macromolecules* **36**, 2661–2667.

Li, J., Li, X., Ni, X., Wang, X., Li, H., and Leong, K. W. (2006). Self-assembled supramolecular hydrogels formed by biodegradable PEO-PHB-PEO triblock copolymers and cyclodextrin for controlled drug delivery. *Biomaterials* **27**, 4132–4140.

Li, J., Ni, X., and Leong, K. W. (2003). Injectable drug-delivery systems based on supramolecular hydrogels formed by poly(ethylene oxide)s and cyclodextrin. *J. Biomed Mater. Res., Part A* **65**, 196–202.

Li, Z., Ning, W., Wand, J., Choi, A., Lee, P. Y., Tyagi, P., and Huang, L. (2003). Controlled gene delivery system based on thermosensitive biodegradable hydrogel. *Pharm. Res.* **20**, 884–888.

Liu, C. B., Gong, C. Y., Huang, M. J., Wang, J. W., Pan, Y. F., Zhang, Y. D., Li, G. Z., Gou, M. L., Wang, K., Tu, M. J., Wei, Y. Q., and Qian, Z. Y. (2008). Thermoreversible gel-sol behavior of biodegradable PCL-PEG-PCL triblock copolymer in aqueous solutions. *J. Biomed. Mater. Res. B. Appl. Biomater.* **84**(1), 165–175.

Liu, C. B., Gong, C. Y., Pan, Y. F., Zhang, Y. D., Wang, J. W., Huang, M. J., Wang, Y. S., Wang, K., Gou, M. L., Tu, M. J., Wei, Y. Q., and Qian, Z. Y. (2007). Synthesis and characterization of a thermosensitive hydrogel based on biodegradable amphiphilic PCL-Pluronic(L35)-PCL block copolymers. *Colloids Surfaces A*. **302**, 430–438.

Miyta, T., Asami, N., and Uragami, T. (1999). A reversibly antigen-responsive hydrogel. *Nature* **399**, 766–769.

Nanjawade, B. K., Manvi, F. V., and Manjappa, A. S. (2007). *In situ*-forming hydrogels for sustained ophthalmic drug delivery. *J. Control Rel.* **122**, 119–134.

Qiu, Y. and Park, K. (2001). Environment-sensitive hydrogels for drug delivery. *Adv. Drug Deliver Rev.* **51**, 321–339.

Rangelov, S., Dimitrov, P., and Tsvetanov, C. B. (2005). Mixed block copolymer aggregates with tunable temperature behavior. *J. Phys. Chem. B.* **109**, 1162–1167.

Suzuki, A. and Tanaka, T. (1990). Phase transition in polymer gels induced by visible-light. *Nature* **346**, 345–347.

Xiong, X. Y., Tam, K. C., and Gan, L. H. (2003). Synthesis and aggregation behavior of Pluronic F127/Poly(lactic acid) block copolymers in aqueous solutions. *Macromolecules* **36**, 9979–9985.

Zhou, S. B., Deng, X. M., and Yang, H. (2003). Biodegradable poly(ε-caprolactone)-poly(ethylene glycol) block copolymers: Characterization and their use as drug carriers for a controlled delivery system. *Biomaterials* **24**, 3563–3570.

16

Athanasopoulos, T., Owen, J. S., Hassall, D., Dunckley, M. G., Drew, J., Goodman, J., Tagalakis, A. D., Riddell, D. R., and Dickson, G. (2000). Intramuscular injection of a plasmid vector expressing human apolipoprotein E limits progression of xanthoma and aortic atheroma in apoE-deficient mice. *Hum. Mol. Genet.* **9**, 2545–2551.

Bales, K. R., Dodart, J. C., DeMattos, R. B., Holtzman, D. M., and Paul, S. M. (2002). Apolipoprotein E, amyloid, and alzheimer disease. *Mol. Inter.* **2**(6), 363–375.

Bannwarth, B., Schaeverbeke, T., Péhourcq, F., Vernhes, J. P., D'Yvoire, M. B., and Dehais, J. (1997). Prednisolone concentrations in cerebrospinal fluid after oral prednisone. Preliminary data. *Rev. Rhum. Engl. Ed.* **64**, 301–304.

Birmingham, M. K., Sar, M., and Stumpf, W. E. (1984). Localization of aldosterone and corticosterone in the central nervous system, assessed by quantitative autoradiography. *Neurochem. Res.* **9**, 333–350.

Boisvert, W. A., Spangenberg, J., and Curtiss, L. K. (1995). Treatment of severe hypercholesterolemia in apolipoprotein E-deficient mice by bone marrow transplantation. *J. Clin. Invest.* **96**, 1118–1124.

Cedazo-Minguez, A. (2007). Apolipoprotein E and Alzheimer's disease: Molecular mechanisms and therapeutic opportunities. *J. Cell Mol. Med.* **11**(6), 1227–1238.

Czock, D., Keller, F., Rasche, F. M., and Häussler, U. (2005). Pharmacokinetics and pharmacodynamics of systemically administered glucocorticoids. *Clin. Pharmacokinet.* **44**, 61–98.

Deng, J., Petersen, B. E., Steindler, D. A., Jorgensen, M. L., and Laywell, E. D. (2006). Mesenchymal stem cells spontaneously express neural proteins in culture and are neurogenic after transplantation. *Stem. Cells* **24**, 1054–1064.

Desai, B. S., Monahan, A. J., Carvey, P. M., and Hendey, B. (2007). Blood-brain barrier pathology in Alzheimer's and Parkinson's disease: Implications for drug therapy. *Cell Transplant* **16**, 285–299.

Dodart, J. C., Marr, R. A., Koistinaho, M., Gregersen, B. M., Malkani, S., Verma, I. M., and Paul, S. M. (2005). Gene delivery of human apolipoprotein E alters brain Abeta burden in mouse model of Alzheimer's disease. *Proc. Natl. Acad. Sci.* **102**(4), 1211–1216.

Donahue, J. E. and Johanson, C. E. (2008). Apolipoprotein E, amyloid-beta, and blood-brain barrier permeability in Alzheimer disease. *J. Neuropathol. Exp. Neurol.* **67**, 261–270.

Friedenstein, A. J., Chailakhyan, R. K., and Gerasimov, U. V. (1987). Bone marrow osteogenic stem cells: *In vitro* cultivation and transplantation in diffusion chambers. *Cell Tissue Kinet* **20**, 263–272.

Friedenstein, A. J., Chailakhjan, R. K., and Lalykina, K. S. (1970). The development of fibroblast colonies in monolayer cultures of guinea-pig bone marrow and spleen cells. *Cell Tissue Kinet* **3**, 393–403.

Friedenstein, A. J., Chailakhyan, R. K., Latsinik, N. V., Panasyuk, A. F., and Keiliss-Borok, I. V. (1974a). Stromal cells responsible for transferring the microenvironment of the hemopoietic tissues. Cloning *in vitro* and retransplantation *in vivo*. *Transplantation* **17**, 331–340.

Friedenstein, A. J., Deriglasova, U. F., Kulagina, N. N., Panasuk, A. F., Rudakowa, S. F., Luria, E. A., and Ruadkow, I. A. (1974b). Precursors for fibroblasts in different populations of hematopoietic cells as detected by the *in vitro* colony assay method. *Exp. Hematol.* **2**, 83–92.

Gough, P. J. and Raines, E. W. (2003). Gene therapy of apolipoprotein E-deficient mice using a novel macrophage-specific retroviral vector. *Blood* **101**, 485–491.

Gregory, C. A. and Prockop, D. J. (2007). Fundamentals of culture and characterization of mesenchymal stem cells from bone marrow stroma. In *Culture of Human Stem Cells*. R. I. Freshney, G. N. Stacey, and J. M. Auerbach (Eds.). Wiley-Liss, New Jersey, pp. 207–232.

Gregory, C. A., Prockop, D. J., and Spees, J. L. (2005). Non-hematopoietic bone marrow stem cells: Molecular control of expansion and differentiation. *Exp. Cell Res.* **306**, 330–335.

Gregory, C. A., Reyes, E., Whitney, M. J., and Spees, J. L. (2006). Enhanced engraftment of mesenchymal stem cells in a cutaneous wound model by culture in allogenic species specific serum and administration in fibrin constructs. *Stem. Cells* **24**, 2232–2243.

Gregory, C. A., Singh, H., Perry, A. S., and Prockop, D. J. (2003). Dkk-1 is required for re-entry into the cell cycle of human adult stem cells from bone marrow stroma (hMSCs). *J. Biol. Chem.* **278**, 28067–28078.

Gretch, D. G., Sturley, S. L., Friesen, P. D., Beckage, N. E., and Attie, A. D. (1991). Baculovirus-mediated expression of human apolipoprotein E in Manduca sexta larvae generates particles that bind to the low density lipoprotein receptor. *Proc. Natl. Acad. Sci. USA* **88**, 8530–8533.

Harris, J. D., Evans, V., and Owen, J. S. (2006). ApoE gene therapy to treat hyperlipidemia and atherosclerosis. *Curr. Opin. Mol. Ther.* **8**, 275–287.

Hasty, A. H., Linton, M. F., Brandt, S. J., Babaev, V. R., Gleaves, L. A., and Fazio, S. (1999). Retroviral gene therapy in ApoE-deficient mice: ApoE expression in the artery wall reduces early foam cell lesion formation. *Circulation* **99**, 2571–2576.

Hatters, D. M., Peters-Libeu, C. A., and Weisgraber, K. H. (2006). Apolipoprotein E structure: Insights into function. *TRENDS Biochem. Sci.* **31**(8), 445–454.

Haynesworth, S. E., Baber, M. A., and Caplan, A. I. (1992a). Cell surface antigens on human marrow-derived mesenchymal cells are detected by monoclonal antibodies. *Bone* **13**, 69–80.

Haynesworth, S. E., Goshima, J., Goldberg, V. M., and Caplan, A. I. (1992b). Characterization of cells with osteogenic potential from human marrow. *Bone* **13**, 81–88.

Hernandez-Nazara, Z. H., Ruiz-Madrigal, B., Martinez-Lopez, E., Roman, S., and Panduro, A. (in press). Association of the Epsilon2 Allele of Apoe Gene to hypertriglyceridemia and to early-onset alcoholic cirrhosis. *Alcohol. Cli. Exp. Res.*

Horejsi, B. and Ceska, R. (2000). Apolipoproteins and atherosclerosis. apolipoprotein E and apolipoprotein(a) as candidate genes of premature development of atherosclerosis. *Physiol. Res.* **49**(Suppl 1), S63–S69.

Isakova, I. A., Baker, K., DuTreil, M., Dufour, J., Gaupp, D., and Phinney, D. G. (2007). Age- and dose-related effects on MSC engraftment levels and anatomical distribution in the central nervous systems of nonhuman primates: Identification of novel MSC subpopulations that respond to guidance cues in brain. *Stem. Cells* **25**, 3261–3270.

Joëls, M. (1997). Steroid hormones and excitability in the mammalian brain. *Front. Neuroendocrinol.* **18**, 42–48.

Kantarci, O. H. (2008). Genetics and natural history of multiple sclerosis. *Semin. Neurol.* **28**(1), 7–16.

Kashyap, V. S., Santamarina-Fojo, S., Brown, D. R., Parrott, C. L., Applebaum-Bowden, D., Meyn, S., Talley, G., Paigen, B., Maeda, N., and Brewer, H. B. Jr. (1995). Apolipoprotein E deficiency in mice: Gene replacement and prevention of atherosclerosis using adenovirus vectors. *J. Clin. Invest.* **96**, 1612–1620.

Kopen, G. C., Prockop, D. J., and Phinney, D. G. (1999). Marrow stromal cells migrate throughout forebrain and cerebellum, and they differentiate into astrocytes after injection into neonatal mouse brains. *Proc. Natl. Acad. Sci. USA* **96**, 10711–10716.

Lei, P., Wu, W. H., Li, R. W., Ma, J. W., Yu, Y. O., Cui, W., Zhao, Y. F., and Li, Y. M. (2008). Prevention and promotion effects of apolipoprotein E4 on amylin aggregation. *Biochem. Biophys. Res. Commun.* **368**(2), 414–418.

Lin, R. C. (1988). Effects of Hormones on apolipoprotein secretion in cultured rat hepatocytes. *Metabolism* **37**(8), 745–751.

Lusis, J. A., Fogelman, A. M., and Fonarow, G. C. (2004). Genetic basis of atherosclerosis: Part I, new gene and pathways. *Circulation* **110**, 1868–1873.

Mahley, R. W. (1988). Apolipoprotein E: Cholesterol transport proetin with expanding role in cell biology. *Science* **240**, 622–629.

Martin-Sanz, P., Vance, J. E., and Brindley, D. N. (1990). Stimulation of apolipoprotein secretion in very-low-density and high-density lipoproteins from cultured rat hepatocytes by dexamethasone. *Biochem. J.* **271**, 575–583.

McColl, B. W., McGregor, A. L., Wong, A., Harris, J. D., Amalfitano, A., Magnoni, S., Baker, A. H., Dickson, G., and Horsburgh, K. (2007). APOE epsilon3 gene transfer attenuates brain damage after experimental stroke. *J. Cereb. Blood Flow Metab.* **27**, 477–487.

Meijer, O. C., de Lange, E. C., Breimer, D. D., de Boer, A. G., Workel, J. O., and de Kloet, E. R.

(1998). Penetration of dexamethasone into brain glucocorticoid targets is enhanced in mdr1A P-glycoprotein knockout mice. *Endocrinology* **139**, 1789–1793.

Munoz, J. R., Stoutenger, B. R., Robinson, A. P., Spees, J. L., and Prockop, D. J. (2005). Human stem/progenitor cells from bone marrow promote neurogenesis of endogenous neural stem cells in the hippocampus of mice. *Proc. Natl. Acad. Sci. USA* **102**, 18171–18176.

Owen, M. and Friedenstein, A. J. (1988). Stromal stem cells: Marrow-derived osteogenic precursors. *Ciba. Found. Symp.* **136**, 42–60.

Peister, A., Zeitouni, S., Pfankuch, T., Reger, R. L., Prockop, D. J., and Raber, J. (2006). Novel object recognition in Apoe-/- mice improved by neonatal implantation of wild-type multipotential stromal cells. *Exp. Neurol.* **201**, 266–269.

Peskind, E. R., Wilkinson, C. W., Petrie, E. C., Schellenberg, G. D., and Raskind, M. A. (2001). Increased CSF cortisol in AD is a function of APOE genotype. *Neurology* **56**, 1094–1098.

Phinney, D. G., Baddoo, M., Dutreil, M., Gaupp, D., Lai, W. T., and Isakova, I. A. (2006). Murine mesenchymal stem cells transplanted to the central nervous system of neonatal versus adult mice exhibit distinct engraftment kinetics and express receptors that guide neuronal cell migration. *Stem Cells Dev.* **15**, 437–447.

Pluta, R. (2006). Is the ischemic blood-brain barrier insufficiency responsible for full-blown Alzheimer's disease? *Neurol. Res.* **28**, 665–671.

Prockop, D. J. (1997). Marrow stromal cells as stem cells for nonhematopoietic tissues. *Science* **276**, 71–74.

Prockop, D. J., Gregory, C. A., and Spees, J. L. (2003). One strategy for cell and gene therapy: Harnessing the power of adult stem cells to repair tissues. *PNAS* **100**(Suppl 1), 11917–11923.

Rinaldi, M., Catapano, A. L., Parrella, P., Ciafrè, S. A., Signori, E., Seripa, D., Uboldi, P., Antonini, R., Ricci, G., Farace, M. G., and Fazio, V. M. (2000). Treatment of severe hypercholesterolemia in apolipoprotein E-deficient mice by intramuscular injection of plasmid DNA. *Gene. Ther.* **7**, 1795–1801.

Sakai, Y., Kim, D. K., Iwasa, S., Liang, J., Watanabe, T., Onodera, M., and Nakauchi, H. (2002). Bone marrow chimerism prevents atherosclerosis in arterial walls of mice deficient in apolipoprotein E. *Atherosclerosis* **161**, 27–34.

Sekiya, I., Larson, B. L., Vuoristo, J. T., Cui, J., and Prockop, D. J. (2004). Adipogenic differentiation of human adult stem cells from bone marrow stroma (MSCs). *J. Bone Miner. Res.* **19**(2), 256–264.

Sekiya, I., Vuoristo, J. T., Larson, B. L., and Prockop, D. J. (2002). *In vitro* cartilage formation by human adult stem cells from bone marrow stroma defines the sequence of cellular and molecular events during chondrogenesis. *Proc. Natl. Acad. Sci. USA* **99**(7), 4397–4402.

Signori, E., Rinaldi, M., Fioretti, D., Iurescia, S., Seripa, D., Perrone, G., Norata, G. D., Catapano, A. L., and Fazio, V. M. (2007). ApoE gene delivery inhibits severe hypercholesterolemia in newborn ApoE-KO mice. *Biochem. Biophys. Res. Commun.* **361**, 543–548.

Stevenson, S. C., Marshall-Neff, J., Teng, B., Lee, C. B., Roy, S., and McClelland, A. (1995). Phenotypic correction of hypercholesterolemia in apoE-deficient mice by adenovirus-mediated *in vivo* gene transfer. *Arterioscler Thromb. Vasc. Biol.* **15**, 479–484.

Uccelli, A., Moretta, L., and Pistoia, V. (2006). Immunoregulatory function of mesenchymal stem cells. *Eur. J. Immunol.* **36**, 2566–2573.

Utermann, G. (1988). Apolipoprotein polymorphism and multifactorial hyperlipidaemia. *J. Inher. Metab. Dis.* **11**(Suppl 1), 74–86.

van Eck, M., Herijgers, N., Yates, J., Pearce, N. J., Hoogerbrugge, P. M., Groot, P. H., and van Berkel, T. J. (1997). Bone marrow transplantation in apolipoprotein E-deficient mice. Effect of ApoE gene dosage on serum lipid concentrations, (beta)VLDL catabolism, and atherosclerosis. *Arterioscler Thromb. Vasc. Biol.* **17**, 3117–3126.

Vogel, T., Weisgraber, K. H., Zeevi, M. I., Ben-Artzi, H., Levanon, A. Z., Rall, S. C. Jr., Innerarity, T. L., Hui, D. Y., Taylor, J. M., Kanner, D., et al. (1985). Human apolipoprotein E expression in Escherichia coli: structural and functional identity of the bacterially produced protein with plasma apolipoprotein E. *Proc. Natl. Acad. Sci. USA* **82**, 8696–8700.

Yue, L., Rasouli, N., Ranganathan, G., Kern, P. A., and Mazzone, T. (2004). Divergent effects of peroxisome proliferator-activated receptor γ agonists and tumor necrosis factor α on adipocyte ApoE expression. *J. Biol. Chem.* **279**, 47626–47632.

Zhao, L., Duan, W., Reyes, M., Keene, C. D., Verfaillie, C. M., and Low, W. C. (2002). Human bone marrow stromal cells exhibit neuronal phenotypes and ameriolate neurological deficits after grafting into the ischemic brain of rats. *Exp. Neurol.* **174**, 11–20.

Zoorob, R. J. and Cender, D. (1998). A different look at corticosteroids. *Am. Fam. Physician.* **58**, 443–445.

Zuckerman, S. H., Evans, G. F., and O'Neal, L. (1993). Exogenous glucocorticoids increase macrophage secretion of apo E by cholesterol-independent pathways. *Atherosclerosis* **103**, 43–54.

17

Araújo, F. P., Petri, D. F. S., and Carmona-Ribeiro, A. M. (2005). Colloid stability of sodium dihexadecyl phosphate/poly(diallyldimethylammonium chloride) decorated latex. *Langmuir* **21**, 9495–9501.

Booser, D. J., Esteva, F. J., Rivera, E., Valero, V., Esparza-Guerra, L., Priebe, W., and Hortobagyi, G. N. (2002). Phase II study of liposomal annamycin in the treatment of doxorubicin-resistant breast cancer. *Can. Chem. Pharm.* **50**, 6–8.

Campanhã, M. T. N., Mamizuka, E. M., and Carmona-Ribeiro, A. M. (1999). Interactions between cationic liposomes and bacteria: The physical-chemistry of the bactericidal action. *J. Lipid. Res.* **40**, 1495–1500.

Campanhã, M. T. N., Mamizuka, E. M., and Carmona-Ribeiro, A. M. (2001). Interactions between cationic vesicles and Candida albicans. *J. Phys. Chem. B.* **105**, 8230–8236.

Carmona-Ribeiro, A. M. (1992). Synthetic amphiphile vesicles. *Chem. Soc. Rev.* **21**, 209–214.

Carmona-Ribeiro, A. M. (2003). Bilayer-forming synthetic lipids: drugs or carriers? *Curr. Med. Chem.* **10**, 2425–2446.

Carmona-Ribeiro, A. M. (2006). Lipid bilayer fragments and disks in drug delivery. *Curr. Med. Chem.* **13**, 1359–1370.

Carmona-Ribeiro, A. M., Castuma, C. E., Sesso, A., and Schreier, S. (1991). Bilayer structure and stability in dihexadecyl phosphate dispersions. *J. Phys. Chem.* **95**, 5361–5366.

Carmona-Ribeiro, A. M. and Chaimovich, H. (1983). Preparation and characterization of large dioctadecyldimethylammonium chloride liposomes and comparison with small sonicated vesicles. *Biochim. Biophys. Acta* **733**, 172–179.

Carmona-Ribeiro, A. M., Vieira, D. B., and Lincopan, N. (2006). Cationic surfactants and lipids as anti-infective agents. *Anti-Infect. Agents. Med. Chem.* **5**, 33–54.

Cocquyt, J., Olsson, U., Olofsson, G., and Meeren, P. (2004). Temperature quenched DODAB dispersions: Fluid and solid state coexistence and complex formation with oppositely charged surfactant. *Langmuir* **20**, 3906–3912.

Correia, F. M., Petri, D. F. S., and Carmona-Ribeiro, A. M. (2004). Colloid stability of lipid/polyelectrolyte decorated latex. *Langmuir* **20**, 9535–9540.

de Verdiere, A. C., Dubernet, C., Nemati, F., Soma, E., Appel, M., Ferte, J., Bernard, S., Puisieux, F., and Couvreur, P. (1997). Reversion of multidrug resistance with polyalkylcyanoacrylate nanoparticles: Towards a mechanism of action. *Br. J. Can.* **76**, 198–205.

Decher, G. and Hong, J. D. (1991). Buildup of ultrathin multilayer films by a self-assembly process: II. Consecutive adsorption of anionic and cationic bipolar amphiphiles and polyelectrolytes on charged surfaces. *Berichte der Bunsen-Gesellschaft* **95**, 1430–1434.

Grabowski, E. and Morrison, I. (1983). Particle size distribution from analysis of quasi-elastic light scattering data. In *Measurements of Suspended Particles by Quasi-Elastic Light Scattering*. Dahneke B. (Ed.). Wiley-Interscience, New York, pp. 199–236.

Hammarstroem, L., Velikian, I., Karlsson, G., and Edwards, K. (1995). Cryo-tem evidence––sonication of dihexadecyl phosphate does not produce closed bilayers with smooth curvature. *Langmuir* **11**, 408–410.

Helmerhorst, E. J., Reijnders, I. M., van't Hof, W., Veerman, E. C. I., and Nieuw Amerongen, A.V. (1999). A critical comparison of the hemolytic and fungicidal activities of cationic antimicrobial peptides. *FEBS Lett.* **449**, 105–110.

Lamprecht, A., Yamamoto, H., Takeuchi, H., and Kawashima, Y. (2005). Nanoparticles enhance therapeutic efficiency by selectively increased local drug dose in experimental colitis in rats. *J. Pharmacol Exp. Ther.* **315**, 196–202.

Lee, K. D., Hong, K., and Papahadjopoulos, D. (1992). Recognition of liposomes by cells: *In vitro* binding and endocytosis mediated by specific lipid headgroups and surface charge density. *Biochim. Biophys. Acta* **1103**, 185–197.

Lincopan, N. and Carmona-Ribeiro, A. M. (2006). Lipid-covered drug particles: Combined action of dioctadecyldimethylammonium bromide and amphotericin B or miconazole. *J. Antimicrob. Chemother.* **58**, 66–75.

Lincopan, N., Mamizuka, E. M., and Carmona-Ribeiro, A. M. (2003). *In vivo* activity of a novel amphotericin B formulation with synthetic cationic bilayer fragments. *J. Antimicrob. Chemother.* **52,** 412–418.

Lincopan, N., Mamizuka, E. M., and Carmona-Ribeiro, A. M. (2005). Low nephrotoxicity of an effective amphotericin B formulation with cationic bilayer fragments. *J. Antimicrob. Chemother.* **55**, 727–734.

Liu, Z., Bendayan, R., and Wu, X. Y. (2000). Triton-X-100-modified polymer and microspheres for reversal of multidrug resistance. *J. Pharm. Pharmacol.* **53**, 1–12.

Lvov, Y., Decher, G., and Moehwald, H. (1993). Assembly, structural characterization, and thermal behavior of layer-by-layer deposited ultrathin films of poly(vinyl sulfate) and poly(allylamine). *Langmuir* **9**, 481–486.

Martins, L. M. S., Mamizuka, E. M., and Carmona-Ribeiro, A. M. (1997). Cationic vesicles as bactericides. *Langmuir* **13**, 5583–5587.

Moghimi, S. M. and Hunter, A. C. (2000). Poloxamers and poloxamines in nanoparticle engineering and experimental medicine. *Trend Biotechnol.* **18**, 412–420.

Nori, A., Jensen, K. D., Tijerina, M., Kopeckova, P., and Kopecek, J. (2003). Subcellular trafficking of HPMA copolymer-TAT conjugates in human ovarian carcinoma cells. *J. Control. Release* **91**, 53–59.

Pacheco, L. F. and Carmona-Ribeiro, A. M. (2003). Effects of synthetic lipids on solubilization and colloid stability of hydrophobic drugs. *J. Colloid Interface Sci.* **258**, 146–154.

Romsicki, Y. and Sharom, F. J. (1999). The membrane lipid environment modulates drug interactions with the P-glycoprotein multidrug transporter. *Biochemistry* **38**, 6887–6896.

Schales, O. and Schales, S. S. (1941). A simple and accurate method for the determination of chloride in biological fluids. *J. Biol. Chem.* **140**, 879–884.

Sicchierolli, S. M., Mamizuka, E. M., and Carmona-Ribeiro, A. M. (1995). Bacteria flocculation and death by cationic vesicles. *Langmuir* **11**, 2991–2995.

Soloviev, M. (2007). Nanobiotechnology today: Focus on nanoparticles. *J. Nanobiotechnol.* **5**, 11–13.

Soma, C. E., Dubernet, C., Barratt, G., Nemati, F., Appel, M., Benita, S., and Couvreur, P. (1999). Ability of doxorubicin-loaded nanoparticles to overcome multidrug resistance of tumor cells after their capture by macrophages. *Pharm. Res.* **16**, 1710–1716.

Tapias, G. N., Sicchierolli, S. M., Mamizuka, E. M., and Carmona-Ribeiro, A. M. (1994). Interactions between cationic vesicles and Escherichia coli. *Langmuir* **10**, 3461–3465.

Tiyaboonchai, W. and Limpeanchob, N. (2007). Formulation and characterization of amph otericin B-chitosan-dextran sulfate nanoparticles. *Int. J. Pharm.* **329**, 142–149.

Tiyaboonchai, W., Woiszwillo, J., and Middaugh, C. R. (2001). Formulation and characterization of amphotericin B-polyethylenimine-dextran sulfate nanoparticles. *J. Pharm. Sci.* **90**, 902–914.

Vieira, D. B. and Carmona-Ribeiro, A. M. (2001). Synthetic bilayer fragments for solubilization of amphotericin B. *J. Colloid Interface Sci.* **244**, 427–431.

Vieira, D. B. and Carmona-Ribeiro, A. M. (2006). Cationic lipids and surfactants as antifungal agents: mode of action. *J. Antimicrob Chemother* **58**, 760–767.

Vieira, D. B., Lincopan, N., Mamizuka, E. M., Petri, D. F. S., and Carmona-Ribeiro, A. M. (2003). Competitive adsorption of cationic bilayers and chitosan on latex: Optimal biocidal action. *Langmuir* **19**, 924–932.

Vieira, D. B., Pacheco, L. F., and Carmona-Ribeiro, A. M. (2006). Assembly of a model hydrophobic drug into cationic bilayer fragments. *J. Colloid. Interface Sci.* **293**, 240–247.

Wei, G. X. and Bobek, L. A. (2004). *In vitro* synergic antifungal effect of MUC7 12-mer with histatin-5 12-mer or miconazole. *J. Antimicrob Chemother* **53**, 750–758.

Wong, H. L., Bendayan, R., Rauth, A. M., Li, Y., and Wu, X. Y. (2007). Chemotherapy with anticancer drugs encapsulated in solid lipid nanoparticles. *Adv. Drug Deliver Rev.* **59**, 491–504.

Wong, H. L., Bendayan, R., Rauth, A. M., and Wu, X. Y. (2004). Development of solid lipid nanoparticles containing ionically-complexed chemotherapeutic drugs and chemosensitizers. J. *Pharm. Sci.* **93**, 1993–2004.

Index

B

C

D

E